Advanced
EXERCISES IN DIAGNOSTIC RADIOLOGY

19

RHEUMATOLOGIC DISORDERS

LAWRENCE F. LAYFER, M.D.
Assistant Professor of Medicine

JERRY PETASNICK, M.D.
Professor of Radiology

ROBERT S. KATZ, M.D.
Associate Professor of Medicine

All of Rush-Presbyterian-St. Luke's Medical Center
Chicago, Illinois

W. B. SAUNDERS COMPANY • 1988
Harcourt Brace Jovanovich, Inc.
Philadelphia • London • Toronto • Montreal • Sydney • Tokyo

W. B. SAUNDERS COMPANY
Harcourt Brace Jovanovich, Inc.

The Curtis Center
Independence Square West
Philadelphia, PA 19106

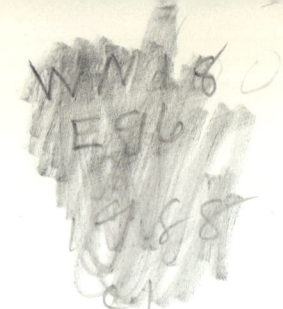

Library of Congress Cataloging-in-Publication Data

Layfer, Lawrence F.

Rheumatologic disorders.

(Advanced exercises in diagnostic radiology; 19)

Includes index.

1. Arthritis—Diagnosis—Problems, exercises, etc.
   2. Rheumatism—Diagnosis—Problems, exercises, etc.
   3. Diagnosis, Radioscopic—Problems, exercises, etc.
I. Petasnick, Jerry.   II. Katz, Robert S.
III. Title. IV. Series. [DNLM: 1.
   Arthritis—radiography. W1 AD402E v. 19/WE 344 L427r]

RC78.E89 vol. 19   616.07'57s   88–3166

[RC933]   [616.7'230757]

ISBN 0–7216–2385–9

Editor: William Lamsback
Designer: Karen O'Keefe
Production Manager: Bill Preston
Manuscript Editor: Jodi Von Hagen
Illustration Coordinator: Walt Verbitski
Indexer: Linda Caravelli

Rheumatologic Disorders—Volume 19   ISBN 0–7216–2385–9

© 1988 by W. B. Saunders Company. Copyright under the Uniform Copyright Convention. Simultaneously published in Canada. All rights reserved. This book is protected by copyright. No part of it may be reproduced, stored in a retrieval system, or transmitted in any form or by any means, electronic, mechanical, photocopying, recording, or otherwise, without written permission from the publisher. Made in the United States of America. Library of Congress catalog card number 88–3166.

Last digit is the print number: 9 8 7 6 5 4 3 2 1

To our wives and children

PREFACE

The roentgenographic examination has three primary purposes in rheumatic illness: (1) to aid in the differential diagnosis by confirming or denying clinical impressions, or suggesting new ones; (2) to assist in judging the severity and extent of an arthritic process at a particular location; and (3) to provide serial assessment of structural joint abnormalities. The objective of this book is to introduce you to the interpretive skills required to use radiographs in this manner, with the hope that it will become a routine part of your evaluation of patients with rheumatic diseases.

The first section in this volume presents a systematic approach to data collection in articular radiography and provides advice on the assimilation of these data into patterns consistent with major rheumatic diagnostic categories.

The second section contains radiographs that demonstrate the major rheumatic illnesses with which you can practice and develop your interpretive skills. The case study method so successfully used in previous volumes in this series will again be used here. As with other volumes, this book is not intended to be a comprehensive anthology of rheumatic radiology, but rather a concise workbook to be used in conjunction with other supplemental readings in the study of rheumatology.

CONTENTS

Section One
APPROACH 3
   Soft Tissue Changes 4
   Bone and Bone Density 9
   Articular Surface Changes 12
   Bone Alignment 16

DISEASE CATEGORIES 20
   Inflammatory Arthritis 21
   Degenerative Arthritis 24
   Infectious Arthritis 27
   Spinal Radiography 30
   Crystal-Induced Arthritis 42

Section Two
EXERCISES 51
   Hands 51
   Knees and Hips 77
   Foot and Ankle 110
   Shoulder 131
   Spine 142

Index 181

SECTION I

APPROACH

Table 1. APPROACH TO RADIOGRAPHIC EXAMINATION

Look for:
  Soft tissue changes
  Bone and bone density changes
  Articular surface changes
  Bone alignment

APPROACH

The radiographic examination should be approached in a systematic fashion so that all aspects of the radiograph are interpreted and nothing is overlooked. The order followed by the interpreter should become routine so that subtle abnormalities are not overlooked in favor of more obvious radiographic changes. Resist the temptation to lunge at a diagnosis! We have divided our routine of observation into four categories, which should be performed in sequence. Table 1 presents our approach in list form. For now, why not try it our way?

Figure 1 is a drawing of a normal hand. We have labeled some of the joints with their abbreviations so that you can get used to their location and terminology. Figure 2 is a radiograph of a normal hand. Spend a moment looking at the four categories: soft tissues, bone

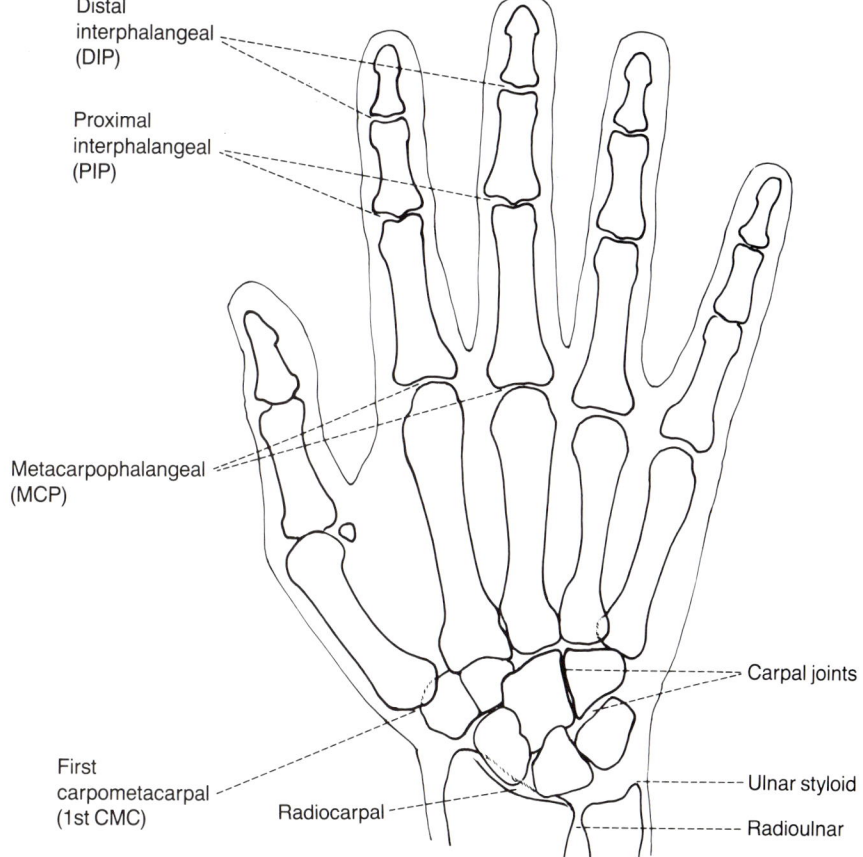

Figure 1

SECTION I—APPROACH

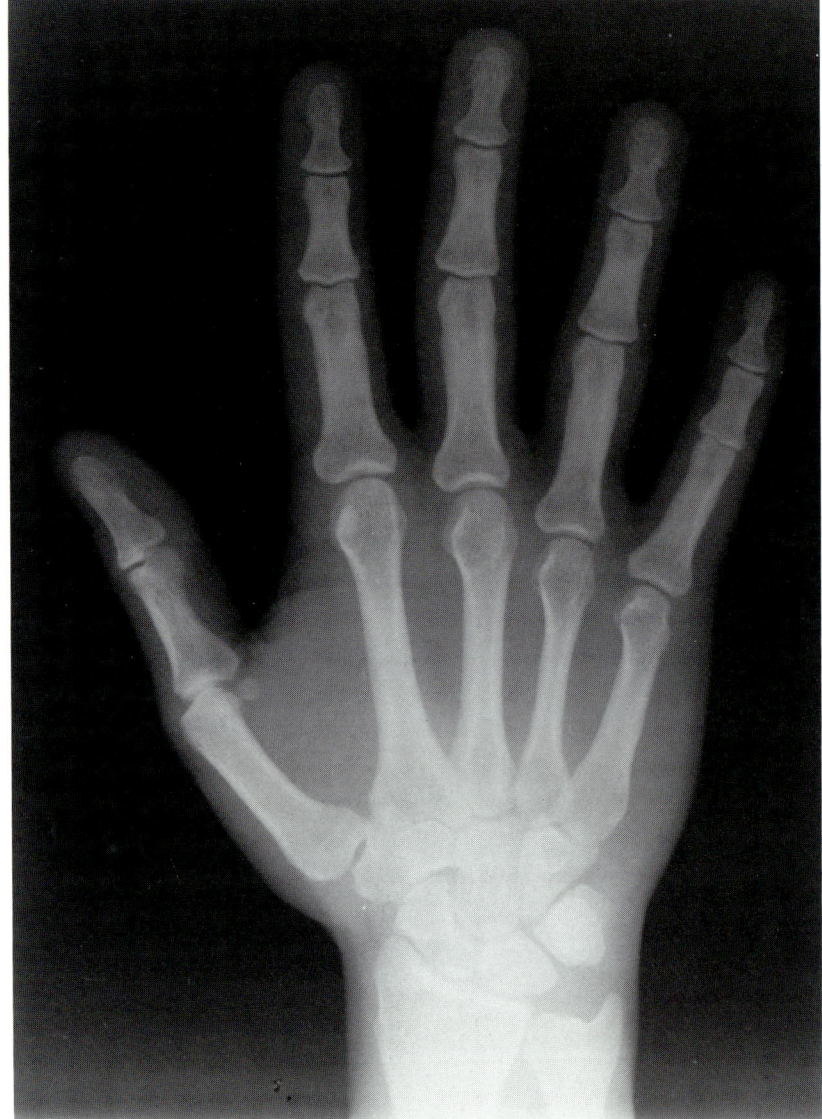

Figure 2

density, articular surface and bone alignment. You may find this a useful reference when viewing the abnormal radiographs depicted in the rest of the book. When you are ready, let's begin by demonstrating some of the changes you should look for in the four basic categories.

Soft Tissue Changes

Examine the soft tissue shadows surrounding the bony structures on the normal hand displayed in Figure 2. The initial step in evaluating any roentgenographic examination of a joint is to look for deviation from the normal contour. Ask yourself these questions: Is there soft tissue swelling? If there is, is it localized to the periarticular region or is it spread more diffusely? If it is periarticular, is it fusiform, as in synovial or capsular swelling, or is it nodular and asymmetric, as in a soft tissue mass? Does it bulge only around an underlying bony abnormality, such as an osteophyte? Comparison of one joint with another on the same radiograph may make it easier to decide whether or not soft tissue swelling is present. Finally, observe the soft tissues for evidence of atrophy or loss of tissue and for soft tissue deposits such as foreign bodies or calcium. Got the idea? Some examples to practice on follow.

Compare the soft tissues in Figure 3 with those in Figure 2. You should notice the fusiform swelling around the proximal interphalangeal

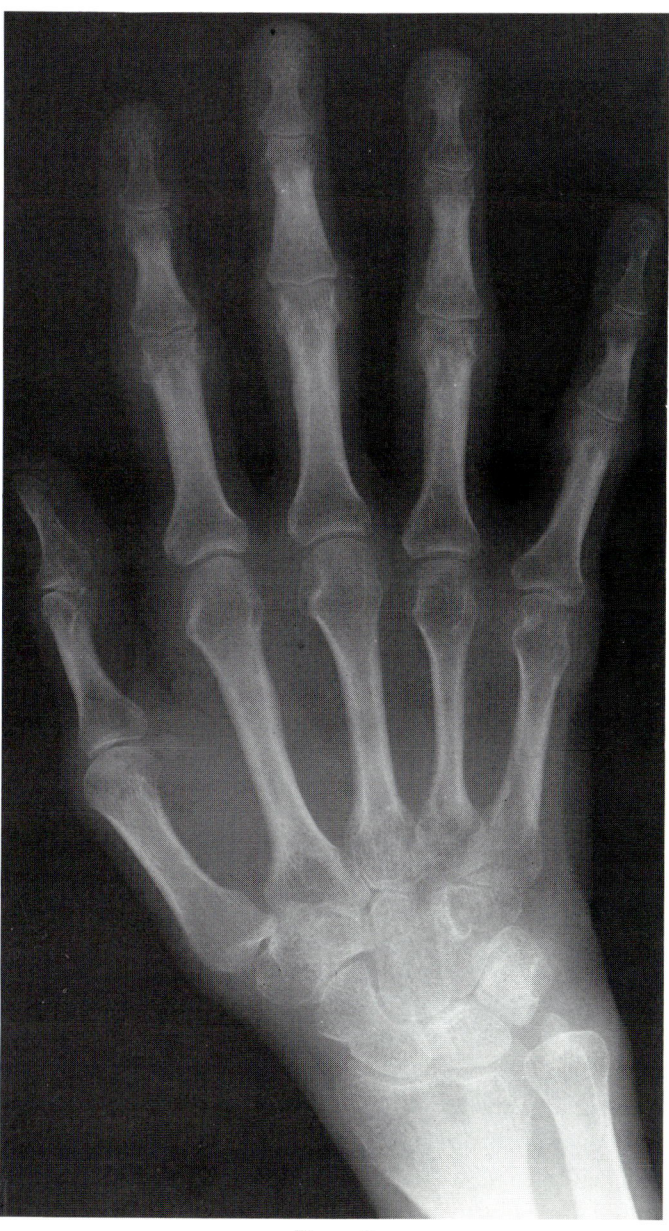

Figure 3

(PIP) joints and the first metacarpophalangeal (MCP) joints. This is the typical capsular enlargement that accompanies active joint disease in rheumatoid arthritis (RA). Note also the swelling around the ulnar styloid, which represents the extensor tendon synovitis seen in this illness. Now look at the soft tissue swellings in Figure 4. Can you see how they differ from those of the previous figure? Although the swelling is around the distal interphalangeal (DIP) and PIP joints and the ulnar styloid, it is asymmetric and nodular instead of fusiform. This does not represent inflamed joints, but rather localized soft tissue masses. These are rheumatoid nodules. Other soft tissue nodules, such as tophi, may have a similar appearance. Note the localized soft tissue masses adjacent to the first and fifth distal phalanges in Figure 5. This patient has gout.

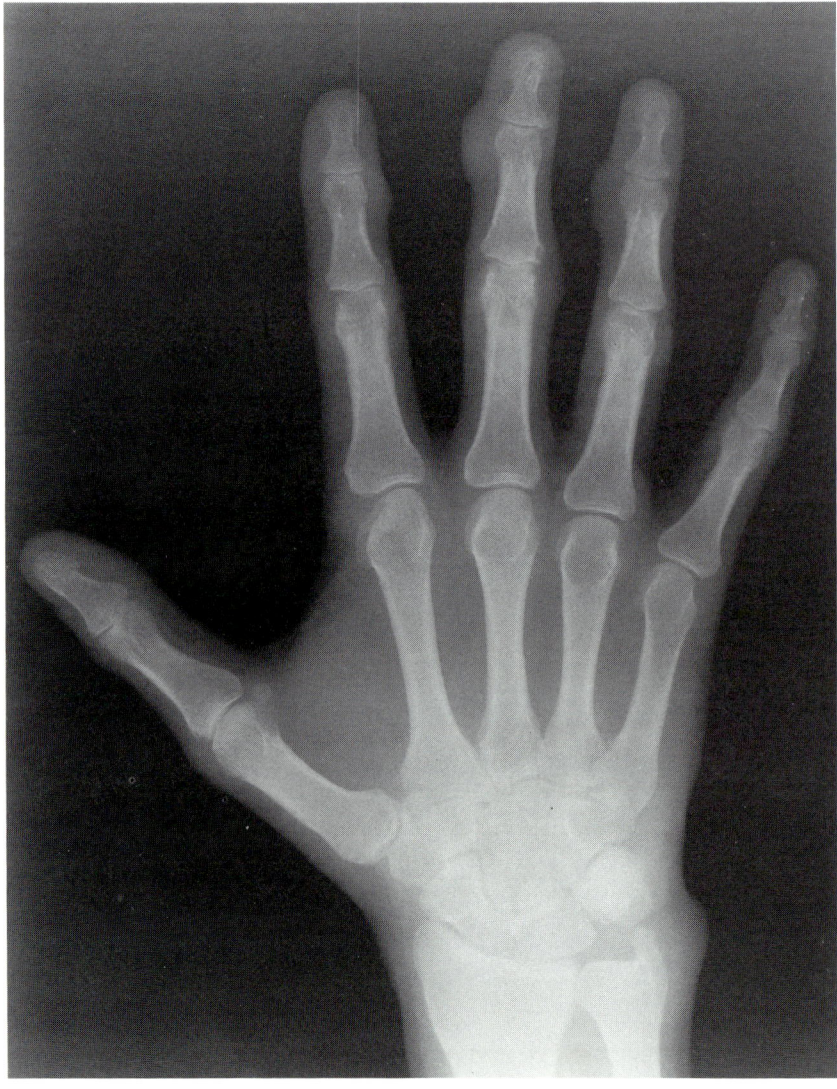

Figure 4

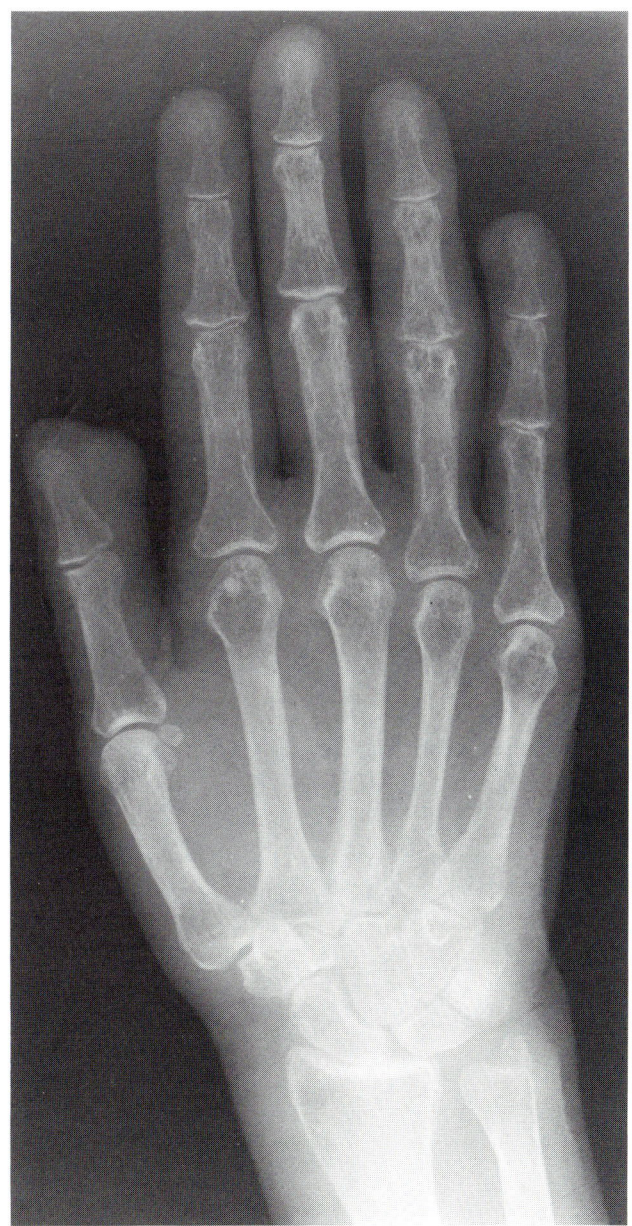

Figure 5

Now look at Figure 6. Did you notice the loss of soft tissue around the distal finger tufts and the deposits of calcium around the soft tissues of the hand? This is the hand of a patient with scleroderma. Tissue is typically lost around the tufts as the vascular disease worsens, and sometimes open ulcerations occur in the area. Calcium deposits are commonly seen in the soft tissues of patients with scleroderma or CREST syndrome but are not specific for the illness. They may also be seen in

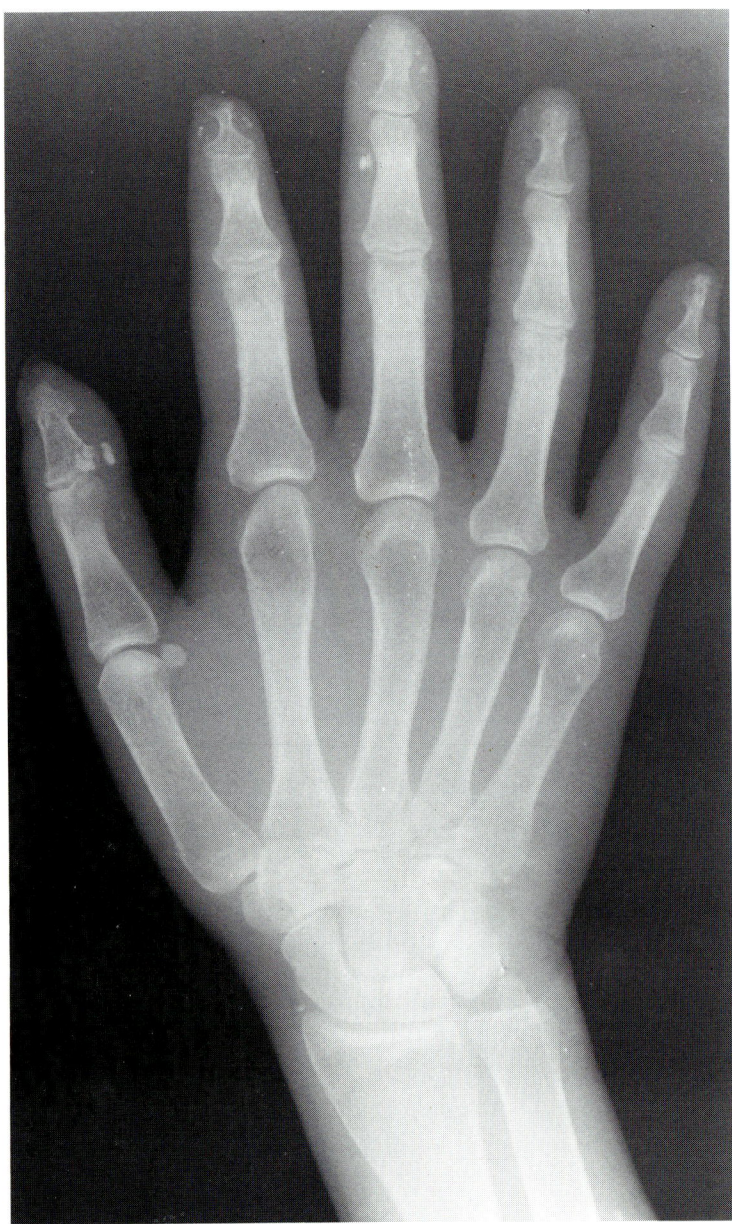

Figure 6

the soft tissues of patients with acute bursitis or tendonitis or in dermatomyositis.

Bone and Bone Density

Now look at the bone density. Ask yourself, Is the radiographic density increased or decreased? If decreased, is it regional or generalized? If regional, is it periarticular? Periarticular density loss often represents inflammation, whereas diffuse density decreases may be due to a number of causes. Osteoporosis, caused by poor mineralization of bone matrix, is the most common cause of diffuse density loss. This is generally seen with aging or as a complication of corticosteroid therapy. Systemic illnesses, such as osteomalacia and hyperparathyroidism, and infiltrative marrow diseases, such as multiple myeloma and metastases, among others, can also cause a generalized decrease in bone density. Focal decreases in density may represent lytic lesions from tumors and must be noted.

Next look for evidence of any increase in density of bone. It is important to note whether an increase in density is in the shaft of the bone or is subchondral in location. Increased bone density in the shaft may be diffuse, as in Paget's disease, or focal, as may be seen in bone infarction. Increases in the subchondral area, often called subchondral sclerosis, represent one of the radiographic hallmarks of degenerative joint disease (DJD).

Finally, look over the contours of the bone, seeking abnormalities such as fracture or periosteal new bone growth. New bone growth may be seen in some inflammatory or infectious illnesses in response to a local or systemic tumor, or it may be present in fracture healing. Now for some examples.

Look at Figure 7. Were you able to see the marked decrease in density around all the MCP joints? If not, compare them with the nearby cortical bone along the metacarpal shaft or to the similar joints in Figure 2. Similar changes may be visible to you around the PIP joints and the carpal area, although these are less obvious. Such periarticular bone loss is typical of inflammatory arthritis. This is an example of early rheumatoid disease. Take a look at Figure 3 again. Do you see similar density changes?

In Figure 8 the density of the bones themselves is normal, and there is no soft tissue swelling. However, solid periosteal new bone growth can be seen along the shafts of all the proximal and middle phalanges, the metacarpal bones and the distal radius and ulna. These findings are characteristic of hypertrophic osteoarthropathy caused by a lung tumor that resulted in polyarticular joint pain, which was this patient's presenting complaint.

In Figure 9, the proximal phalange of the third digit is denser than its neighbors. Note that the cortex is thickened and the trabeculae are prominent. This is Paget's disease. Unfortunately, not all density increases will be as obvious.

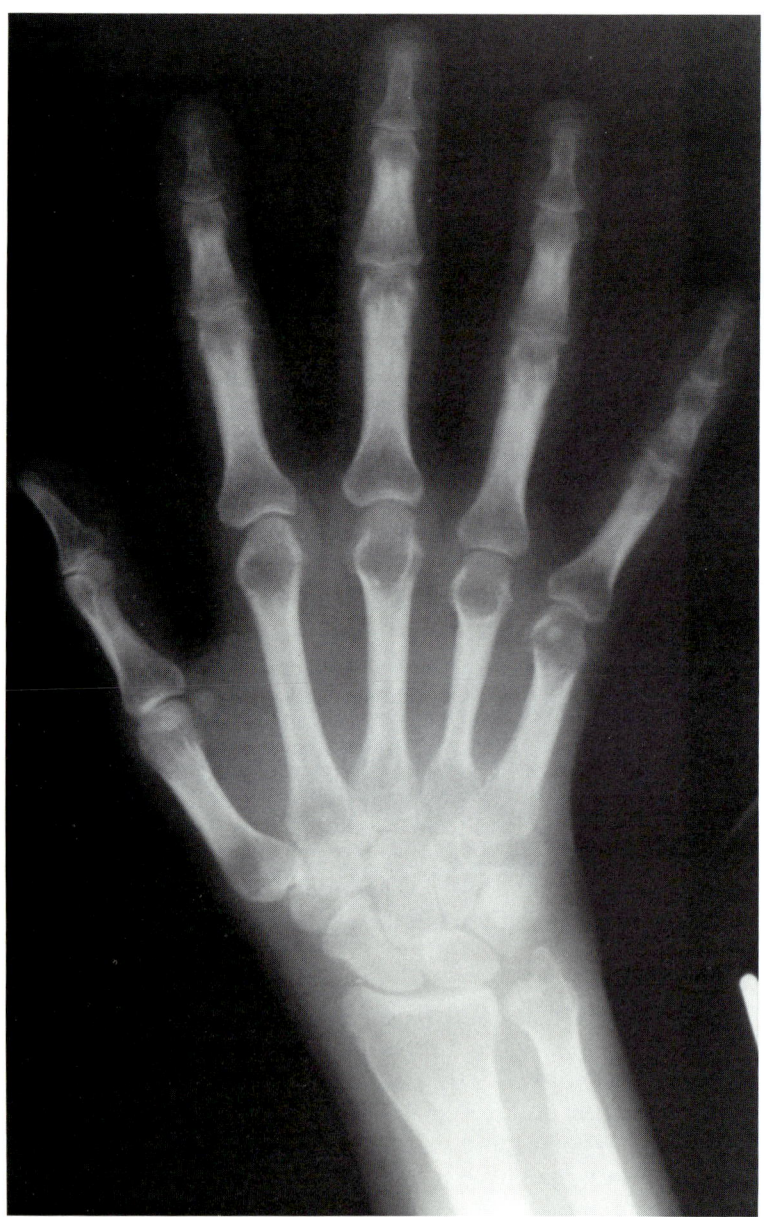

Figure 7

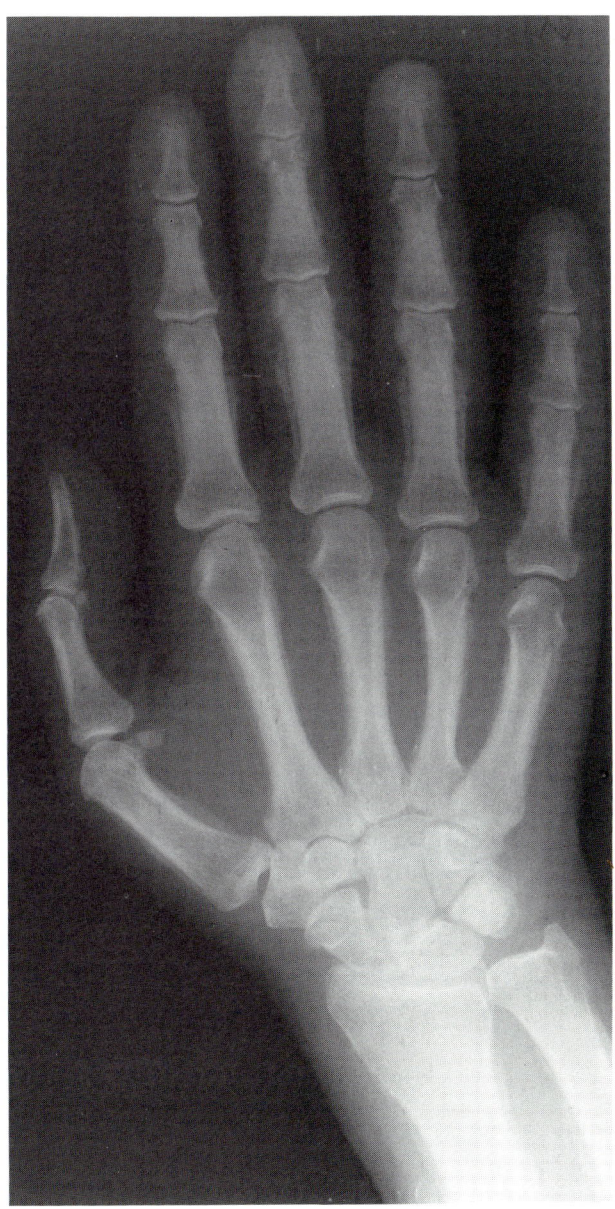

Figure 8

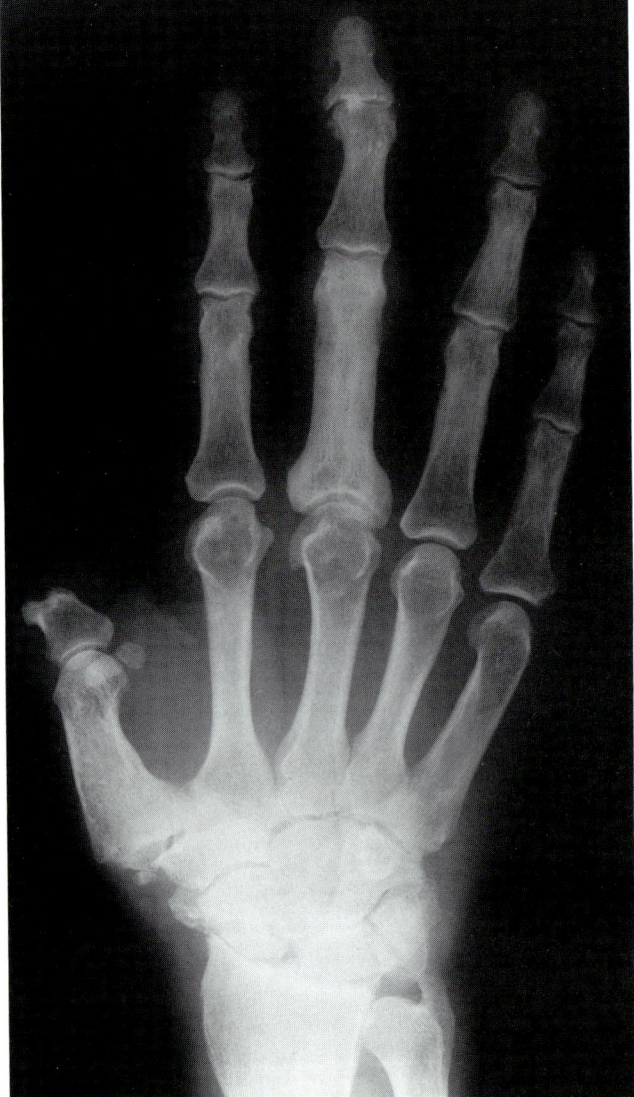

Figure 9

Articular Surface Changes

The third area to concentrate on is the joint itself. First note whether or not the joint space is narrowed. Again, comparison with similar ipsilateral joints or with its mate on the opposite side of the body may aid in such a decision. The joint space represents the radiolucent articular cartilage, and narrowing indicates that the cartilage has been destroyed to some degree. Sometimes the nature of the destruction gives clues to its cause: Inflammatory destruction often causes uniform narrowing across the entire joint, whereas degenerative destruction will usually be nonuniform and asymmetric. Eventually, the whole joint space may be entirely destroyed, with bone abutting on bone. Fusion across a joint may occasionally occur at this point.

While looking at the joint space, also observe the cortical edge of the bone. Note if juxta-articular erosions, subchondral cysts or marginal osteophytes exist. Erosions and cysts represent destruction of subchondral bone in a fashion similar to that which narrows the cartilage space. Marginal osteophytes represent new bone formation and are a radiographic hallmark of degenerative arthritis. When any cartilage or subchondral bone change is noted, always compare it with prior radiographs if possible; the amount of time it takes to develop such changes often gives clues to the nature of the underlying process. Degenerative changes generally develop over several years, whereas inflammatory changes may take only months to occur, and infectious changes may be seen after only a few weeks.

Look at Figure 10. Notice the periarticular decrease in bone density

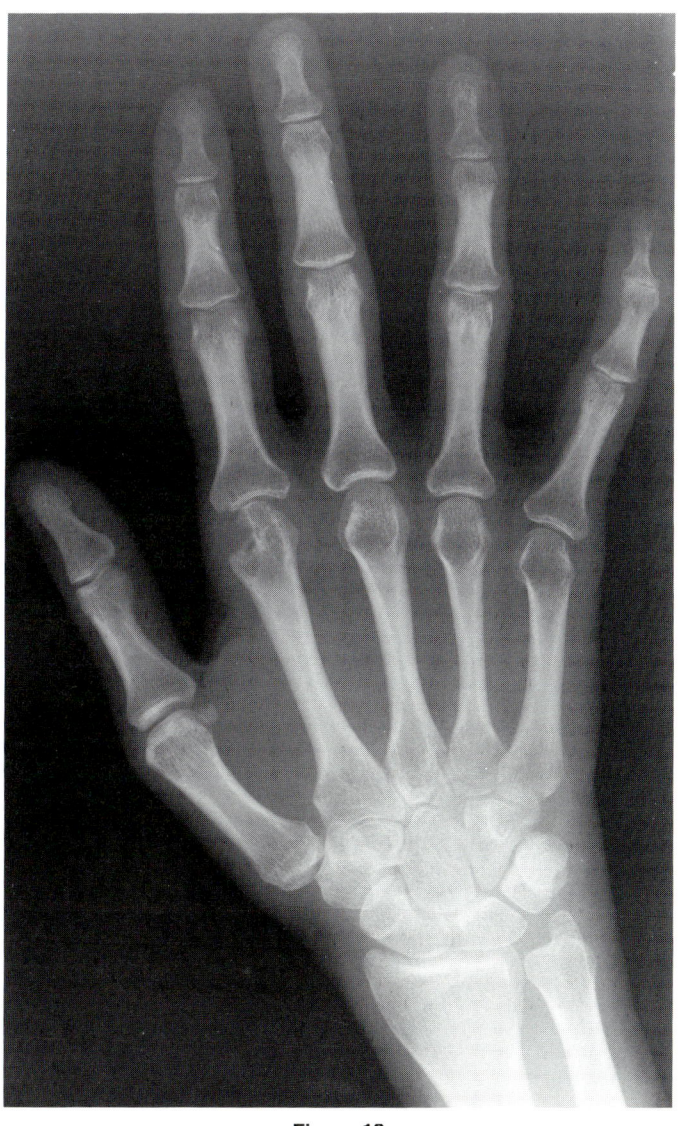

Figure 10

and the large erosion in the distal end of the second metacarpal bone. The second MCP joint is narrowed. This is early inflammatory arthritis, in this case RA with subchondral bone and cartilage destruction. Figure 11 shows the second MCP joint erosion from another view.

Now look at Figure 12. There is soft tissue swelling around several PIP and DIP joints, and the soft tissues are deformed around bony overgrowths, or typical osteophytes, at a few DIP joints. No periarticular demineralization is present. Subchondral cysts are seen around the right first DIP joint. Erosions of subchondral bone are present at some of the PIP and DIP joints. The fourth and fifth DIP joints of the right hand show apparent joint space fusion. Be careful: Other views showed these joints to be overlapping rather than fused and to still have some joint space left. This is a hand with a variant of osteoarthritis (OA) called erosive OA. More on this later.

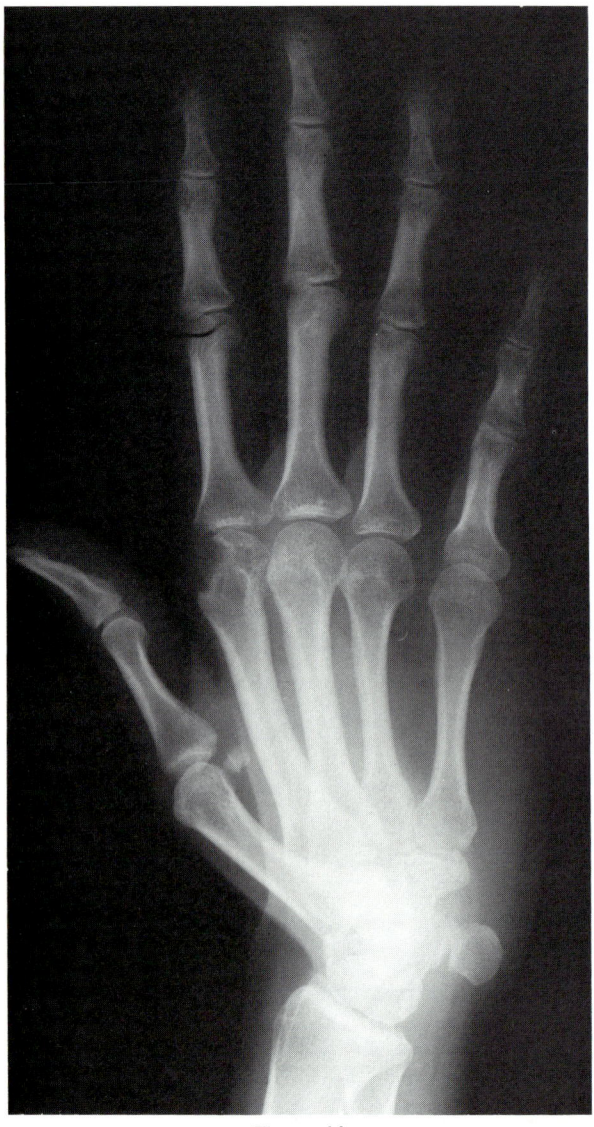

Figure 11

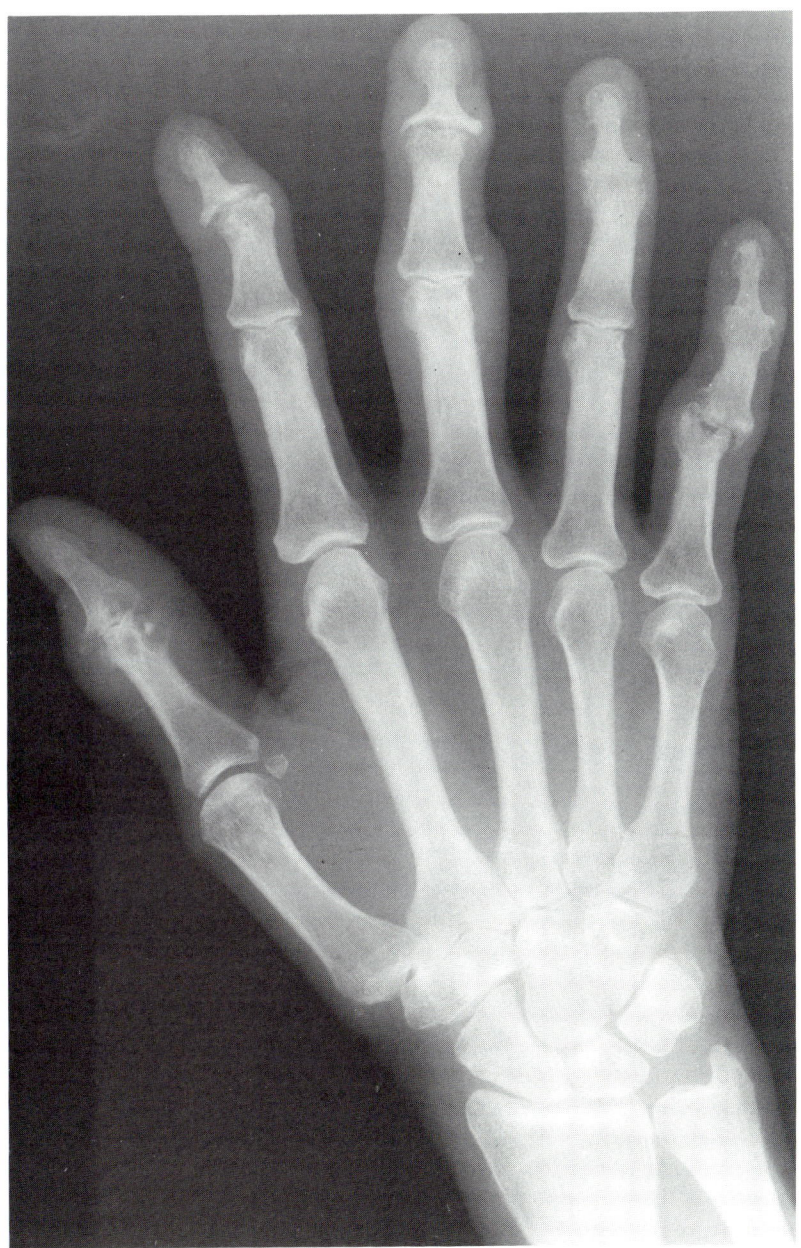

Figure 12

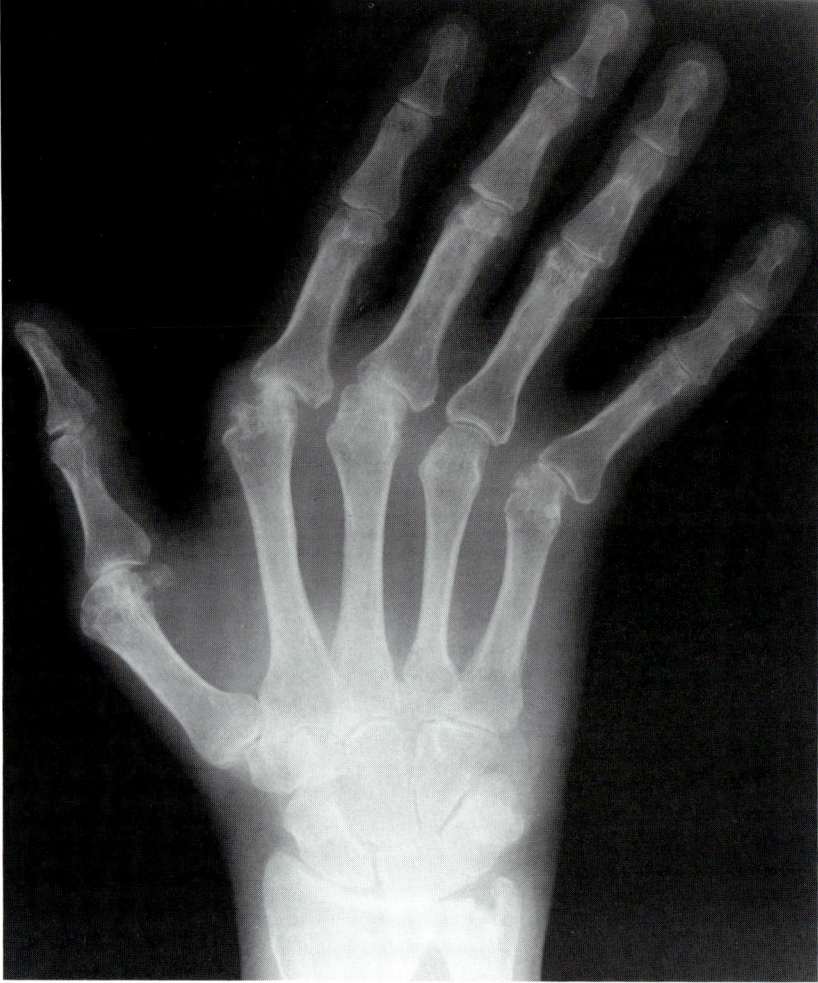

Figure 13

Bone Alignment

Finally, evaluate the alignment of the bones across the joint. Has deformity or subluxation occurred? Alignment changes occur because of laxity of underlying ligaments or because of severe destruction of the articular cartilage. Noting such deformity gives you additional information as to how severe the underlying joint disease is. In addition, the pattern of the deformity may be specific for a particular illness, and thus may help in making a diagnosis. To get you a good start on interpretation, a series of common deformities follows.

Look at Figure 13, which demonstrates ulnar deviation. Note that there are a generalized decrease in bone density, extensive erosive disease at all the MCP joints and ulnar deviation of the second through the fifth digits at the MCP joints. This patient has RA.

Figure 14 demonstrates a boutonnière deformity of the third digit. Boutonnière is the name for flexion at the PIP joint and hyperextension

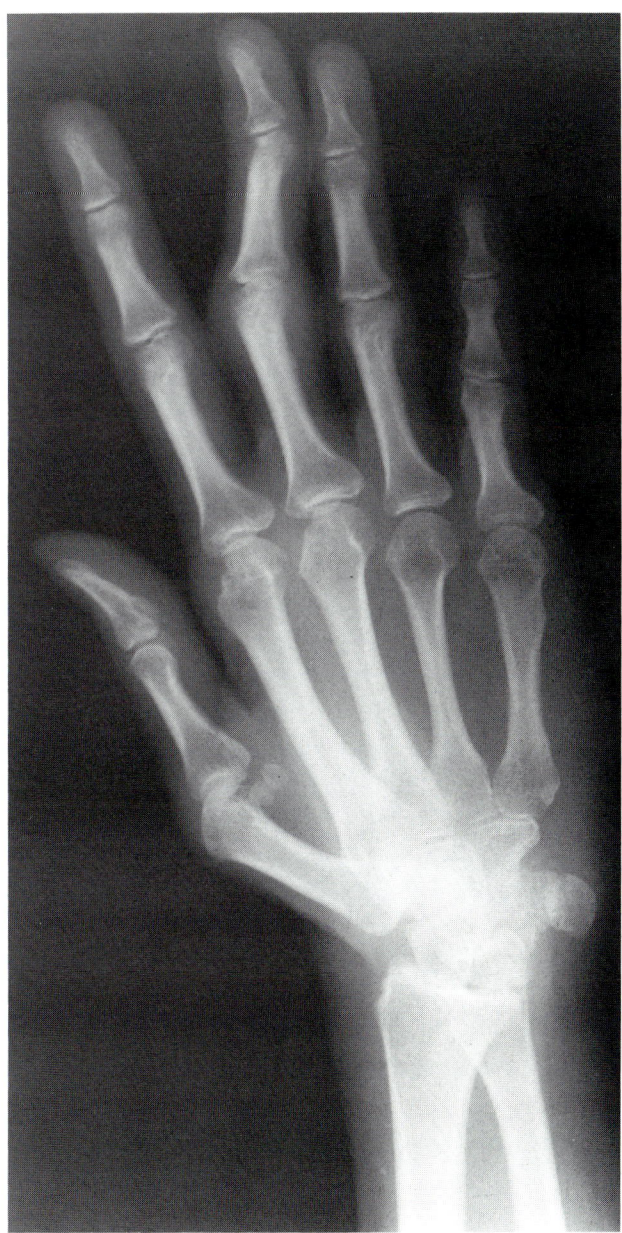

Figure 14

at the DIP joint. This is most commonly seen in RA as a result of an abnormality of the extensor tendons.

Figure 15 demonstrates a swan-neck deformity, or hyperextension at the PIP joints and flexion at the DIP joints of the second through the fifth digits. This is also common in RA.

Figure 16 shows a boutonnière deformity of the thumb. Note the flexion at the PIP joint and the marked hyperextension at the DIP joint. Swan-neck deformities are present at the second through the fifth digits. Ulnar deviation is also present.

Figure 17 demonstrates a varus deformity of the knees: Note that there is narrowing of the medial joint space bilaterally, with more extensive changes on the right, leading to the deformity. A valgus deformity would result from predominantly lateral cartilage narrowing.

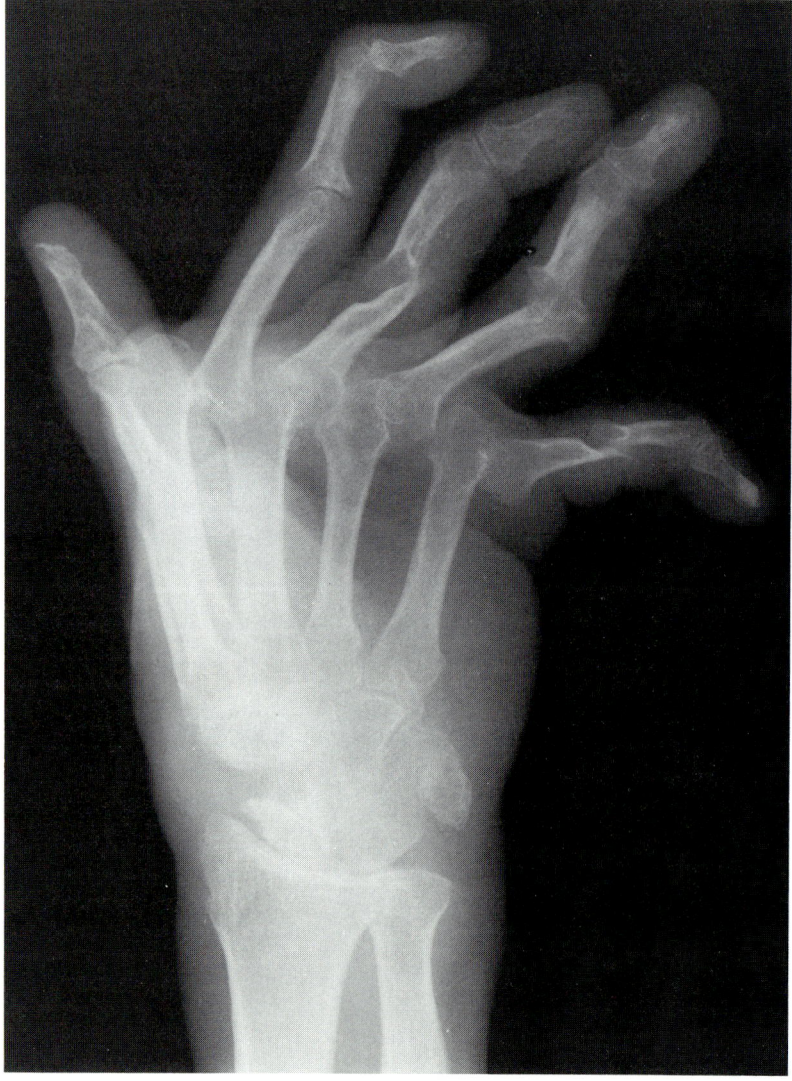

Figure 15

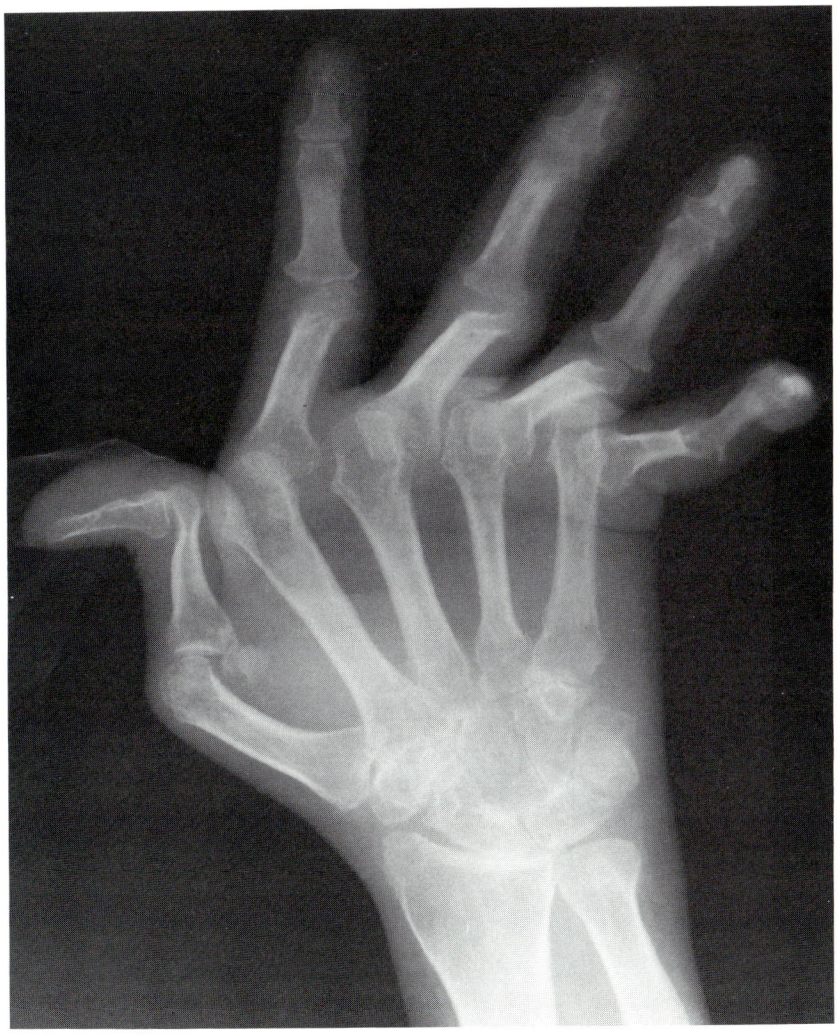

Figure 16

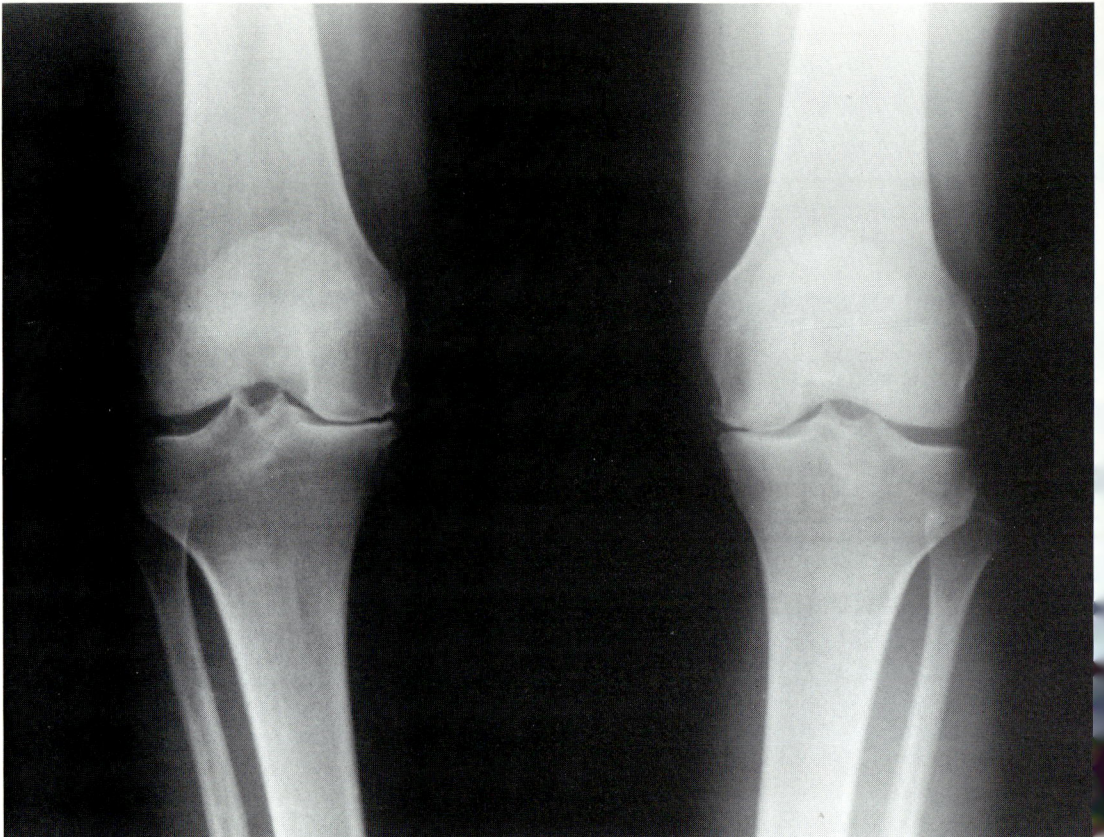

Figure 17

In each of the examples to be given in the remainder of this book, analyze the radiographs in the order we have suggested. Write your observations in each of the four categories we have listed. Force yourself to be complete and to resist the temptation to make a diagnosis based on the most obvious and easily seen abnormality.

DISEASE CATEGORIES

Now that we've discussed the roentgenographic approach, let us turn our attention to using your observations in forming a clinical impression. Table 2 contains a list of the four major diagnostic categories in the rheumatic illnesses. Each category has typical radiographic patterns that you will need to learn. The following sections will provide

Table 2. DIAGNOSTIC CATEGORIES IN RHEUMATIC ILLNESS

Inflammatory Arthritis: Rheumatoid arthritis (RA), systemic lupus erythematosus (SLE), juvenile chronic polyarthritis (JCP), ankylosing spondylitis, psoriatic arthritis, and others
Degenerative Arthritis: Osteoarthritis (OA), both primary and secondary
Infectious Arthritis: Pyogenic, fungal and tubercular arthritis
Crystal-Induced Arthritis: Uric acid, calcium hydroxyapatite, calcium pyrophosphate dihydrate (CPPD)

Table 3. RADIOLOGIC CHANGES IN INFLAMMATORY ARTHRITIS

- Soft tissue swelling and joint effusion
- Periarticular demineralization
- Marginal erosions and subchondral cysts
- Uniform cartilage loss
- Subluxation and deformity
- No new bone formation
- Changes occur over months to years

the basic information you need to categorize the radiographic abnormalities in the cases presented.

Inflammatory Arthritis (Table 3)

The earliest radiographic finding in inflammatory arthritis is soft tissue swelling, which represents capsular distension. Regional osteopenia in the subchondral area (periarticular decrease in bone density or demineralization) soon follows as a result of the increased vascularity. As synovium proliferates, destructive changes become apparent with marginal and articular erosions and subchondral cysts, which represent pannus (inflamed synovium) invasion of bone and cartilage. As destruction progresses, cartilage loss occurs and can be seen as joint space narrowing. Note that when this occurs, it is uniform across the joint space, and no marginal bony proliferation or subchondral sclerosis occurs. Erosive inflammatory changes generally occur over no less than a 3 to 6 month period. More rapid changes should suggest another condition such as infection. As the inflammatory damage continues, ligamentous laxity develops and leads to deformities that are visible on both clinical and radiologic examinations. Such deformities often have recognizable patterns, as was discussed in Figures 13 through 17.

The various inflammatory arthritides have individual characteristics that may help you to distinguish among them when looking at a radiograph. RA generally affects large and small joints in a bilateral symmetric pattern. It is not at all unusual in this illness for radiographs of the MCP and PIP joints and the wrists of the right and left hands to appear as mirror images of each other. In contrast, psoriatic arthritis is generally asymmetric in distribution and will often involve the DIP joint. Systemic lupus erythematosus (SLE), while having a rheumatoid-like pattern of distribution, causes a deforming but often nondestructive pattern of involvement. The case studies in Section II will help you with this concept.

Look at Figure 18. Did you follow the order of observation we suggested in Table 1? If you did, you will have noted the soft tissue swelling around the MCP joints and the ulnar styloid. There is a generalized decrease in bone density. Extensive erosive disease is present in all of the MCP joints, the carpal bones, the distal radius and the radioulnar joint. Once you've decided an inflammatory process is occurring, the pattern of involvement may help you to decide which inflammatory disease it is. The pattern of arthritis in this patient is characteristic of RA. You will encounter other patterns in the cases in Section II.

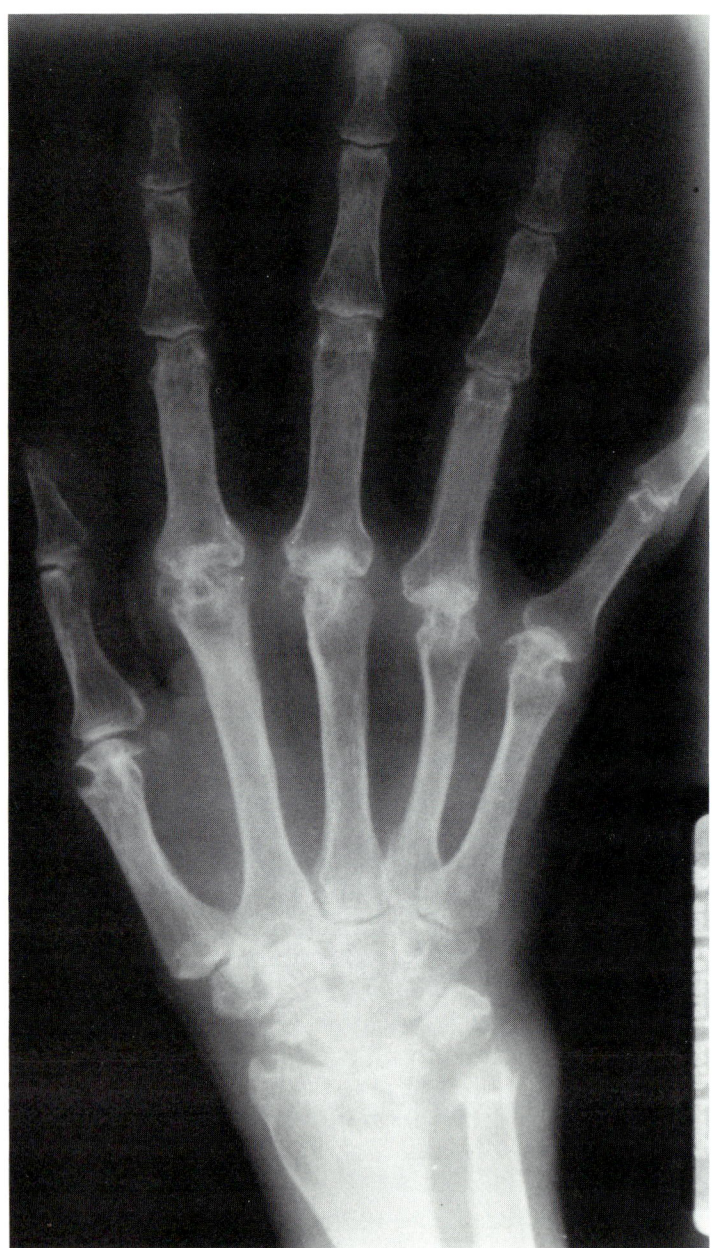
Figure 18

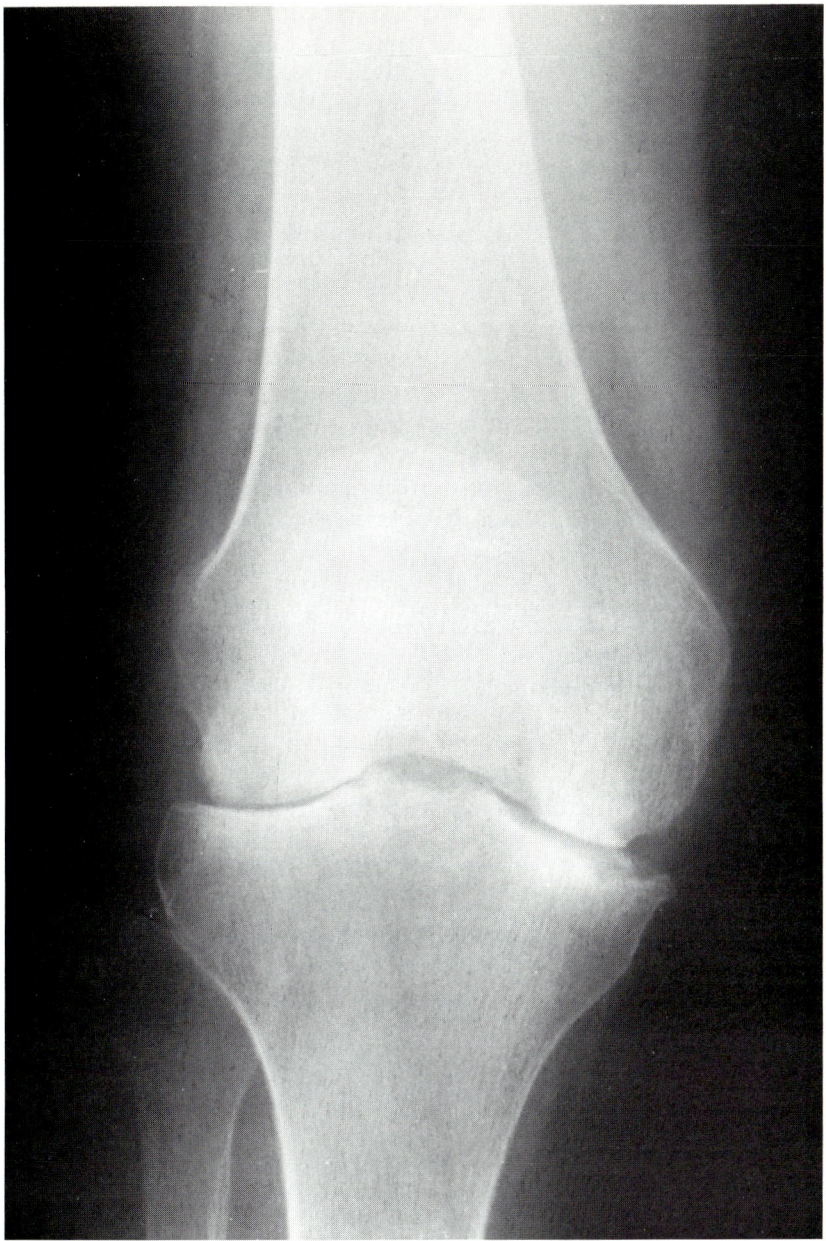

Figure 19

Figure 19 demonstrates inflammatory changes in larger joints. Joints such as hips, knees and shoulders tend not to show soft tissue swelling, and periarticular demineralization may be more difficult to see in such thick bones. Note, however, that the radiograph of this knee shows the typical cartilage changes of an inflammatory arthritis: uniform joint space narrowing without marginal bony proliferation or subchondral sclerosis. This is the knee of a patient with RA, although other types of inflammatory arthritis look similar. Now that you've gotten the feeling for observing an inflammatory joint, let us move on.

Degenerative Arthritis

In degenerative arthritis (Table 4), the pathologic lesion is primary degeneration of articular cartilage rather than inflammatory proliferation of synovium. As a result, narrowing of cartilage is often the earliest finding. The cartilage loss is usually nonuniform and may lead to radiologically or clinically evident joint deformity. Subchondral sclerosis, rather than periarticular osteoporosis, is commonly visible, as is new bone formation in the form of marginal osteophytes. This further distinguishes degenerative arthritis from inflammatory arthritis. These changes occur over many years, and old films should be sought to help confirm such a temporal progression. If cartilage loss occurs over weeks to months, the diagnosis of degenerative arthritis is suspect, and another category of illness must be considered.

Look at Figure 20. There is no fusiform swelling or soft tissue masses. No periarticular demineralization is visible. Rather, there is a generalized decrease in bone density. There is narrowing of the DIP and PIP joints, but sparing of the MCP joints and the wrist. Observation of the articular surface area of the involved joints reveals subchondral sclerosis and marginal osteophytes. The tips of the fingers look deformed by the joint disease. This is the most common form of degenerative arthritis: primary OA. Compare it with the hand showing RA in Figure 19. Can you see the differences? Did you also note the OA changes at the base of the thumb? The pattern of degenerative changes at the DIP and first carpometacarpal (CMC) joints is typical for primary OA, which is a familial degenerative arthritis. Clinically, the marginal osteophytes correlate well with the Heberden's and Bouchard's nodes that are palpable on the fingers of such patients.

Secondary OA, in contrast with primary OA, is usually monoarticular, occurs at any joint, and can usually be traced to some prior joint insult such as an old fracture or trauma. The radiographic changes of secondary OA may also be superimposed on those of a prior septic joint or joint with inactive RA. Look at the knee on the next film.

Figures 21 and 22 demonstrate anteroposterior (AP) and lateral views of the knee. The soft tissues are normal. The density of the bone appears increased in the subchondral areas. There is no periosteal reaction, but marginal osteophytes have formed. The joint space is narrowed medially, and there is a varus deformity of the knee. This is a typical degenerated knee. The patient tore his medial meniscus playing football 10 years earlier and developed secondary OA as a result. Bearing in mind these lessons, let us move on to the next section.

Table 4. RADIOLOGIC CHANGES IN DEGENERATIVE ARTHRITIS

Nonuniform cartilage loss
Subchondral sclerosis
Marginal osteophyte formation
Deformity without subluxation
Changes occur over years to decades

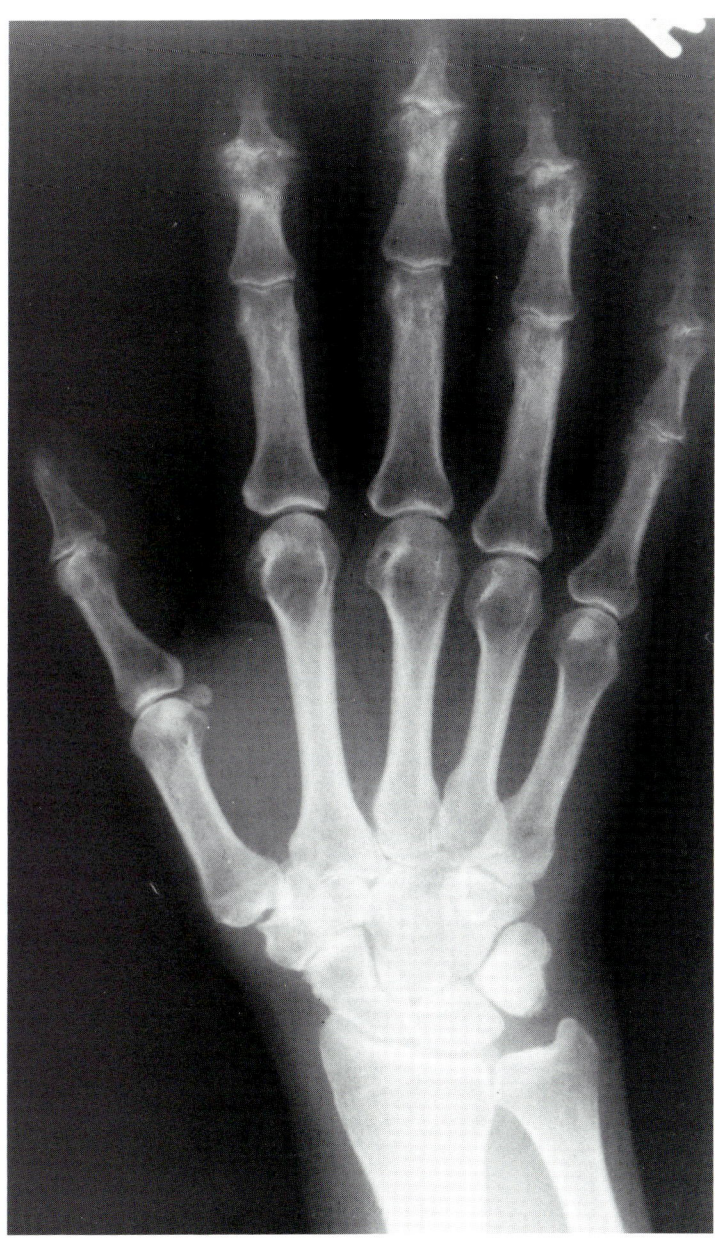

Figure 20

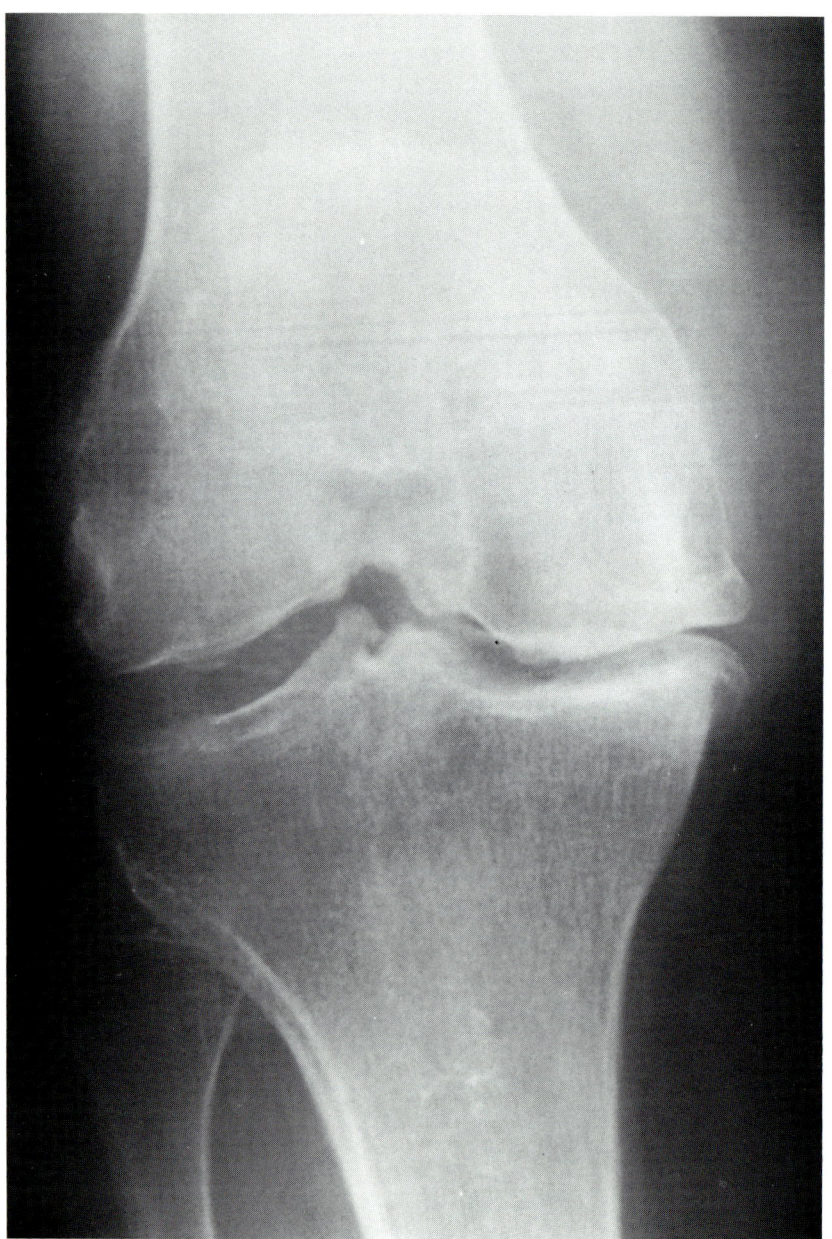

Figure 21

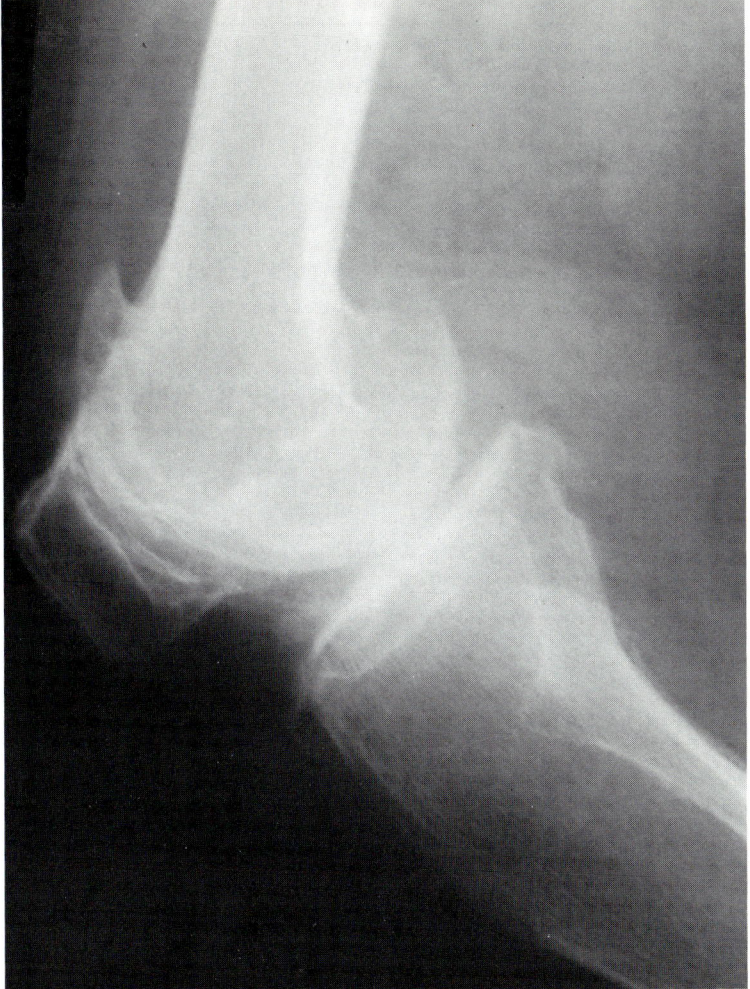

Figure 22

Infectious Arthritis

Initially, radiographic changes seen in infectious arthritis (Table 5) are similar to those seen in early inflammatory arthritis; the radiographs are normal or show evidence of joint effusion and soft tissue swelling. Regional osteoporosis soon follows. Cartilage destruction with erosion and uniform loss of joint space may begin to occur as early as 7 days after the onset of infection, clearly distinguishing pyogenic infections from any other articular process. Bone changes, including periosteal reaction and periarticular osteoporosis, are common in infectious arthritis. Bony sequestrum, or pieces of dead and sclerotic bone in the area of infection, may develop and be visible on radiographs. Nonpyogenic infections, such as those caused by tuberculosis or fungi, show similar radiographic changes but often have a slower onset and less periosteal reaction. Their appearance therefore may more closely mimic an inflammatory noninfectious arthritis. Later, secondary degenerative changes due to abnormal stress on the joint may develop in infectious

SECTION I—APPROACH

Table 5. RADIOLOGIC CHANGES IN INFECTIOUS ARTHRITIS

Soft tissue swelling and effusion
Periarticular osteoporosis
Uniform cartilage erosion with joint space narrowing
Periosteal new bone growth
Bone sequestrum
Onset of changes in 7 to 14 days

arthritis, and radiographs may reflect this. In addition, one must be alert to infectious changes that are superimposed on a degenerative or inflammatory arthritis. Be on your toes!

The next three radiographs are from the same man, an unfortunate soul with swelling of his right knee. The first two radiographs (Figs. 23

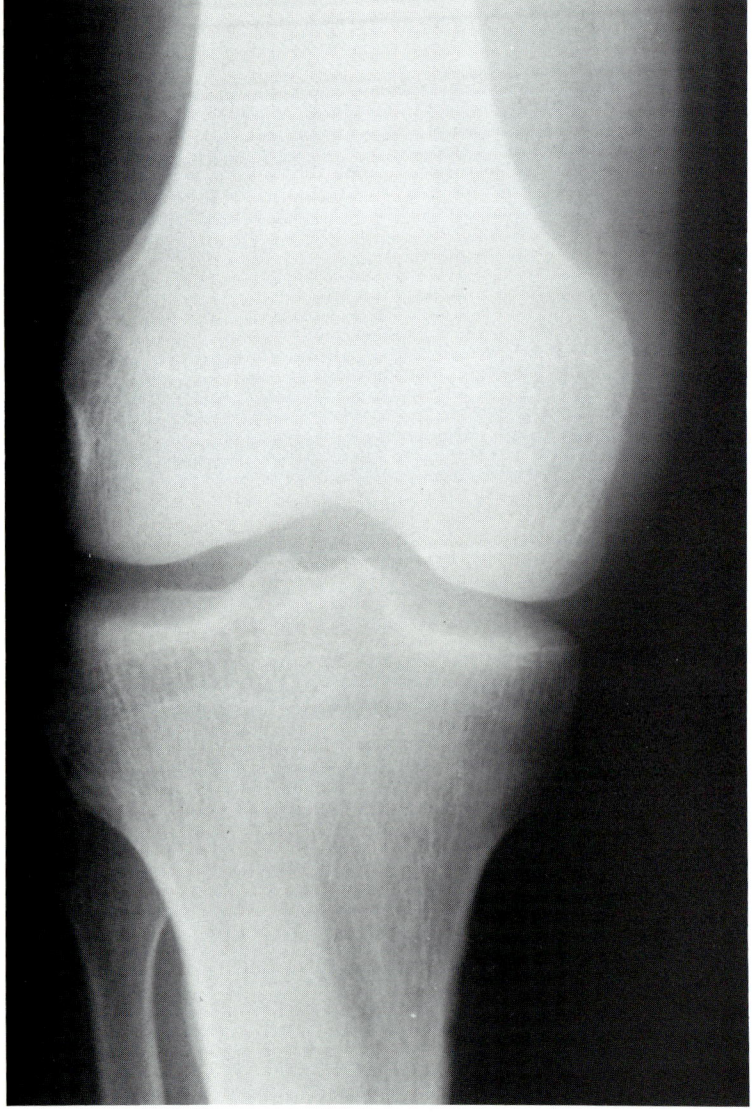

Figure 23

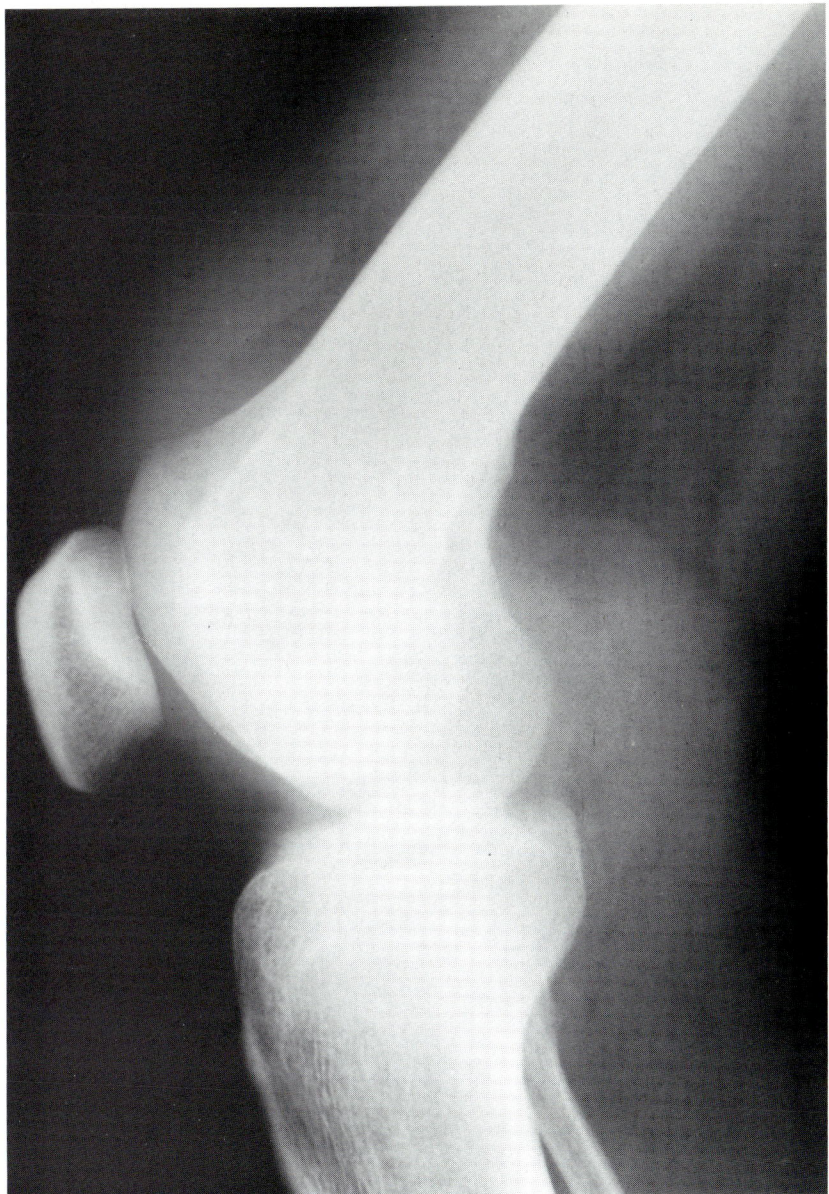

Figure 24

and 24) were taken at the beginning of his illness; the third radiograph (Fig. 25) was taken 1 month later. Can you see a difference? The first two look normal except for the joint effusion visible on the lateral radiograph. The third, however, demonstrates several changes over the intervening month. You should be able to note the loss of bone density around the proximal tibia, which is associated with several subchondral bone erosions on the joint surfaces of the medial and lateral femoral condyles. There is also some joint space narrowing. Although these are characteristics of an inflammatory arthritis, the rapid changes should alert you to consider another category of illness. In fact, *Staphylococcus aureus* was cultured from his joint fluid. This man had a pyogenic

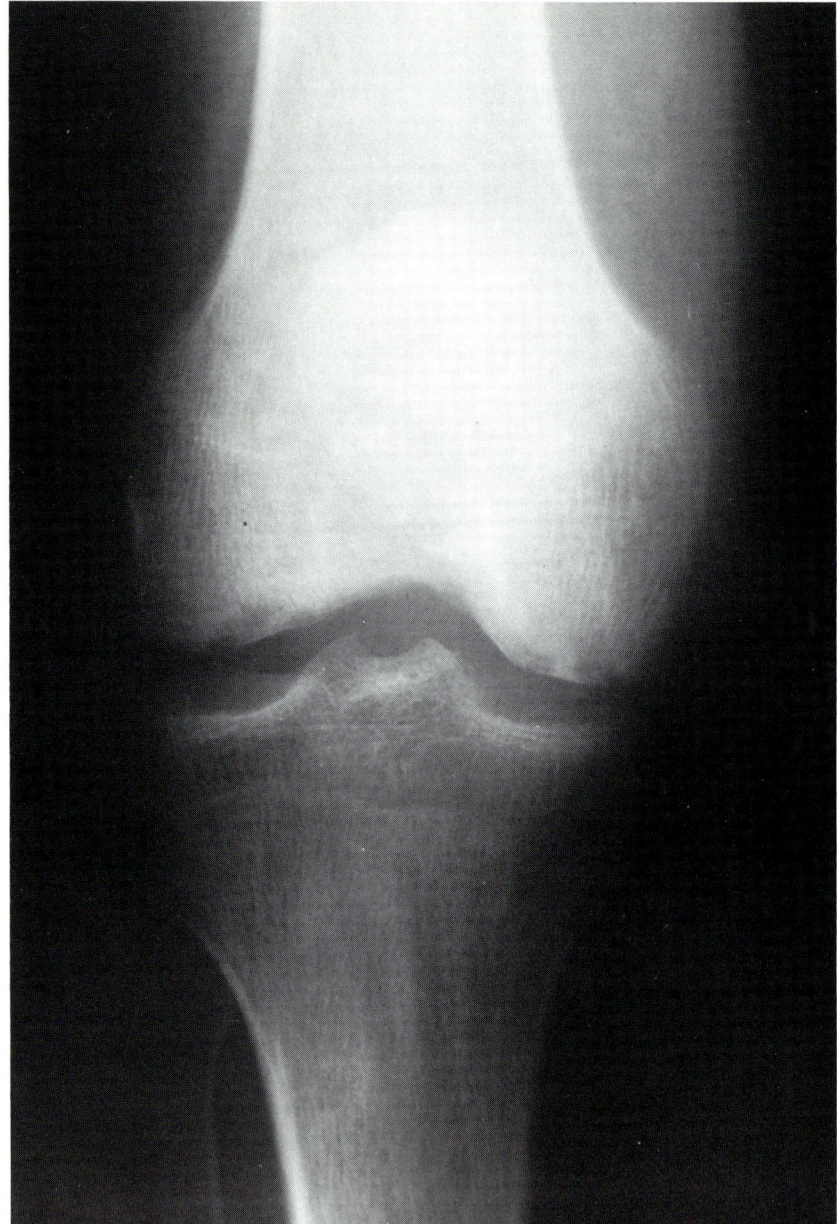

Figure 25

arthritis. Note the absence of periosteal reaction and bone sequestrum, which are late findings and are not present in every case.

SPINAL RADIOGRAPHY

Before we leave these three categories, we need to spend a bit of time discussing the radiologic manifestations that inflammation, degeneration and infection can cause in the spine. Look at the radiographs of the normal lumbosacral spine in Figures 26, 27 and 28. We have labeled some of the important parts you should be able to identify. As before, use these radiographs as references for the abnormal radiographs that follow them.

Figures 26 and 27 demonstrate normal AP and lateral views of the lumbar spine. Note the slight concavity of the anterior surface of each vertebral body. The apophyseal joints (facet joints) can be identified on both the AP and the lateral views (arrows).

Figure 28 shows a normal oblique view of the lumbar spine. The facet joints and the pars articularis (arrow) are best seen in this view. This is the site at which spondylolysis fractures occur.

The inflammatory spinal arthritides include ankylosing spondylitis and the other spondyloarthropathies (i.e., psoriatic spondylitis, reactive arthritis such as Reiter's syndrome and the spondylitis of inflammatory bowel disease). The inflammation involves not only the synovial joints

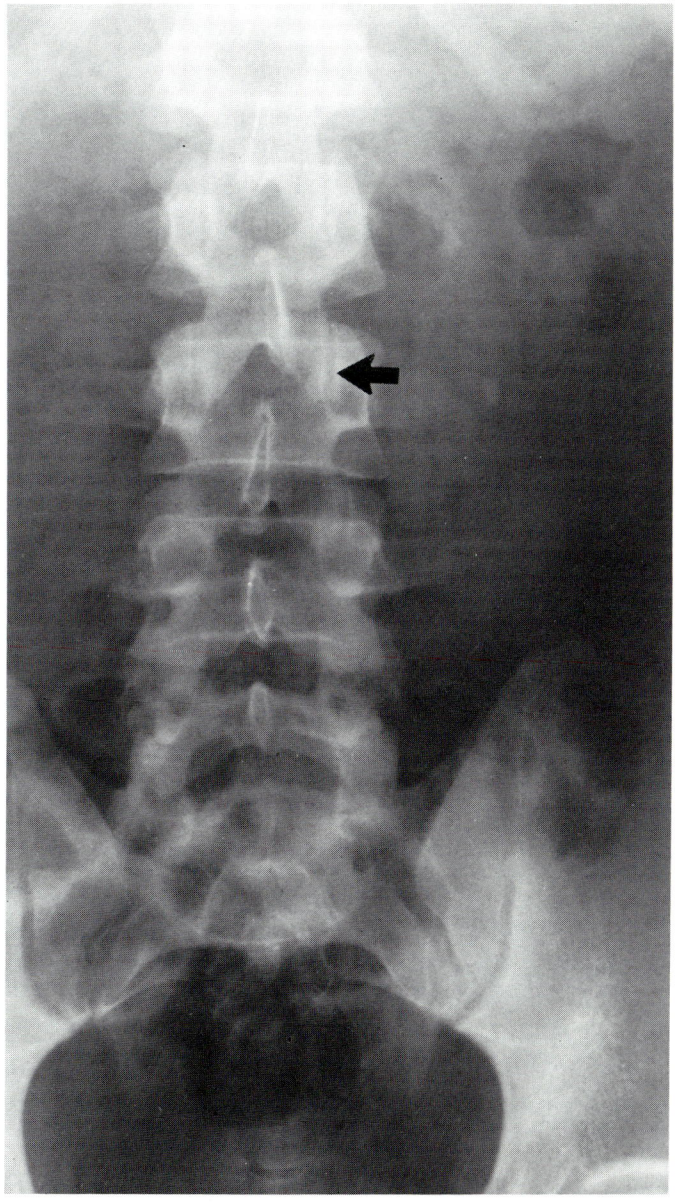

Figure 26

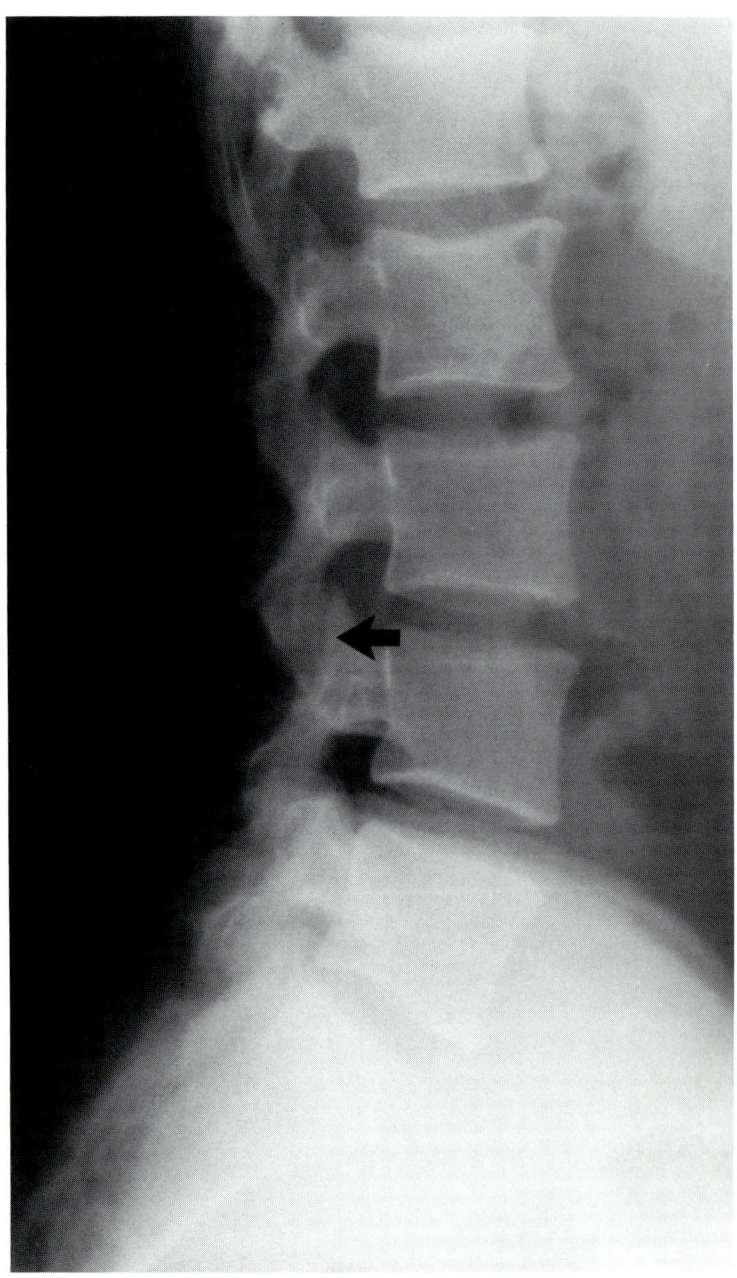

Figure 27

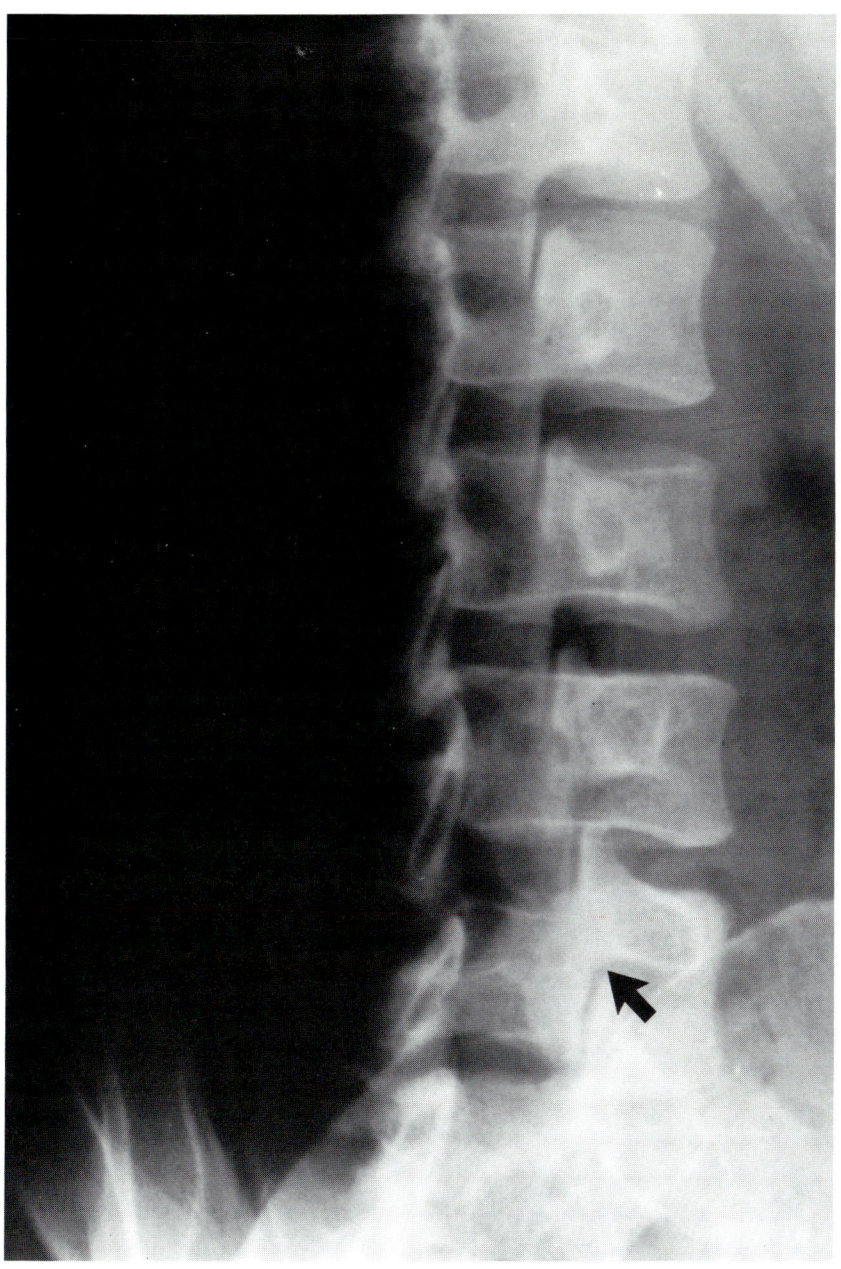

Figure 28

but also the attachments of the spinal ligaments to bone (enthesitis). Changes are seen earliest in the sacroiliac joints, in which initial erosion and narrowing give way to sclerosis and fusion. In the vertebral bodies, inflammation of the spinal ligaments leads to erosion of the tip of the concave vertebral body, changing it into a squared vertebra. Later, calcification of the ligaments occurs, forming the bony bridges known as syndesmophytes. The thin syndesmophytes are a hallmark of inflammatory spondyloarthropathy and must be distinguished from the osteophytes of OA or the bony bridges of the diffuse idiopathic skeletal hypertrophy (DISH) syndrome (more on that later). The spinal apophyseal joints undergo a similar process and eventually erode and fuse. Progression is variable, with some patients exhibiting only sacroiliitis, with or without a few asymmetric syndesmophytes in the lower spine, and some patients having bony bridges extending all the way up to form a completely fused "bamboo" spine.

Figure 29 demonstrates an AP view of the sacroiliac joints. Look at the erosions, marginal sclerosis and symmetric joint space narrowing. This patient has ankylosing spondylitis with moderately advanced changes in the sacroiliac joints. Ankylosing spondylitis begins in the sacroiliac joints in which the abnormalities are usually bilateral and symmetric and are easier to see on the iliac side of the joint.

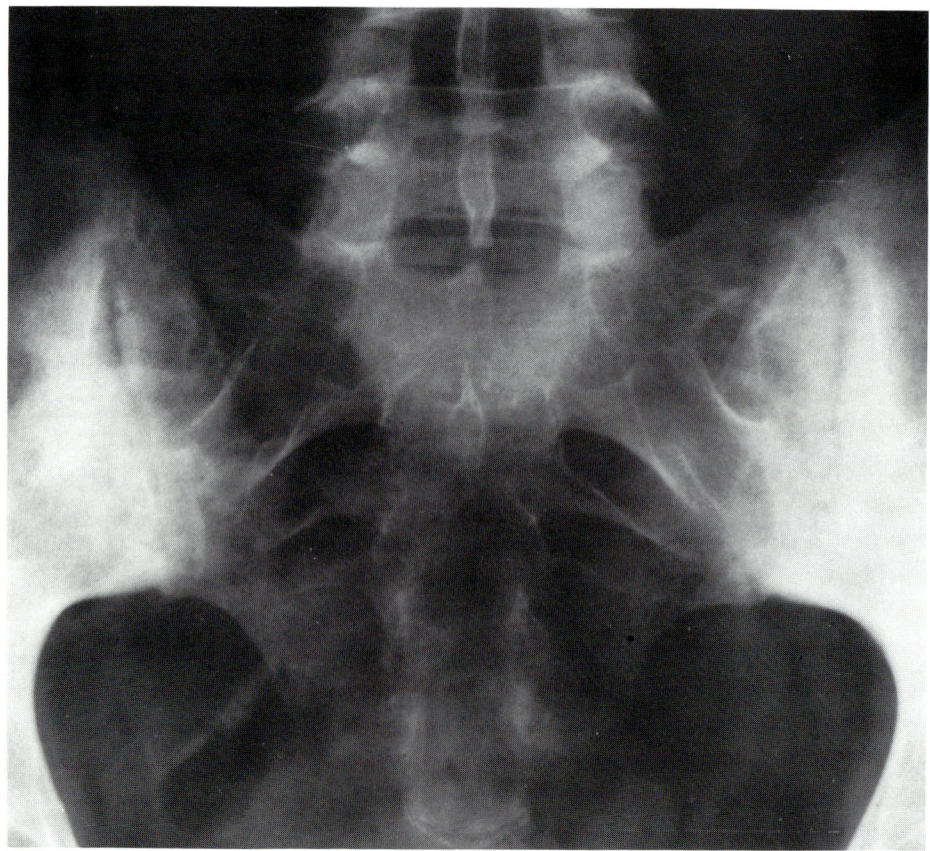

Figure 29

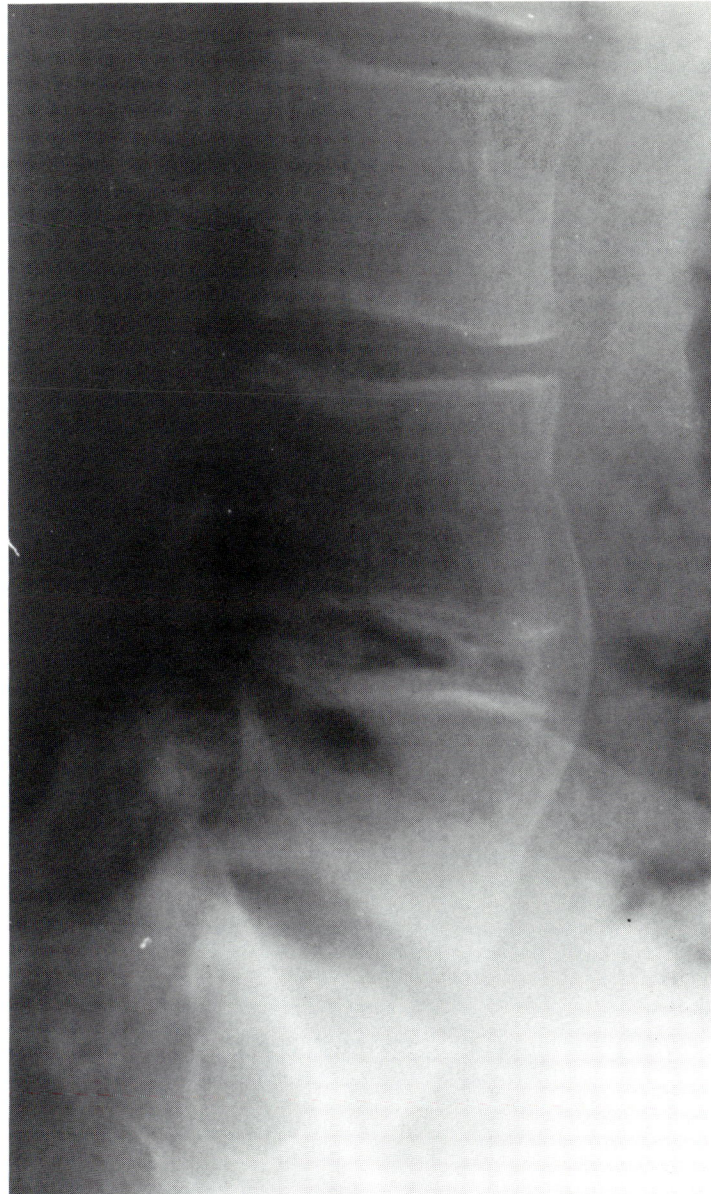

Figure 30

Figure 30 shows a lateral view of the lumbar spine in a young male with psoriatic spondyloarthropathy. The vertically oriented bony overgrowth bridging the L4/L5 intervertebral disc space is a syndesmophyte. Compare this lesion with the osteophytic growth in Figure 32.

Late ankylosing spondylitis is shown in Figure 31. The sacroiliac joints are fused and the syndesmophytes bridge all of the intervertebral disc spaces, producing the so-called bamboo spine. Note also that the apophyseal joints are fused and that there is ligamentous calcification between the spinous processes in the midline lower lumbar region.

Spinal OA shows radiographic changes that are similar to peripheral joint OA. The intervertebral disc degenerates and narrows, bringing the

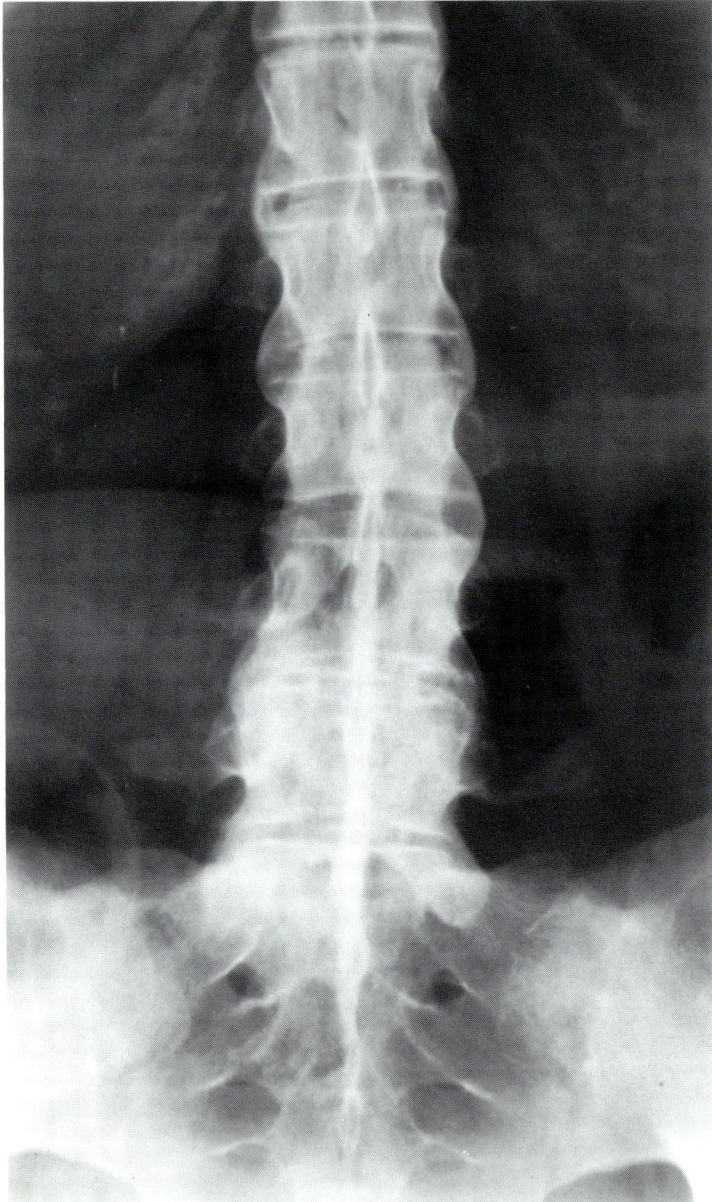

Figure 31

vertebrae closer together. Bony sclerosis and marginal osteophytes develop in the vertebrae above and below the degenerating disc. Severely degenerated discs may appear to have gas in them—the "vacuum disc" phenomenon. Osteoarthritic changes of sclerosis, joint space narrowing and osteophyte formation also occur in the spinal apophyseal joints (facets). Occasionally this may lead to subluxation and slippage of one vertebra on another, or spondylolisthesis. All these changes may cause nerve entrapment, either in the neural foramina or the central canal, causing symptoms of a radiculopathy or a myelopathy, respectively. Of course, below the L1/L2 level, the spinal cord has ended, so even central canal narrowing causes radiculopathy there. These areas are better seen on a computed axial tomography (CAT) scan, a myelogram, or magnetic resonance imaging, some of which will be demonstrated in the next section.

Figure 32 shows spondylitis deformans or spinal OA. The bony outgrowths at the corners of the vertebral bodies are osteophytes. Compare these with the bone growth seen in Figures 29 and 31.

Figure 33 demonstrates spinal stenosis. There is extensive bony overgrowth in the region of the apophyseal joint, in addition to the narrowed disc and posterior vertebral osteophytes at the L4/L5 disc space. These factors will cause a narrowed spinal canal or neuroforamina, or both, and will lead to symptoms of a lumbar radiculopathy.

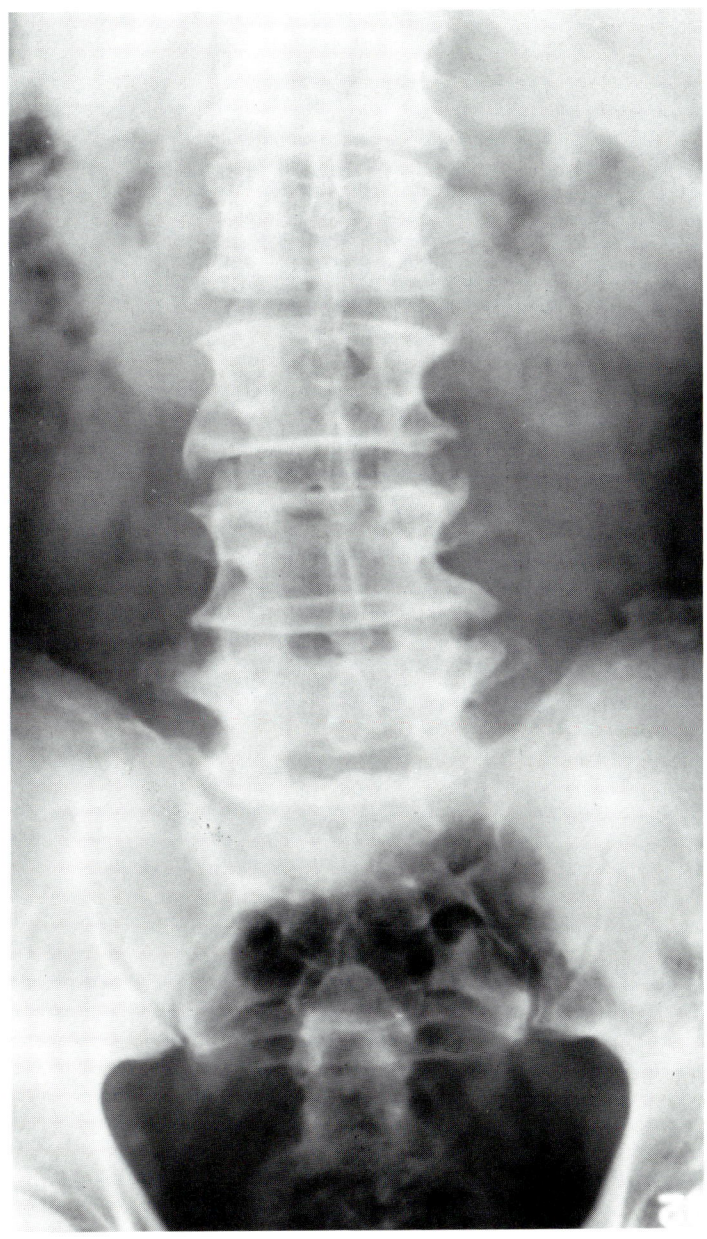

Figure 32

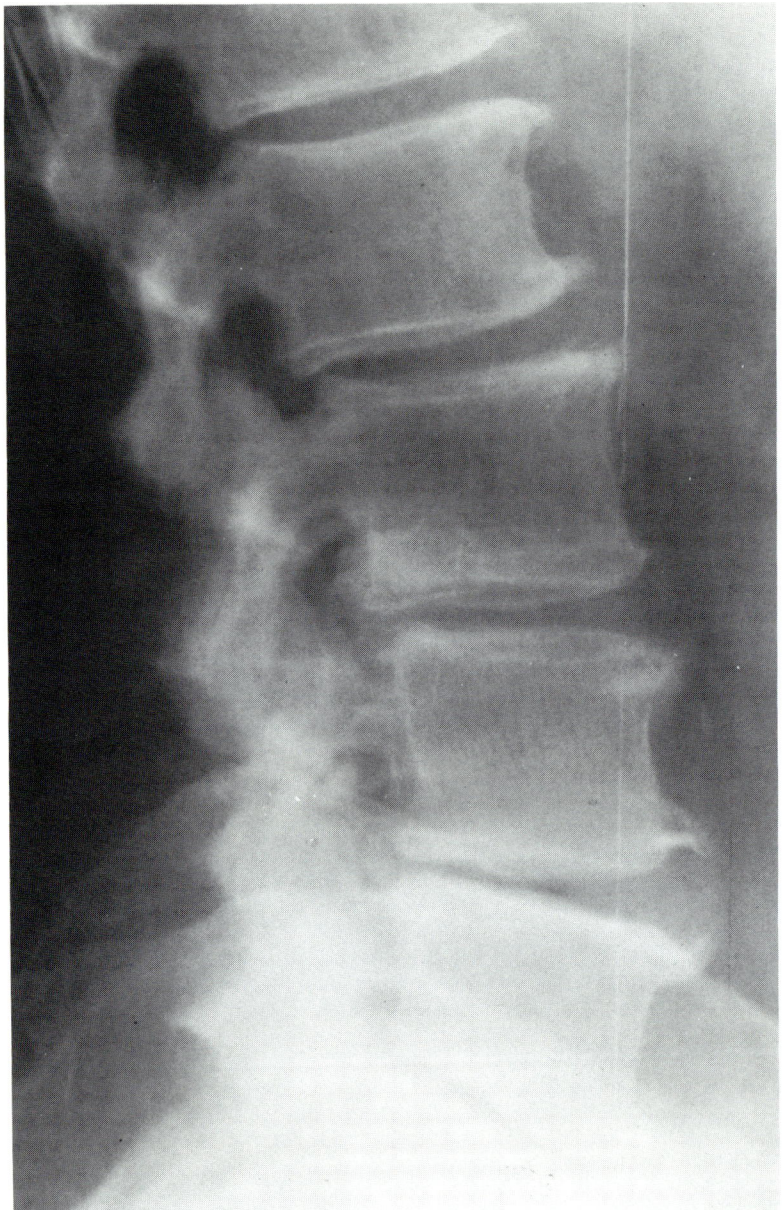

Figure 33

Septic disc infections present a radiographic appearance that is similar to that of peripheral joint infection. Disc space narrowing and vertebral endplate deossification and erosion are the earliest findings and may be associated with a contiguous vertebral osteomyelitis and the attendant bone changes. Ultimately, vertebral collapse and deformity of the spine may be seen. Infection may spread directly to the surrounding soft tissues, leading to a local soft tissue abscess. One common site for this is the psoas muscle. In nonpyogenic infections, such as tuberculous or fungal infections, vertebral endplate sclerosis may occur. Noninfectious traumatic and inflammatory discitis, as seen in the spondyloarthropathies, may have a radiographic appearance that is similar to that of a septic discitis and must be differentiated from infections. These will be discussed further in the next section.

Figure 34 shows a lateral view of the lumbar spine. The radiograph demonstrates moderate hypertrophic disease at all levels. Note particularly the L1/L2 disc space. The disc space is narrowed, and destructive changes are present in the opposing endplates of L1 and L2. This type of change is characteristic of a disc space infection.

Figure 35 is an AP view of the spine in another patient with septic discitis. There is narrowing of the T10/T11 disc space with destruction of the opposing endplates. Note the lateral displacement (arrow) of the paraspinal lines, which is indicative of extension beyond the disc space (paraspinal abscess).

Before we leave the spine, we include in Figures 36, 37 and 38 the standard views of the cervical spine: the AP view (Fig. 36), the lateral view (Fig. 37) and the oblique view (Fig. 38). Most of what we said previously about the lumbar spine is also valid for the cervical spine. Please pay particular attention to two areas. Note on the lateral view the relationship between the odontoid and the anterior part of the body of C1 (arrows), as this will be important later in our study of RA; also

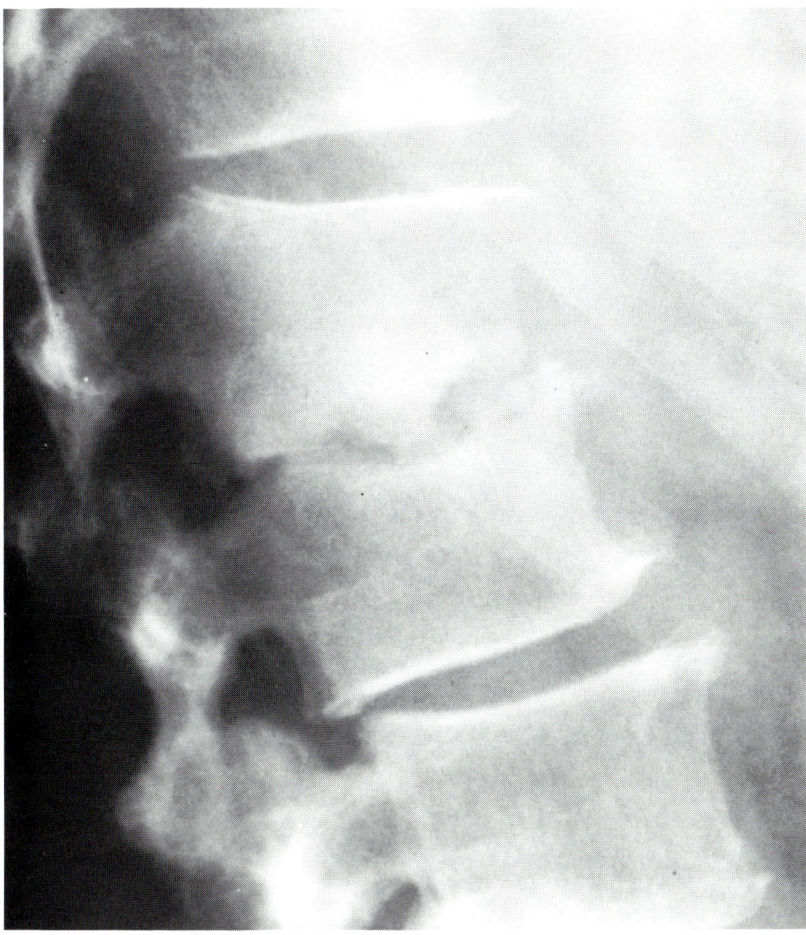

Figure 34

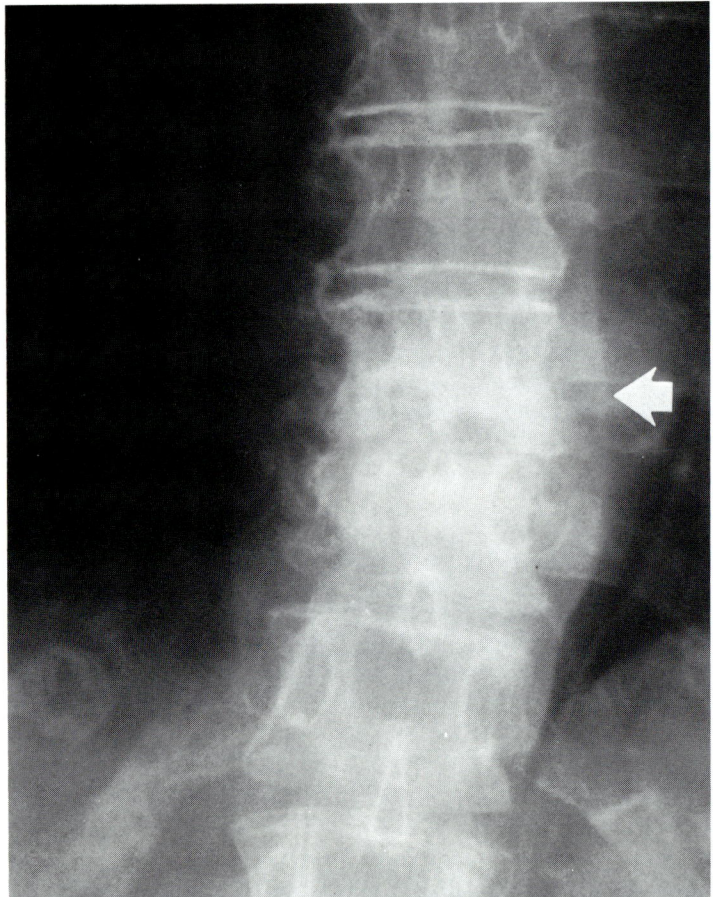

Figure 35

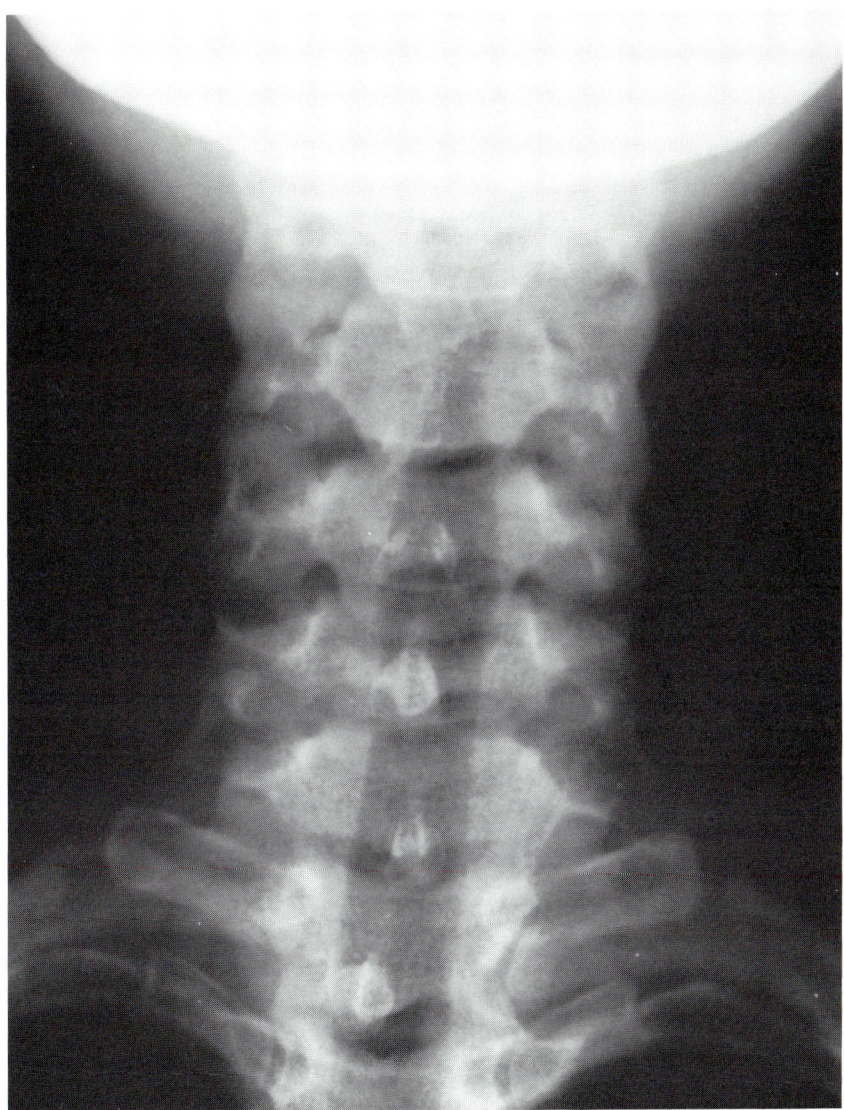

Figure 36

note on the oblique view how nicely the neural foramina are demonstrated (arrow). In the next section, we will show you examples of degenerative disease with osteophyte formation, leading to nerve root compression in this area.

Crystal-Induced Arthritis

Before we leave the section on approaching the radiograph, we need to discuss the crystal arthropathies. They are a heterogeneous group of illnesses, with their clinical and radiologic characteristics dependent on the type of crystal involved. We will discuss the three most commonly seen crystal diseases: uric acid disease, calcium pyrophosphate dihydrate (CPPD) disease, and calcium hydroxyapatite (CHO) disease.

The radiologic manifestations of uric acid arthropathy can be divided into two distinct but related entities: acute gouty attacks and chronic tophaceous deposits (Table 6). Acute gouty attacks are the result of precipitation of uric acid crystals into the synovial space, inciting a

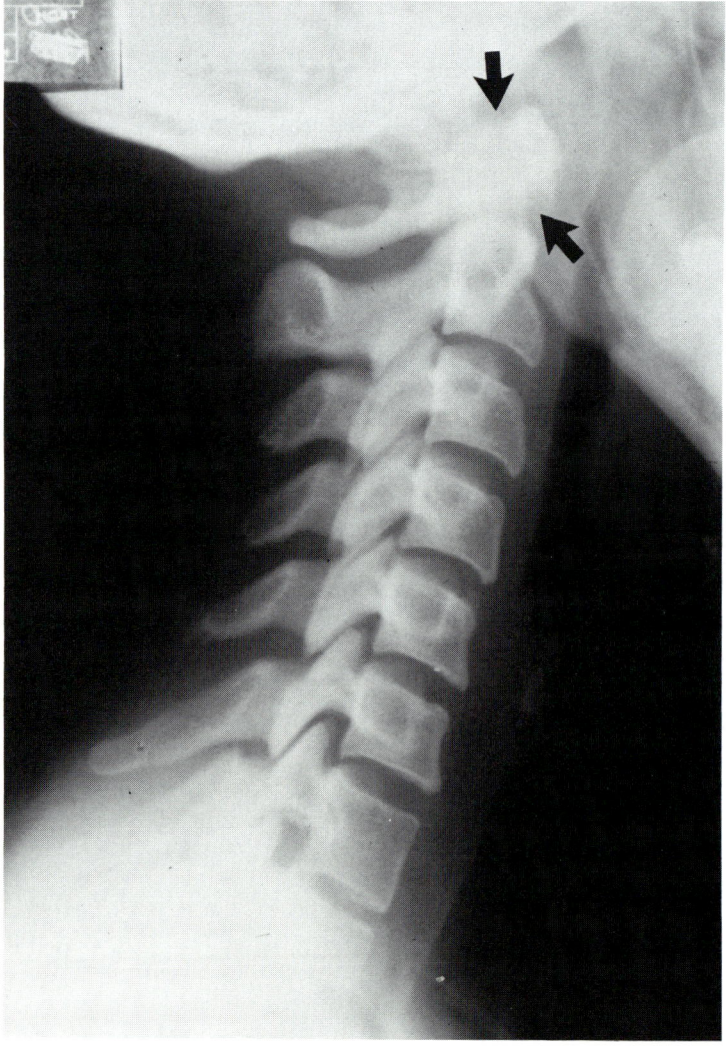

Figure 37

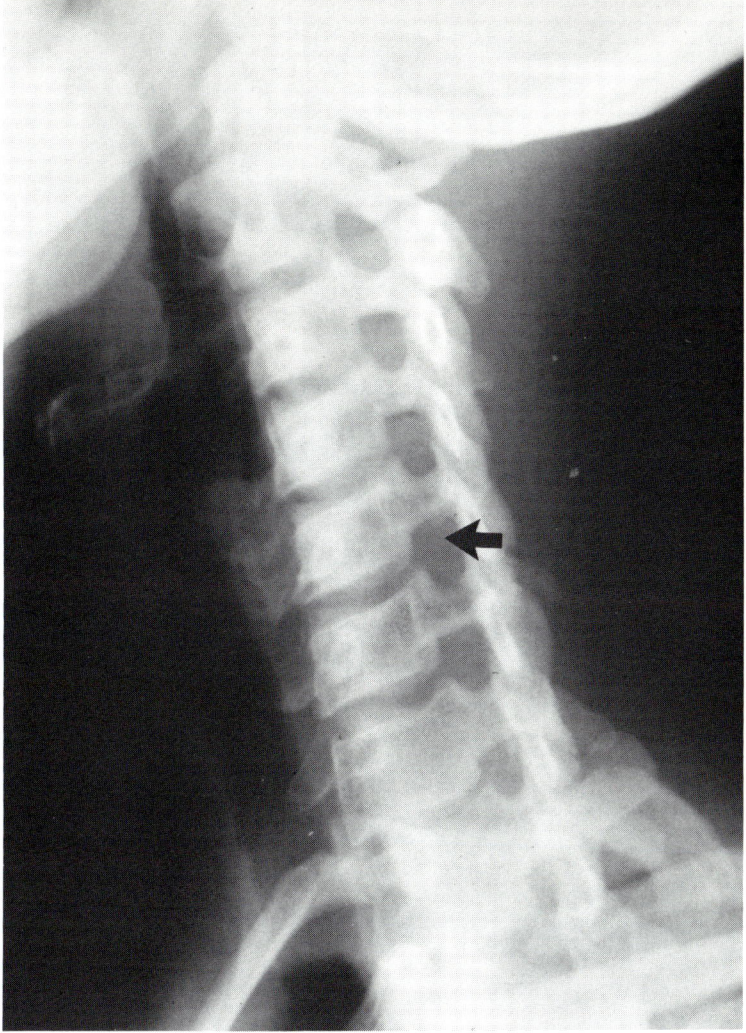

Figure 38

neutrophilic inflammatory response and leading to acute pain, swelling, redness and tenderness. As you would expect in this circumstance, radiographs are nonspecific, revealing only soft tissue swelling or synovial effusions, or both, that are indistinguishable from other causes of such inflammation.

Tophaceous gout results from chronic periarticular and soft tissue deposits of urates that form hard nodules called tophi. When close to the skin they are palpable, often on the pinna of the ear or in the olecranon bursa by the elbow. In a periarticular distribution, the deposits often are visible on radiographs as a soft tissue density. Figure 39 demonstrates tophaceous gout around the first MTP joint. Note also that the deposit contains a small area of calcification and that it is associated with erosion of the metatarsal head, all typical signs of tophaceous deposits. The bone may respond with an osteophyte-like growth around the tophi as if it were trying to encircle it. This growth is called an overhanging lip. Such changes are very specific for long-standing gout.

The second type of crystal we will discuss is that of CPPD (Table 7). CPPD crystals become deposited in articular cartilage around chon-

Table 6. URATE CRYSTALS IN URIC ACID ARTHROPATHY

Acute Gout
  Soft tissue swelling
  Capsular swelling
Chronic Tophaceous Gout
  Soft tissue density
  Fine calcium deposits in density
  Erosions near the deposit
  Overhanging osteophytic lip

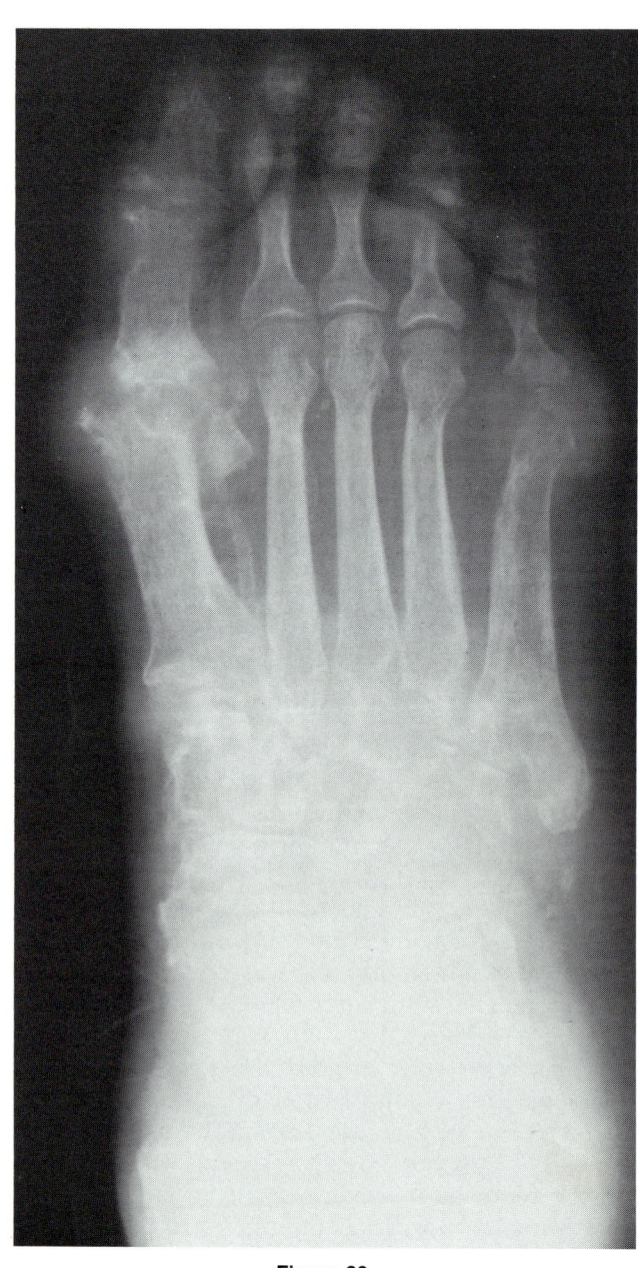

Figure 39

Table 7. CPPD CRYSTALS

Manifestations of CPPD Deposits	States Associated with Chondrocalcinosis
Chondrocalcinosis	Hemochromatosis
Degenerative arthritis	Ochronosis
Acute crystal arthritis–pseudogout	Hyperparathyroidism
	Wilson's disease
	Aging
	Idiopathic states
	Familial conditions
	Hypothyroidism
	Other

drocytes in response to a number of metabolic and other disease states. When enough CPPD crystals have been deposited, three things occur: (1) The crystals become visible on radiographs as thin linear deposits of calcium in the articular hyaline cartilage and the fibrocartilage (chondrocalcinosis); (2) articular cartilage degenerates as chondrocyte death occurs (OA); and (3) crystals may shed cartilage into the intra-articular space, which leads to an acute crystal-induced synovitis (pseudogout).

Chondrocalcinosis has a typical radiologic picture. Look at Figure 40, which demonstrates the fine linear calcification in the triangular

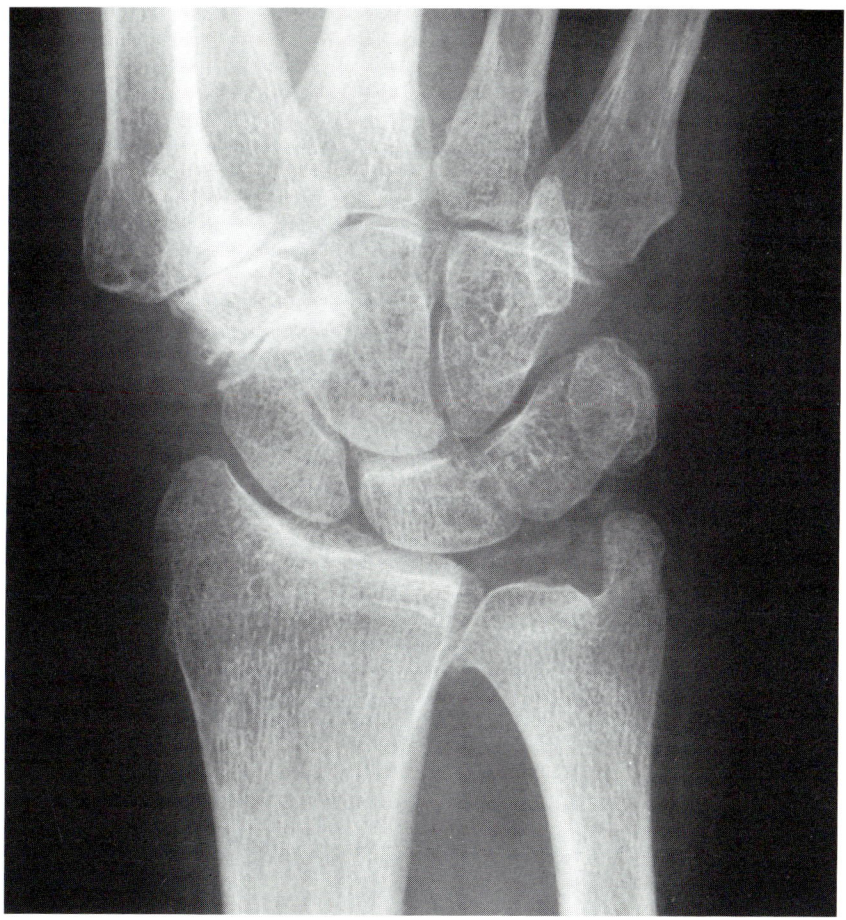

Figure 40

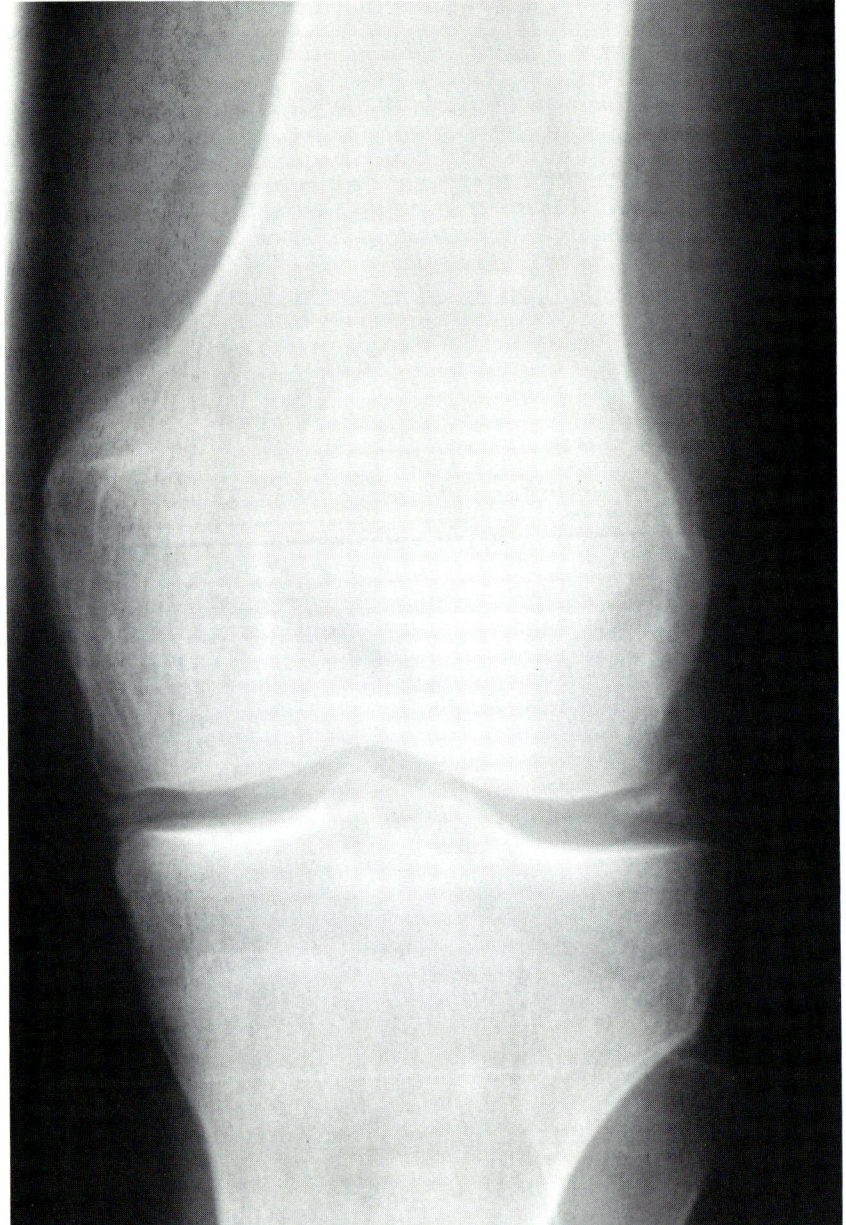

Figure 41

cartilage of the wrist overlying the distal ulna. Figure 41 (AP view) and Figure 42 (lateral view) show similar calcification in the medial and lateral menisci of the knee as well as in the patellofemoral region. Did you notice the joint effusion in the suprapatellar pouch? Another common location for the deposits is in the symphysis pubis, but the deposits can be seen at any cartilage location, including the intervertebral disc.

Radiographically, the degenerative arthritis of CPPD looks similar to that of primary OA, with subchondral sclerosis and cysts, loss of cartilage space and osteophyte formation. The distribution, however, tends to differ. CPPD is more likely to affect the patellofemoral joint than is primary OA and is also more likely to involve all three compartments of the knee simultaneously. It also affects the wrist, the MCP joints and joints around the ankle and foot in places in which primary OA is never found. The destruction is occasionally so severe that it may resemble a neuropathic (Charcot) joint.

Acute pseudogout has a radiographic picture that is similar to that of acute gout, with soft tissue swelling and articular effusion. It often prefers the wrist, knee and ankle to the great toe. Of course, synovial fluid analysis will reveal CPPD crystals rather than urates.

Our final crystal is CHO. This is most commonly found as an amorphous mass deposit around the shoulder tendons or the greater trochanter of the hip, at which point it is often but not invariably associated with acute episodes of inflammatory bursitis. Look at Figure 43, which demonstrates such a deposit in the rotator cuff. This patient presented with a sudden inability to lift his arm because of localized pain at the site of the deposit, which was completely relieved by a local injection of cortisone into the bursa. Such deposits are also seen around

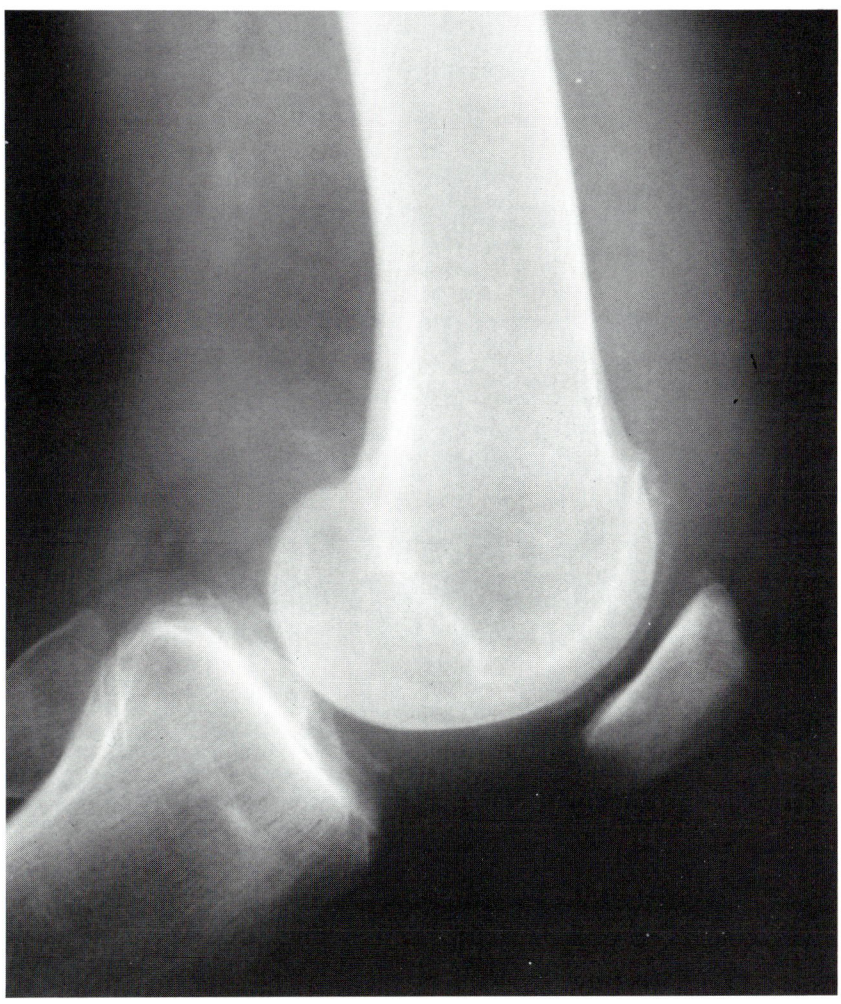

Figure 42

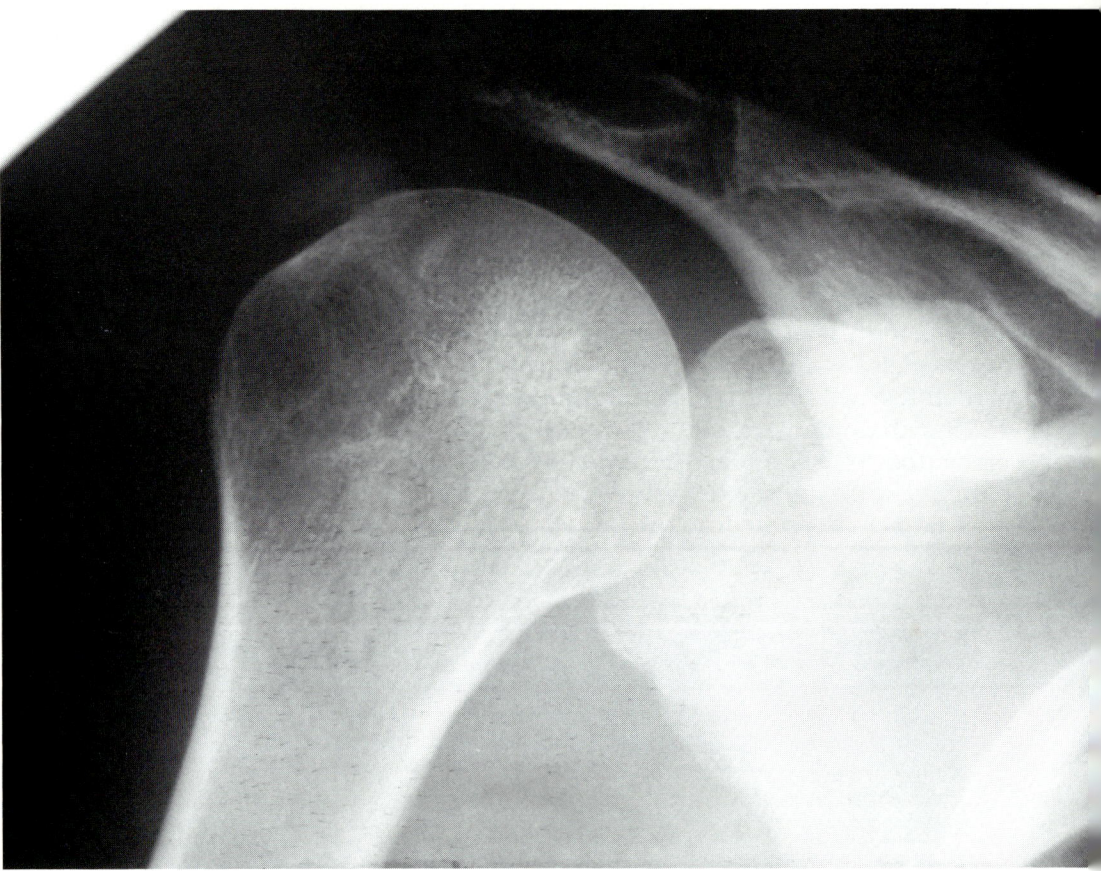

Figure 43

smaller joints or tendons in some patients, particularly those who undergo renal dialysis. These deposits may correlate with areas of clinical tenderness at these points. In the elderly, such deposits may be found around a destroyed, eroded shoulder in which they seem to play a role in initiating the chronic inflammation that leads to such destruction (Milwaukee shoulder). Finally, apatite may be seen in the soft tissues or muscles of patients with scleroderma, dermatopolymyositis or myositis ossificans, in which it seems unassociated with acute inflammation.

SECTION II

EXERCISES

SECTION II—EXERCISES

EXERCISES

Now that we've given you the fundamentals of radiographic interpretation, let us practice on some actual cases. The rest of the book consists of a series of radiographs, often with a case history associated, for you to practice on. Remember to interpret them using the approach we gave you in Table 1 and the guidelines we gave you in the other tables. Refer to these in order to help synthesize your thoughts. Good luck.

Hands

Exercise 1

Compare the two hand radiographs given. Decide which is inflammatory and which is degenerative.

Figure 44 demonstrates soft tissue swelling around areas of osteophyte formation and deformity in a distribution of the DIP and PIP joints. There is no demineralization, and the wrist and MCP joints are spared. This is typical DJD. In contrast, Figure 45 shows a diffuse periarticular decrease in bone density around all joints, especially the wrist, which is eroded. Look at the narrowing of the radiocarpal joint.

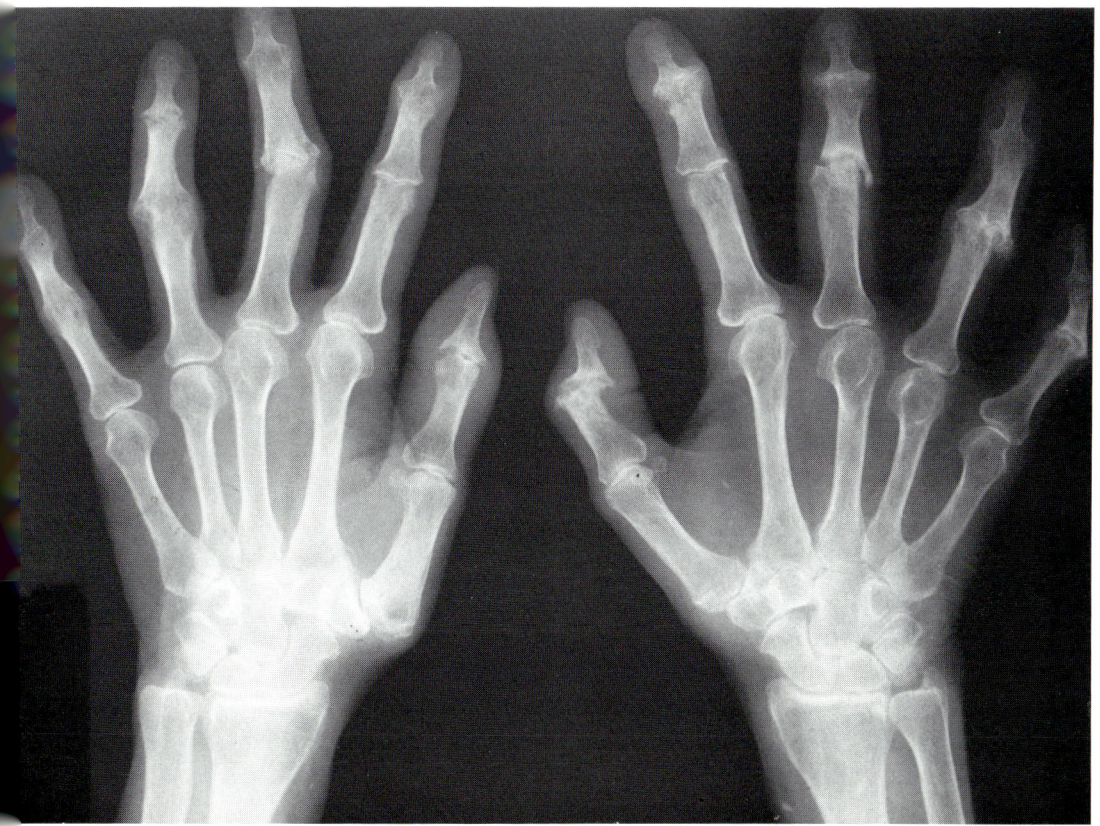

Figure 44

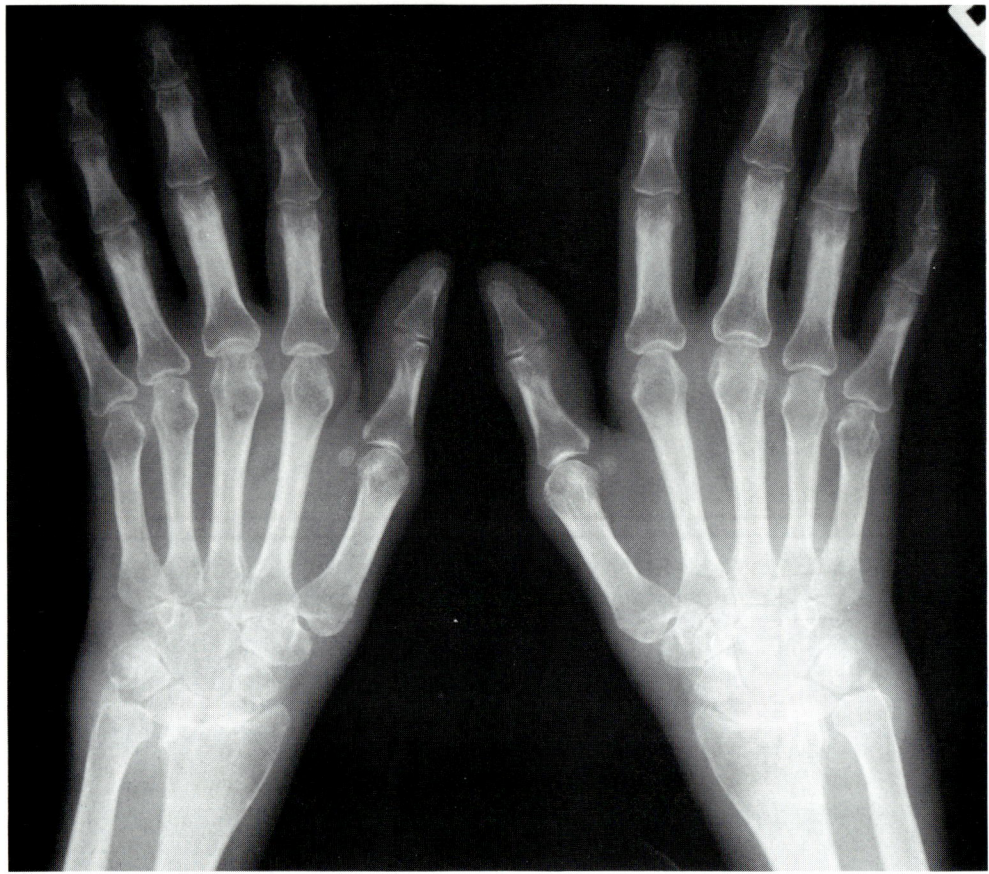

Figure 45

The soft tissue swelling is mostly around the PIP joints, especially the third one, and is diffuse. There is no new bone growth. Did you notice the soft tissue nodular-like swellings on the medial end of the index finger PIP joints? This is RA with nodules.

If you had trouble with this one, review for a moment the difference between inflammatory and degenerative arthritis as given in Tables 2 and 3. In addition, a useful clinical clue to remember is that degenerative arthritis tends to attack the DIP, PIP and first CMC joints, whereas RA attacks the PIP and MCP joints and the wrist. This difference in sites of involvement between the two may be an aid in diagnosis for you.

Exercise 2

Jed, 47 years old, has a history of pain and swelling at several DIP joints. His father, who is with him at the examination, has similar swellings, but he claims they aren't as painful as his son's are. On examination, Jed's DIP joints are red and tender. In addition, his nails look ragged and irregular, and he has a rash. His father's DIP joints are hard and are not tender. Look at their radiographs (Figs. 46 and 47) and decide if they have the same illness or not.

SECTION II—EXERCISES

Jed's radiograph (Fig. 46) demonstrates an inflammatory type of soft tissue swelling around the second, third and fourth DIP joints. There is some widening of the distal bone of the DIP, but with inflammatory erosions in them and in the proximal end. Although the distribution is correct for OA, these are not the Heberden's nodes of OA. His father's radiograph (Fig. 47) shows osteophytes at his DIP and PIP joints with severe joint space narrowing (look especially at the osteophytes off the DIP of the thumb), but without real soft tissue swelling. Jed has psoriatic arthritis, and this explains his nail and skin changes. The DIP joint is a typical site for the inflammatory changes of psoriatic arthritis, which tends to be much more asymmetric than the changes

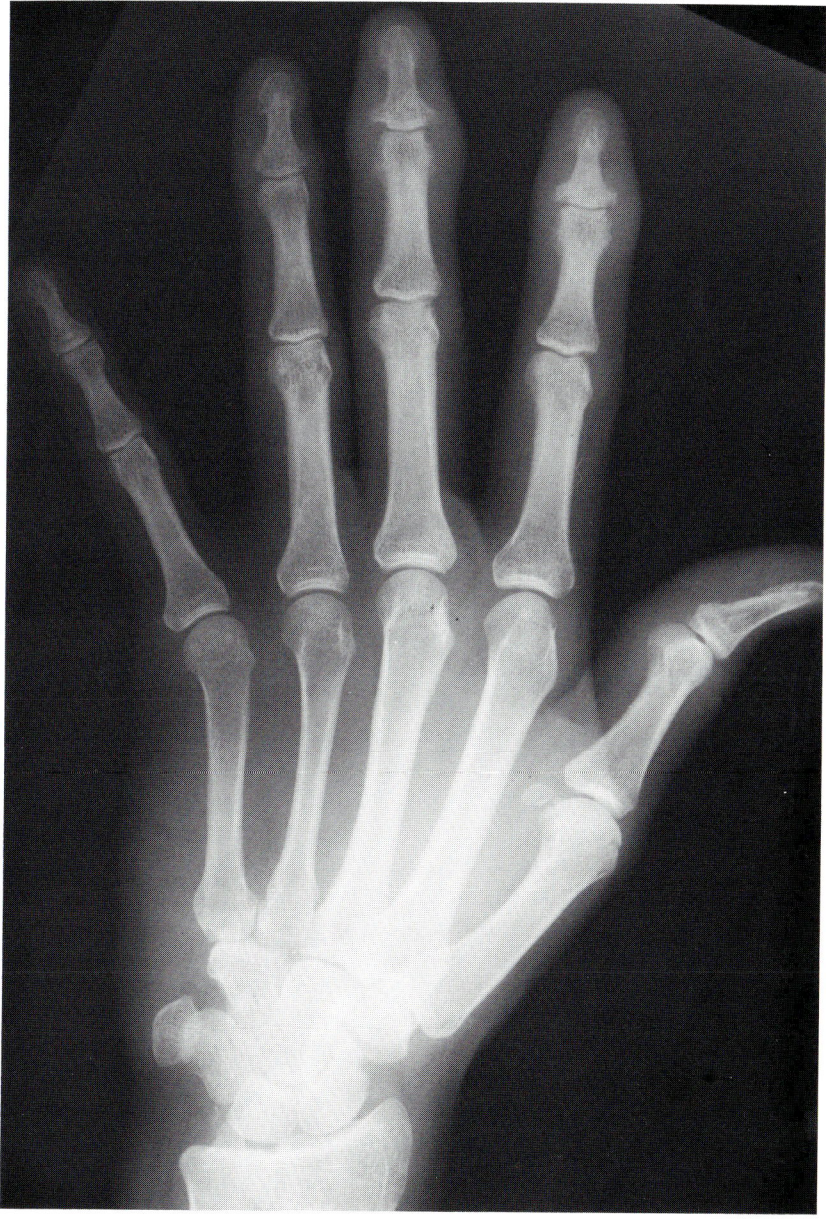

Figure 46

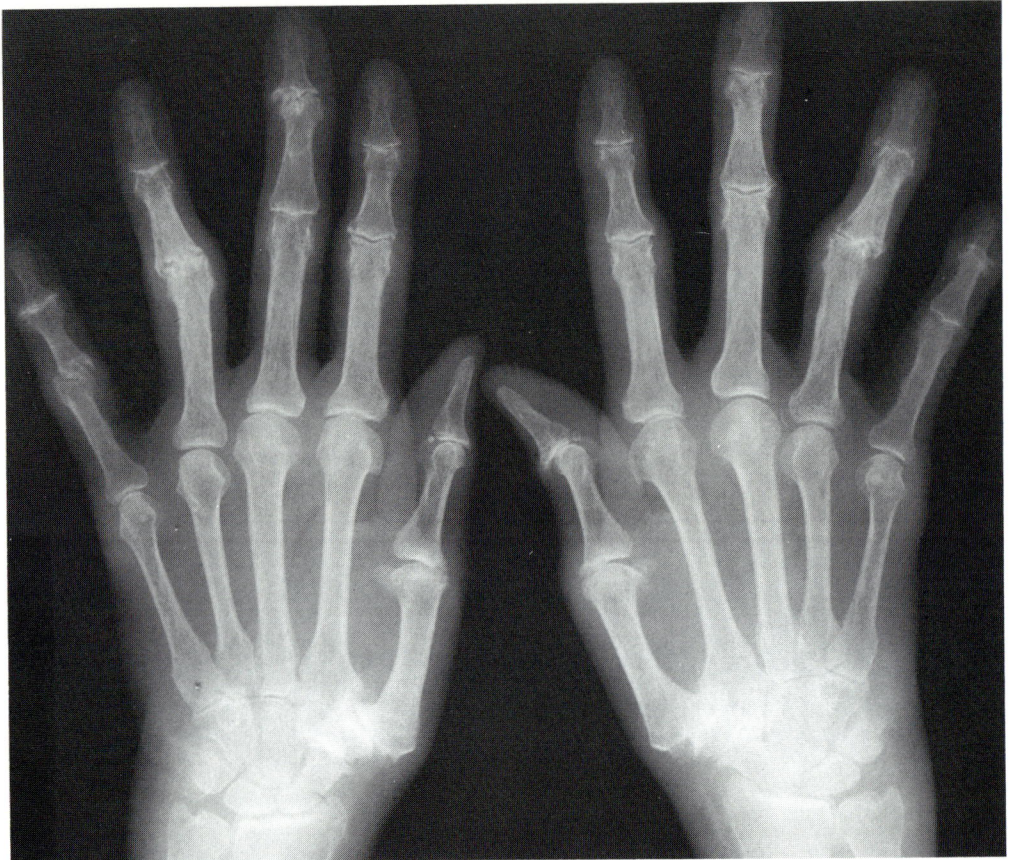

Figure 47

of RA. His father has typical OA. Look at the first CMCs on his father's hands, which manifest similar OA changes.

Exercise 3

Rosa, 58 years old, has striking ulnar deviation at all the MCP joints of her left hand and at most of those on her right hand. You are surprised, therefore, when a radiograph of her hands (Fig. 48) fails to find this subluxation or any erosive disease of the MCP joints at all. The radiograph is not normal however. Can you think of a diagnosis that fits this radiographic and clinical situation?

Rosa demonstrates severe periarticular osteopenia at the MCP, PIP, and DIP joints and at the wrists but no joint erosion or ulnar deviation! Does this surprise you given the clinical description of her hands? It shouldn't. Rosa has SLE, and this is typically a nonerosive but occasionally deforming arthritis. When the radiographic cassette supports the hands, the deformity, which is due to ligamentous laxity rather than bony destruction, may abate, only to return when the hands are lifted from the cassette, as in the Norgaard view in Figure 49. In both films you can see the nonerosive deformity of her thumb. Also notice some OA at the DIP joints of both hands. Rosa is 58 years old and not immune to other illnesses!

SECTION II—EXERCISES

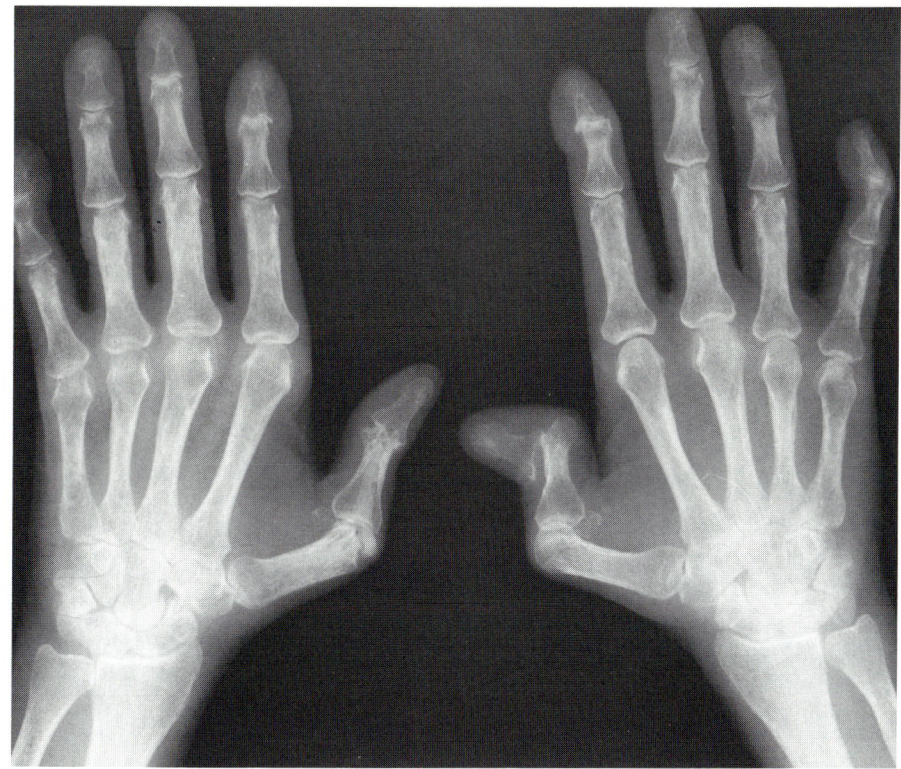

Figure 48

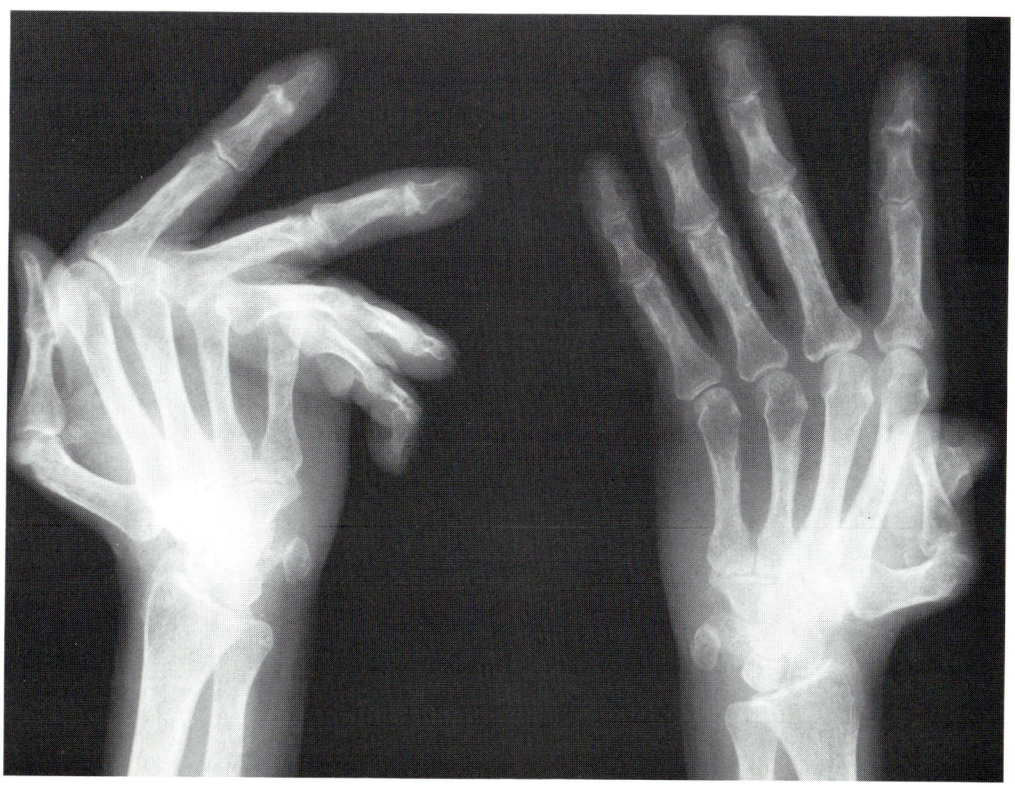

Figure 49

Exercise 4

Henrietta has pain and decreased range of motion in her thumb. She's 68 years old and has noticed knobby fingers developing over the last few years. Look at her radiograph and explain why her thumb hurts (Fig. 50).

The thumb radiograph demonstrates narrowing of the first CPC joint associated with subchondral sclerosis and hypertrophic changes. Henrietta has OA. Figure 51 shows a two-part cemented prosthesis that was placed to relieve her symptoms.

Exercise 5

Irma, 53 years old, complains of pain in both her DIP and PIP joints and around the radial part of her wrist and thumbs. What does the radiograph (Fig. 52) tell you about the nature of her disease?

Irma has an extensive erosive arthritis that at first glance appears to be severe RA. Although there are large erosions around most of the MCP joints, the involvement of the DIP joints and the sparing of the left third MCP joint suggest the pattern and asymmetry of psoriatic arthritis rather than RA. Note the tapering of the proximal bone of

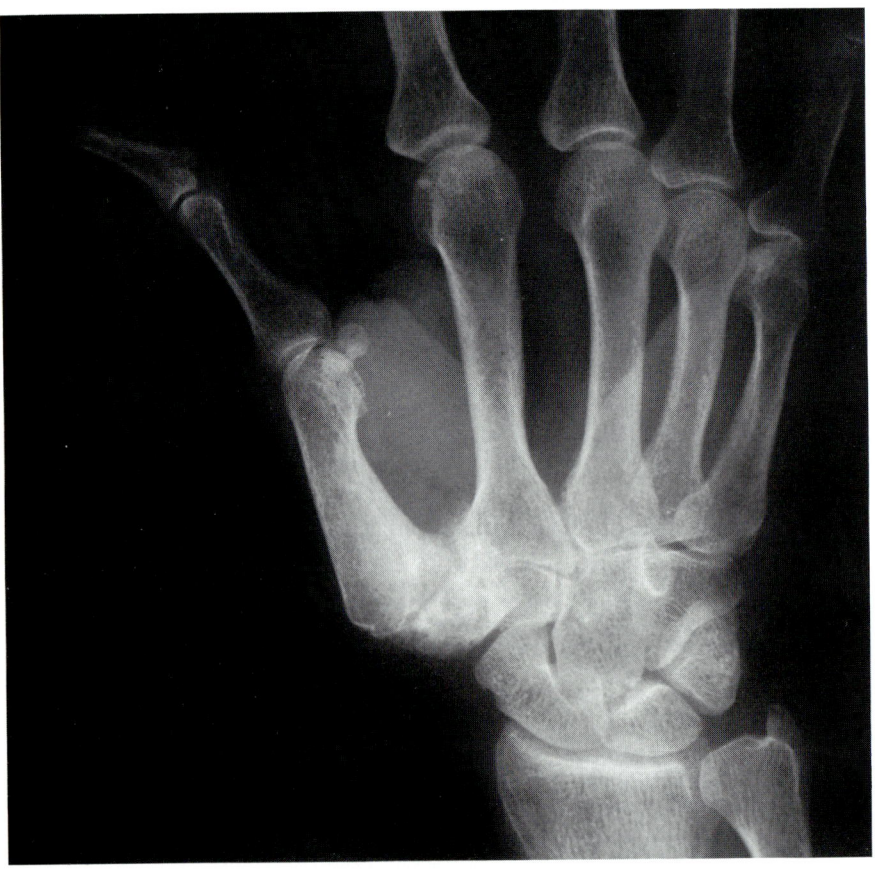

Figure 50

SECTION II—EXERCISES

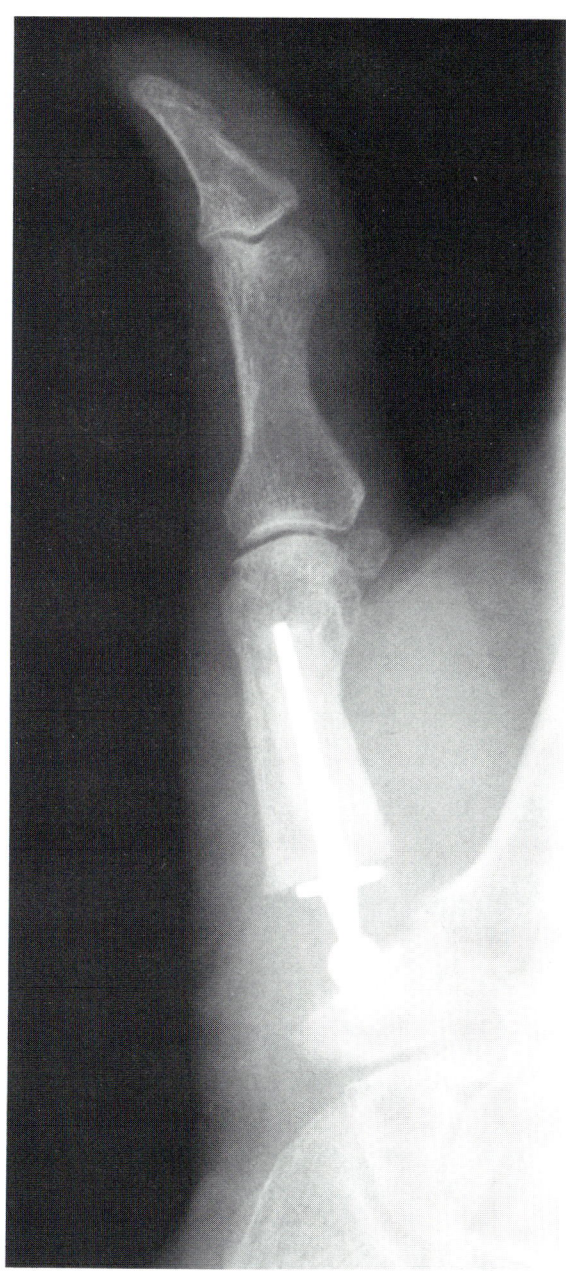

Figure 51

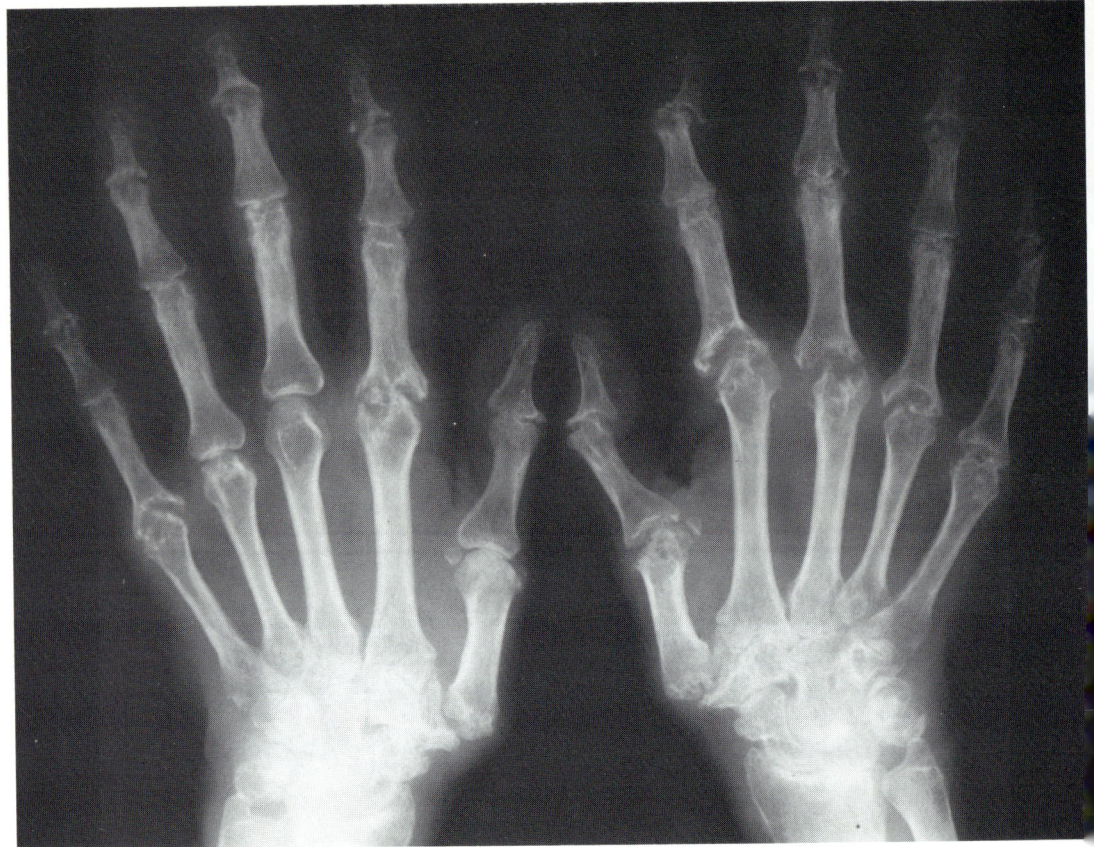

Figure 52

many of her DIP joints, which indent the widened distal end to form a "pencil and cup" deformity, typical of psoriatic arthritis. Irma had a scaling rash around her elbows, scalp and knees and pitting of her nails. She has psoriasis with psoriatic arthritis.

Exercise 6

Marcia has had RA for several years. Look at her hand radiographs. Describe what you see on the first film (Fig. 53) that confirms the diagnosis of RA and then describe what progression occurred over the 3 years that passed until the next film (Fig. 54).

The first radiograph (Fig. 53) demonstrates soft tissue swelling of the right first MCP joint, in which there is an erosion. No other soft tissue swelling is obvious. There is periarticular osteopenia, and erosions are present at the second and third left MCP heads. A few tiny erosions are present in the carpal bones. Three years later (Fig. 54) there is extensive destruction of the left wrist, and there is soft tissue swelling with erosion at several MCP joints. Ulnar deviation of the digits is now present. These changes are characteristic of RA. Marcia's illness has been very active. Look at what happened to her hips over the same period (Figs. 55 and 56). There is uniform narrowing of the joint space of both hips, with periarticular osteopenia. There are no osteophytes.

SECTION II—EXERCISES

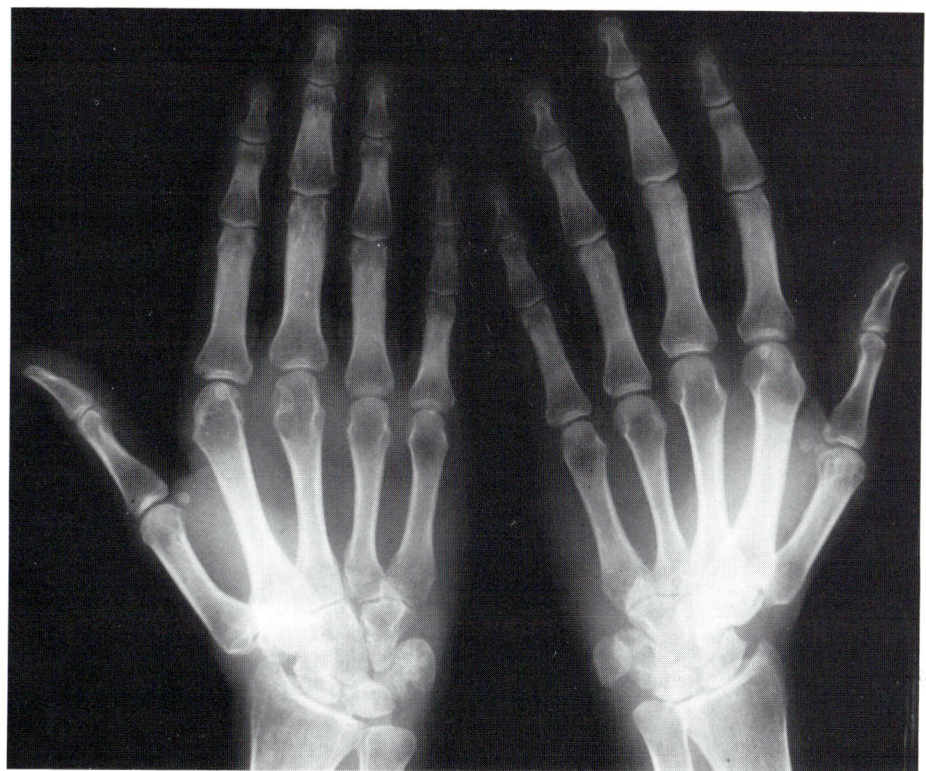

Figure 53

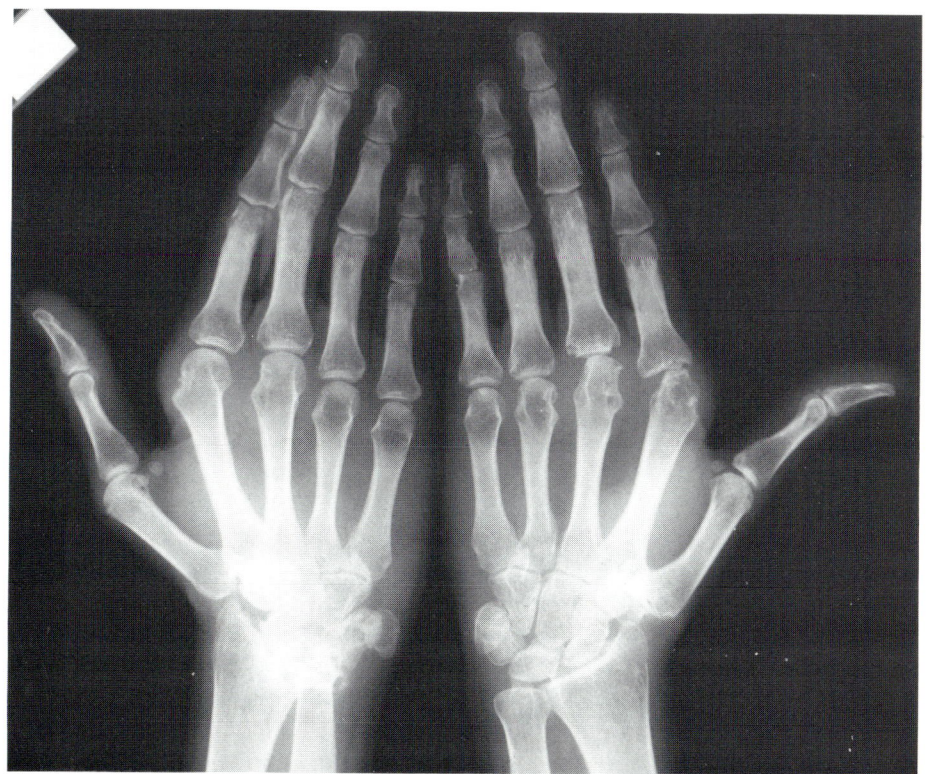

Figure 54

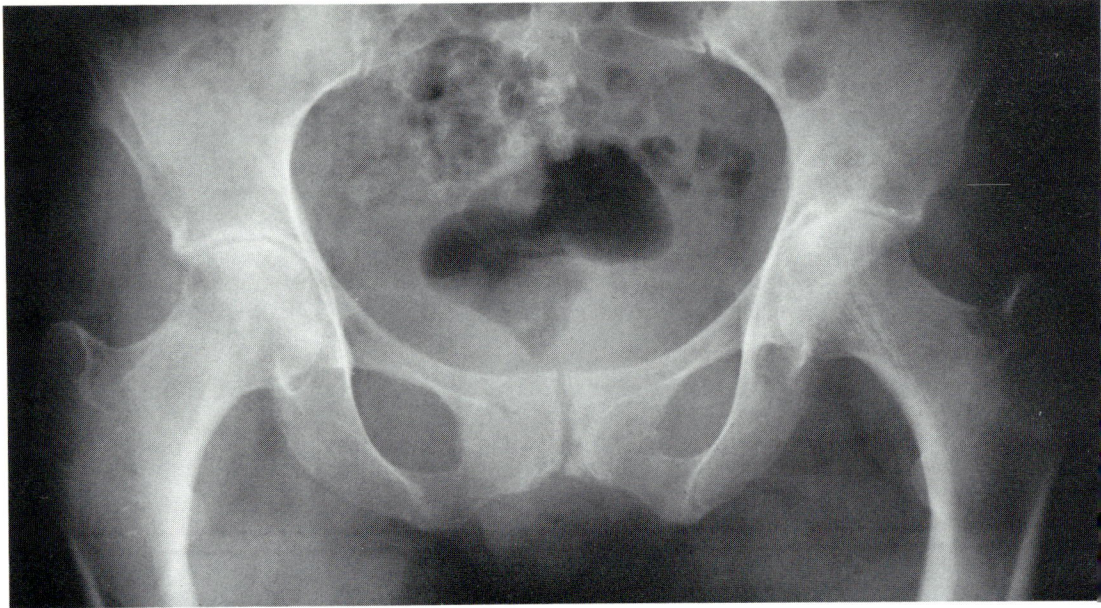

Figure 55

Note the erosions around the pubic symphysis. Three years later, there is worse narrowing and the hips have migrated in toward the pelvis, which is called protrusio acetabuli, a common RA lesion. As can be supposed, she required total hip replacements bilaterally. Look also at her elbow radiographs (Figs. 57 and 58). Destruction and disability were so severe here that a total elbow replacement was indicated (Fig. 59).

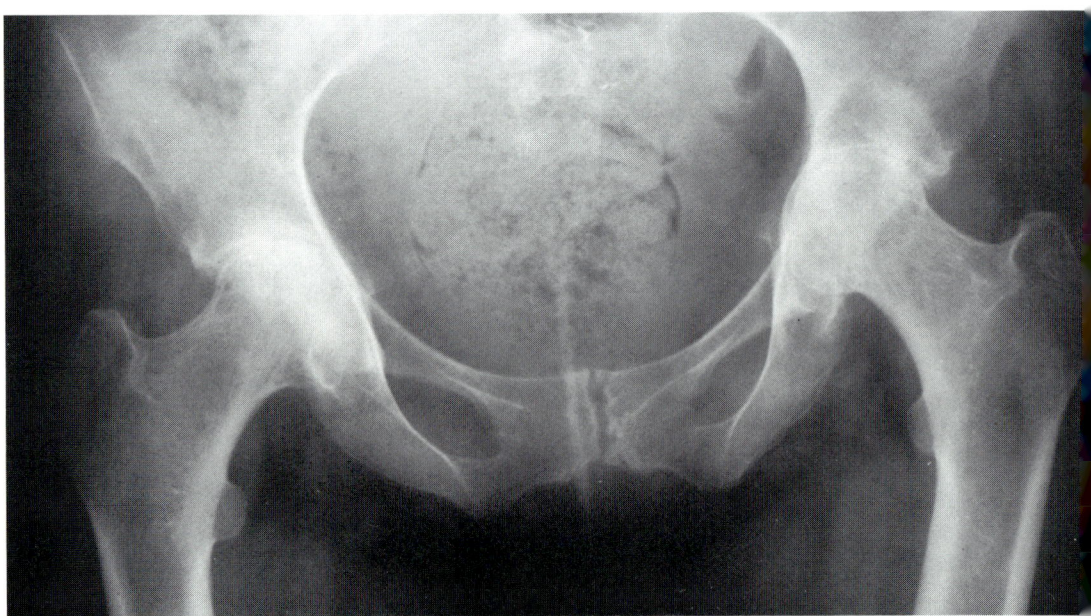

Figure 56

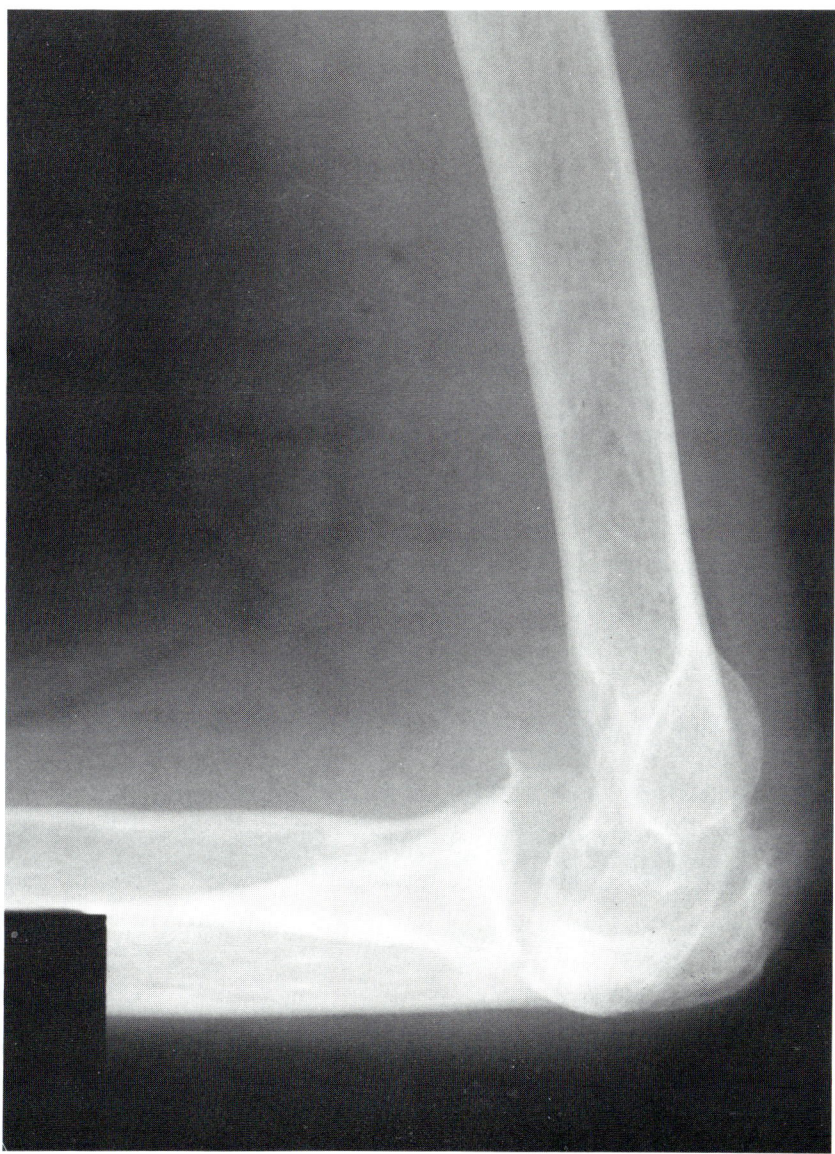

Figure 57

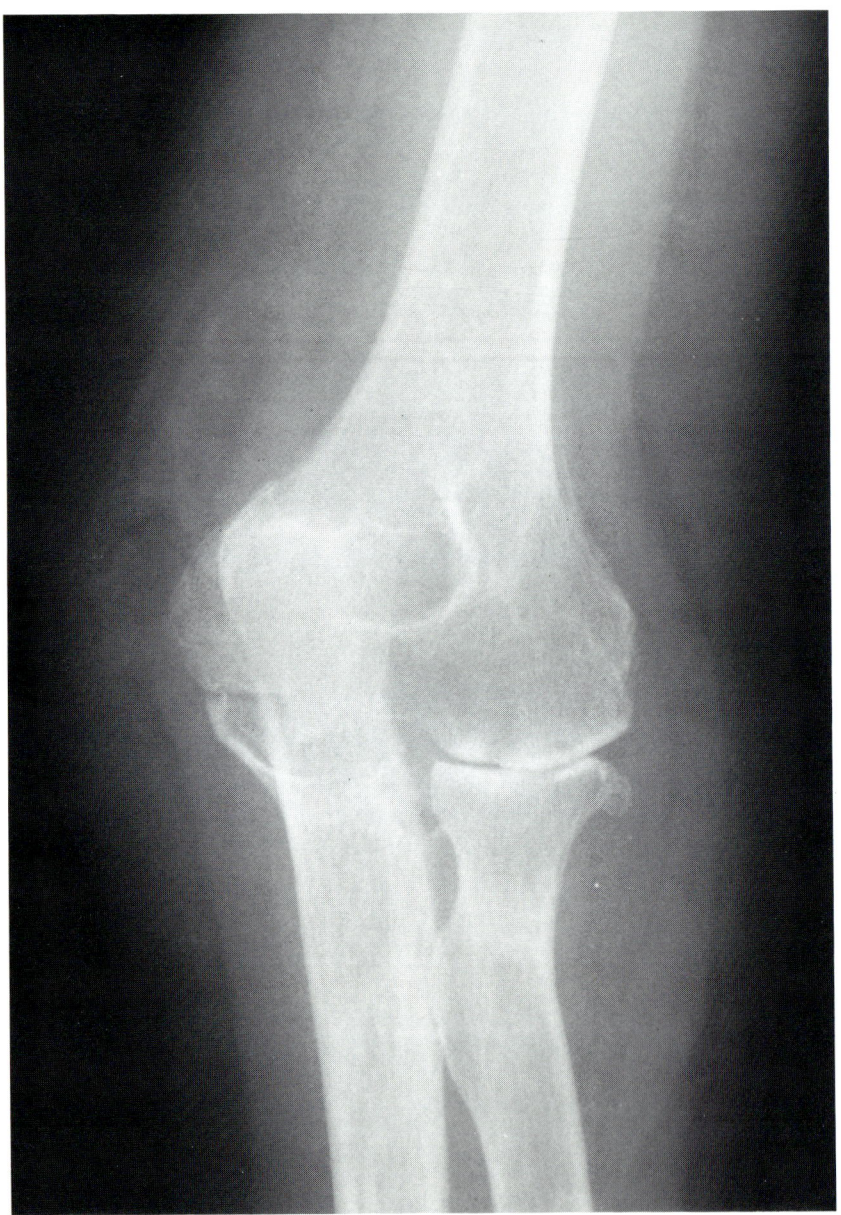

Figure 58

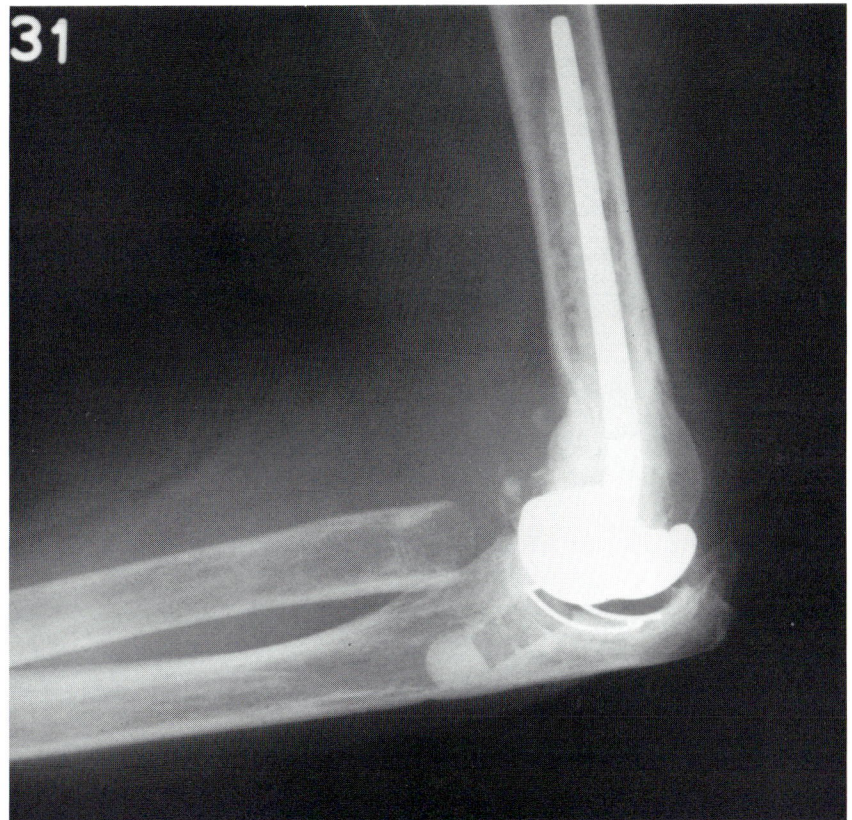

Figure 59

Exercise 7

Sam, 41 years old, has a 2 year history of pain and swelling around his MCP and PIP joints, wrists and knees. His condition has been diagnosed as RA in the past, despite his being seronegative. He tells you he has been recently discovered to be diabetic. You note he has a tan despite it being midwinter. Look at his radiographs (Figs. 60 and 61). Are you satisfied with the diagnosis?

Sam's radiographs reveal changes in a distribution that is consistent with RA, but without the characteristic features of RA. Look at Figure 60. Despite the involvement of the PIP and MCP joints and the wrist, there is an absence of periarticular osteopenia; in fact, there is subchondral sclerosis. Also, there are osteophytes off the MCP joints. This is DJD, but in an unusual location. One would expect DJD to occur in the DIP, PIP, and first CPC joints. DJD changes in unusual locations are often seen in CPPD crystal diseases. Look at Sam's knees (Fig. 61) and note that he has chondrocalcinosis in the meniscus, as well as DJD. Sam has hemochromatosis, which explains his "tan" and his diabetes. This iron deposition disease is often associated with deposits in synovium as well as in skin, heart, pancreas, liver and other organs. In joints, CPPD deposition results, with chondrocalcinosis, DJD and acute pseudogout as consequences.

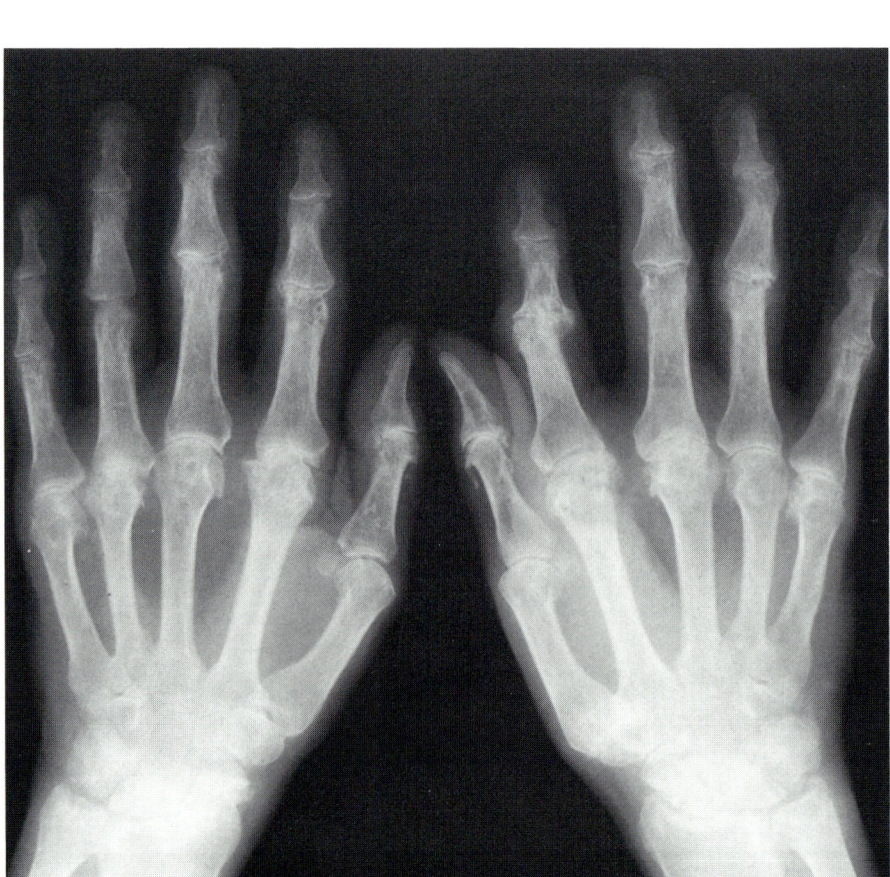

Figure 60

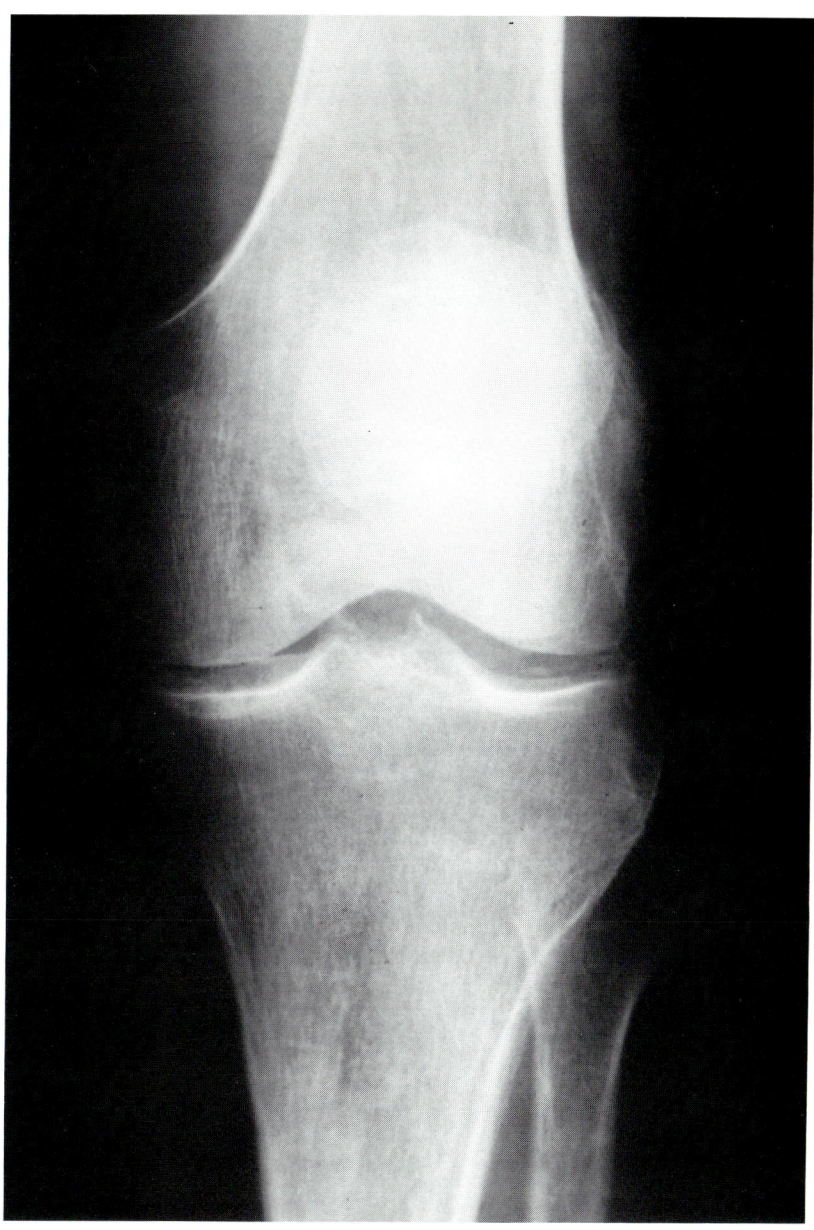

Figure 61

Exercise 8

Look at the hand radiographs in Figures 62 through 65 and decide what you think the diagnosis is.

Figure 62 reveals asymmetric soft tissue swelling around the DIP, PIP and MCP joints of the index finger, associated with narrowing of the DIP joint and narrowing and an early "pencil and cup" configuration of the MCP joint. In addition, there is narrowing of the second PIP joint and soft tissue swelling around the third and fourth PIP joints but not around the fifth. The wrist is spared. This is psoriatic arthritis, demon-

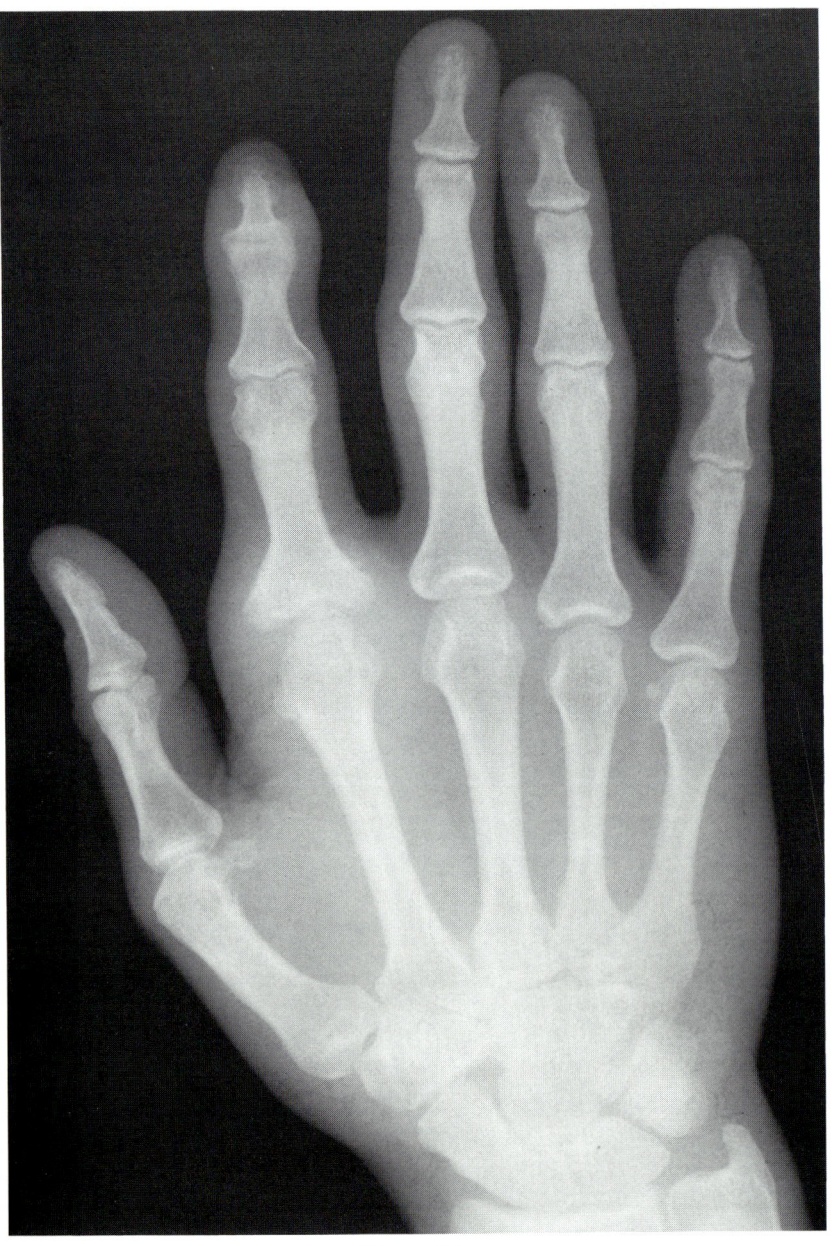

Figure 62

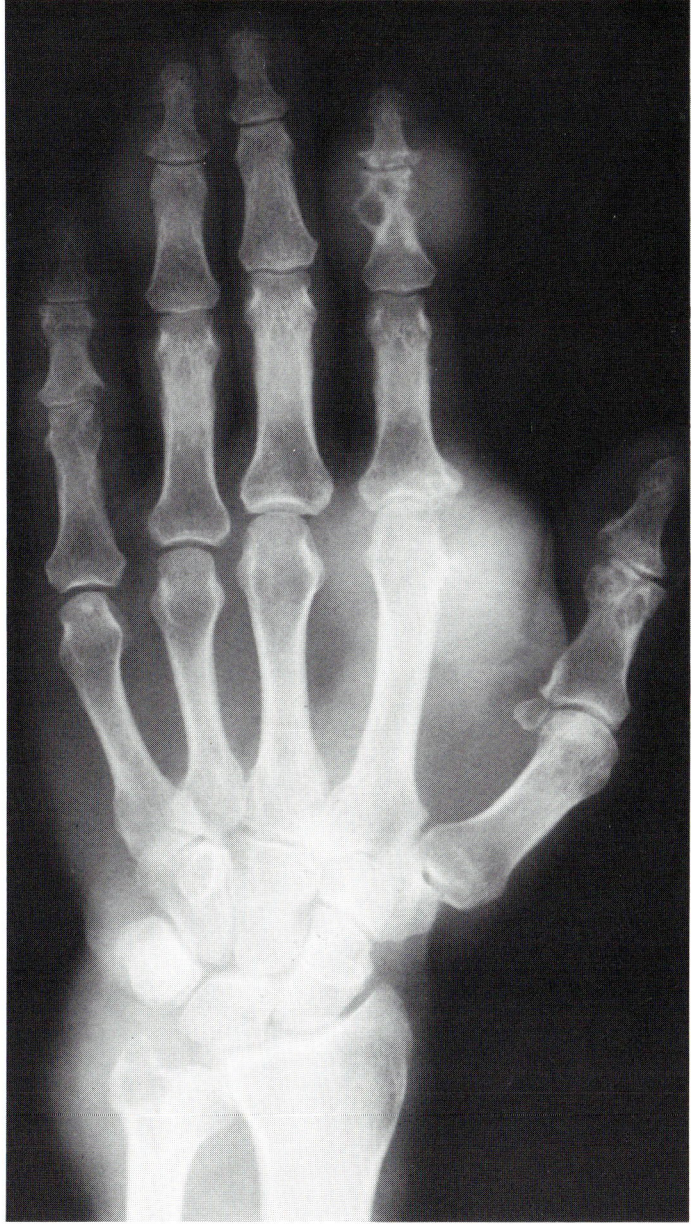

Figure 63

strating many of the typical findings. Clinically the index finger appeared diffusely swollen—the "sausage" digit so characteristic of this illness.

Figure 63 shows massive nodular soft tissue deposits of increased density around several DIP and PIP joints, as well as over the distal ulna. There are erosions and cyst formation around the bones at the points at which these deposits abut, usually in the joint. This is tophaceous gout. Calcium may occasionally be seen in these deposits. The erosions may contain overhanging lips, or osteophytes trying to encircle the tophi, such as seen in the fifth PIP joint.

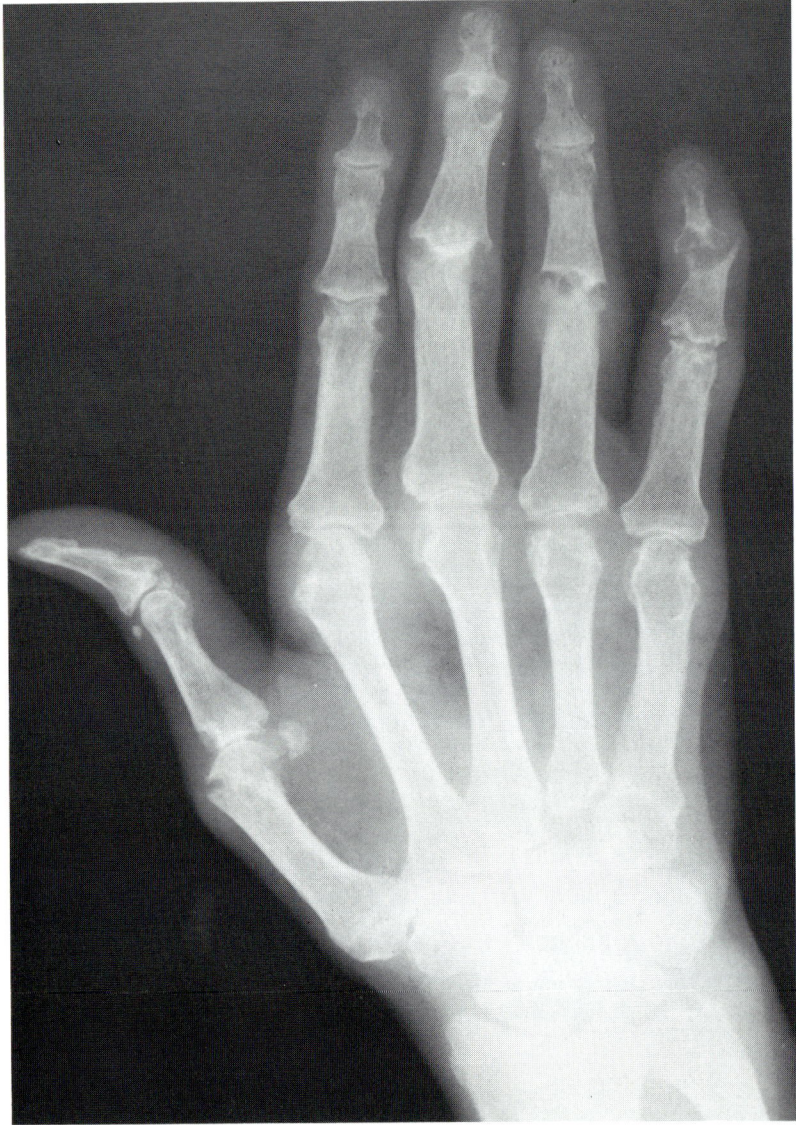

Figure 64

Figure 64 demonstrates erosion, joint space narrowing and periarticular osteopenia of multiple DIP, PIP, MCP and wrist joints. This would suggest an inflammatory arthritis such as RA or psoriatic arthritis. Look at the erosion in the DIP joint of the fifth finger; notice the slight hooking of the overlying bone. This is tophaceous gout! Clinically, one can be fooled into thinking this is RA if one is not careful. Always check the urate levels and get fluid for crystal analysis.

Figure 65 demonstrates loss of the terminal tuft bone in all fingers. This acro-osteolysis is due to scleroderma. Look at the way the skin on the thumbs is flattened and how the other finger tips are in forced flexion. Such skin changes have also been seen in patients with polyvinyl chloride exposure.

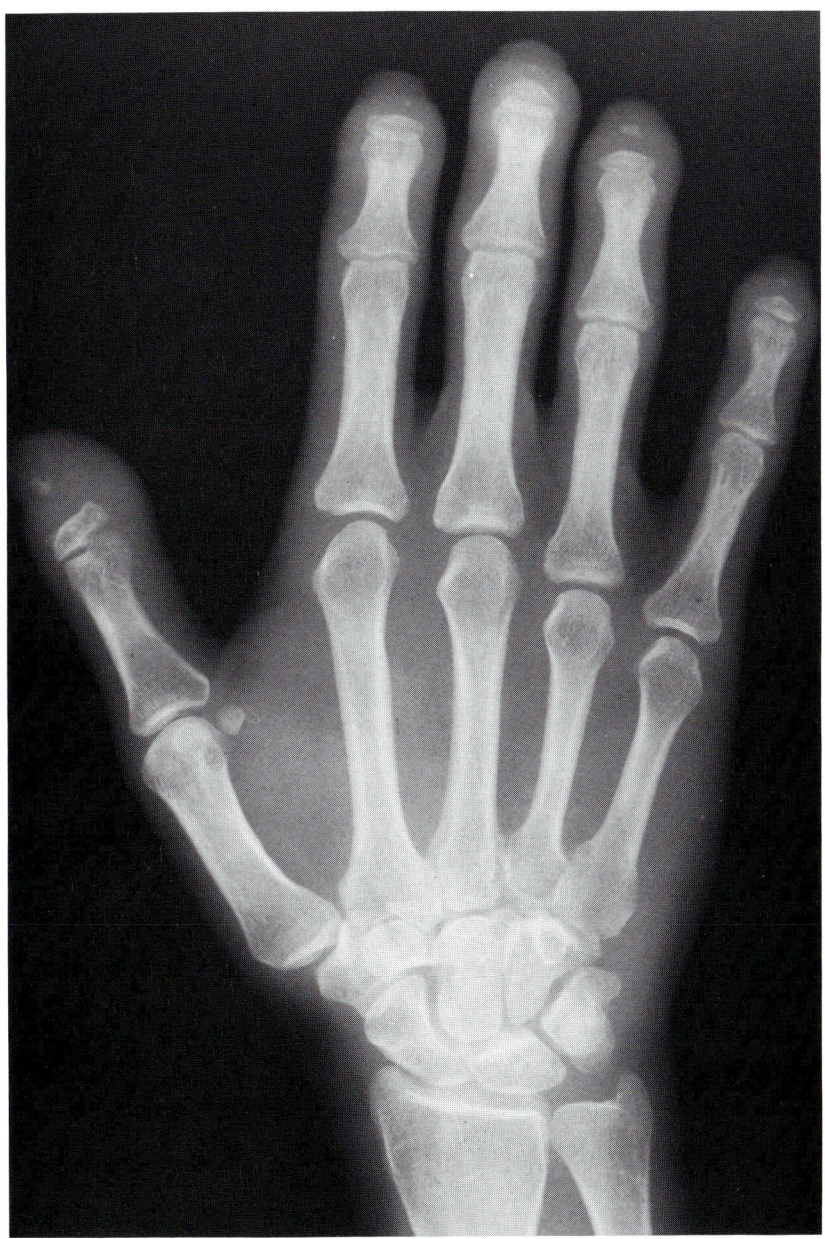

Figure 65

Exercise 9

Joan comes to you saying she has had hand pain for about 8 months. While you are taking her history, she hands you a set of films done elsewhere. After looking at the films (Figs. 66 and 67), you have a pretty good idea what her problem is. What's your diagnosis before the physical examination?

Both hands reveal soft tissue swelling around the PIP and MCP joints of the index finger, the left being worse than the right in both cases. Periarticular osteopenia is probably present in the fingers but not

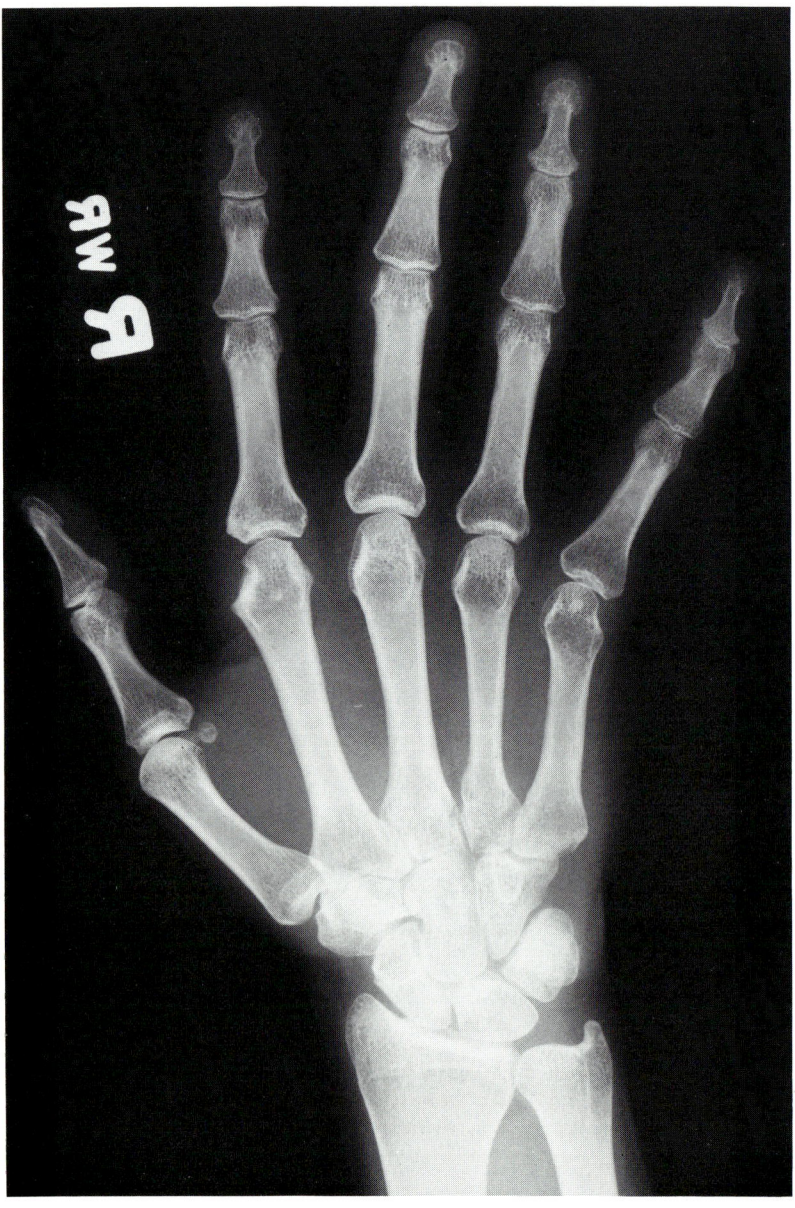

Figure 66

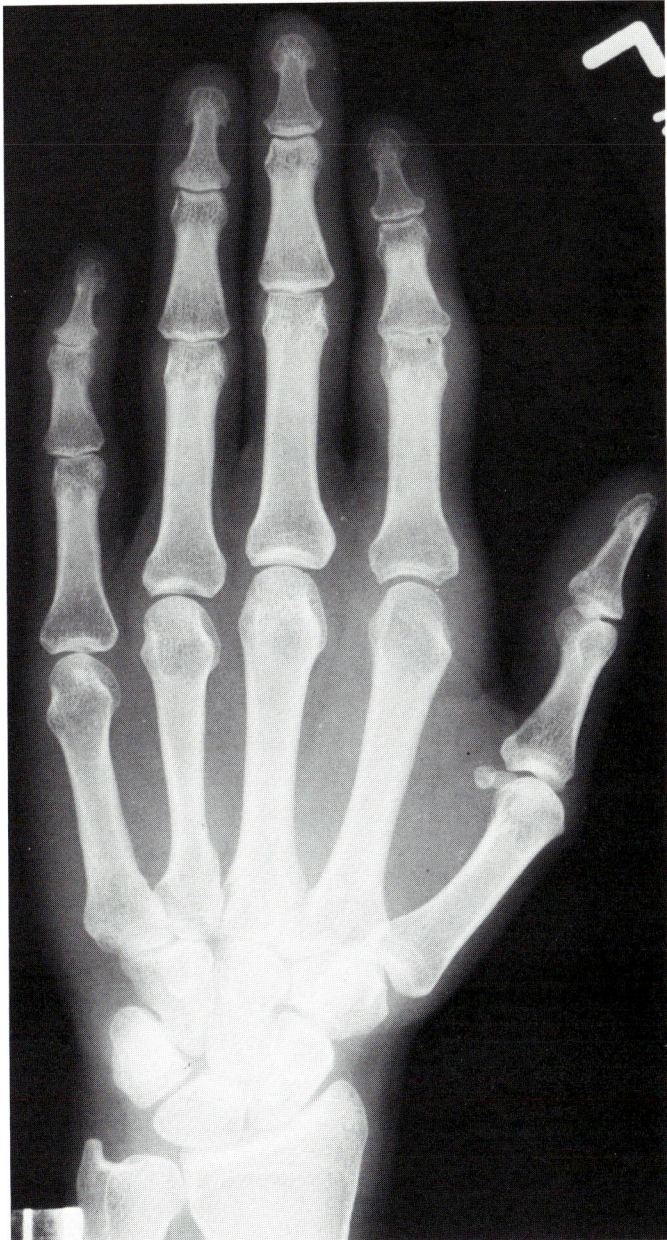

Figure 67

at the wrist. Note the erosion around the right second MCP joint. Look also at the left fifth DIP joint. It not only is slightly deformed (as is its mate on the right) but also has a lateral and medial erosion. The asymmetry of the presentation should make you wonder about Reiter's disease or psoriatic arthritis, which is what you discover when you examine Joan's nails and skin. Look at her bone scan (Fig. 68), which further highlights the asymmetric distribution of activity in the joints.

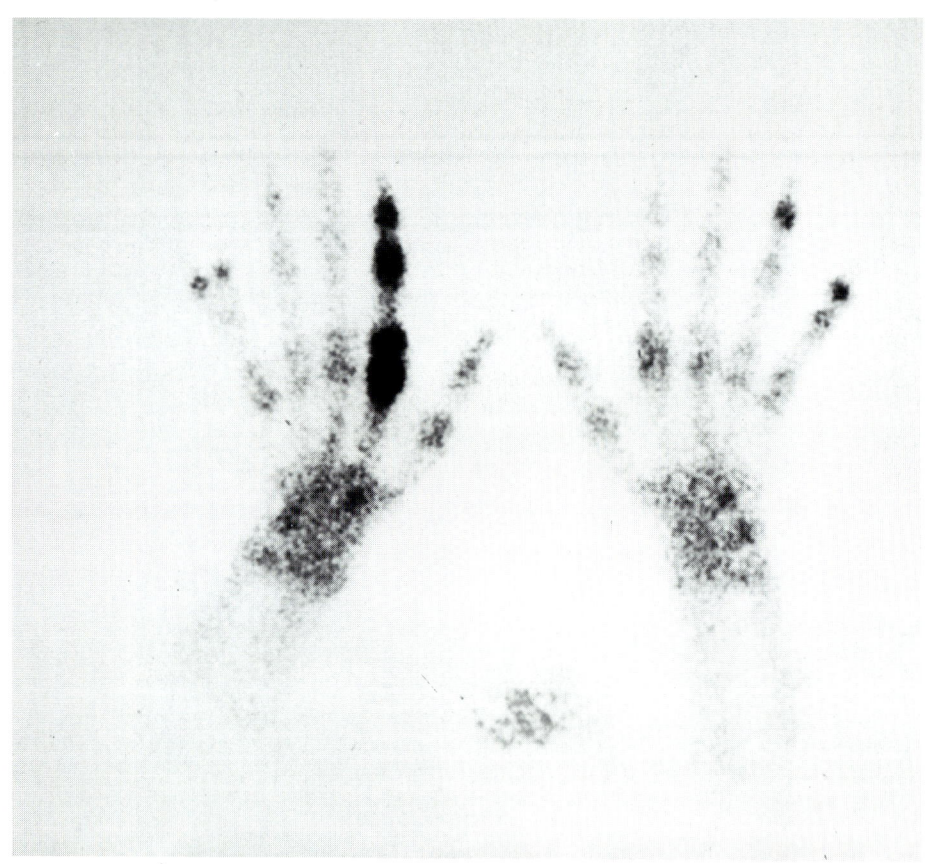

Figure 68

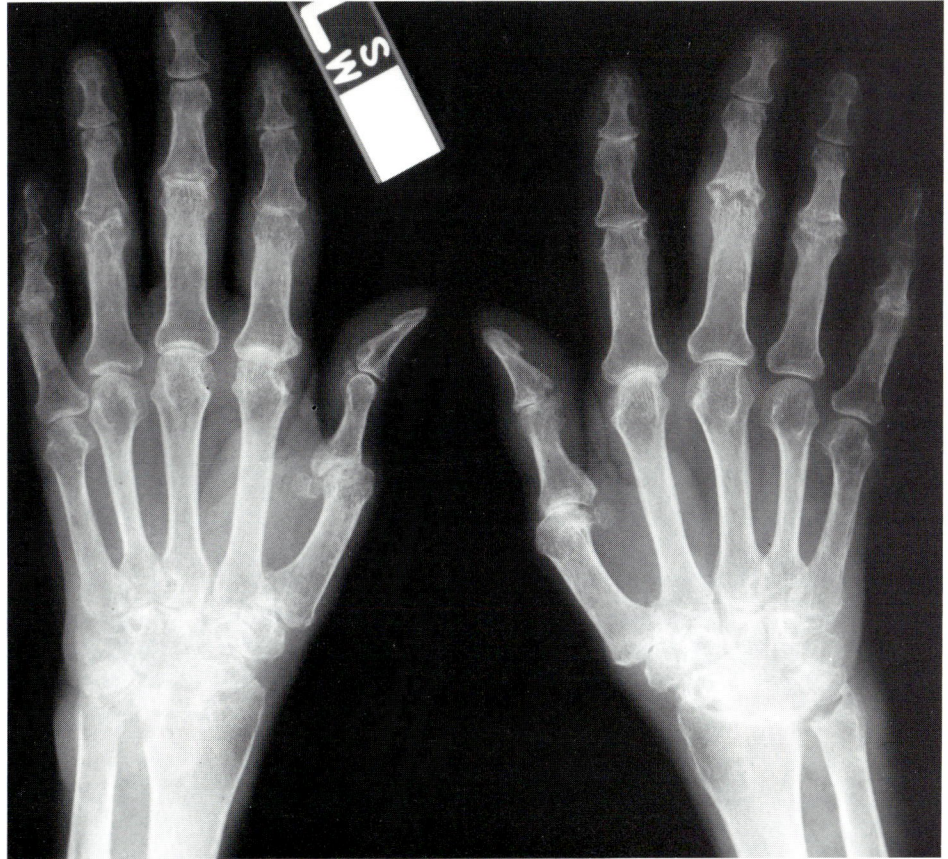

Figure 69

Exercise 10

Annie has RA. Her wrist, always a source of pain, has become increasingly useless because of its instability while holding objects (Fig. 69). She is admitted for wrist surgery. You are asked to review her preoperative chest radiograph (Fig. 70) for the surgical intern, who hears rales and wonders if she's experiencing heart failure. What advice do you give the intern?

Examination of the wrists demonstrates diffuse osteopenia and extensive symmetric destruction of both wrists, which is characteristic of advanced RA. Note the severe destructive changes in the PIP joints. The chest radiograph reveals a diffuse interstitial infiltrate in both lungs, which is most prominent in the lower lobes and has the appearance of honeycombing. Note the normal-sized heart. This is a rheumatoid lung. Old films are found that show no change over the last 2 years, and as the patient is asymptomatic you send her to the operating room—only after she gets flexion and extension neck films to look for cervical spine subluxation (see Exercise 55). The surgeon decides to place a total wrist prosthesis rather than do a fusion. Figures 71 and 72 show a two-part prosthesis placed at the radiocarpal joint.

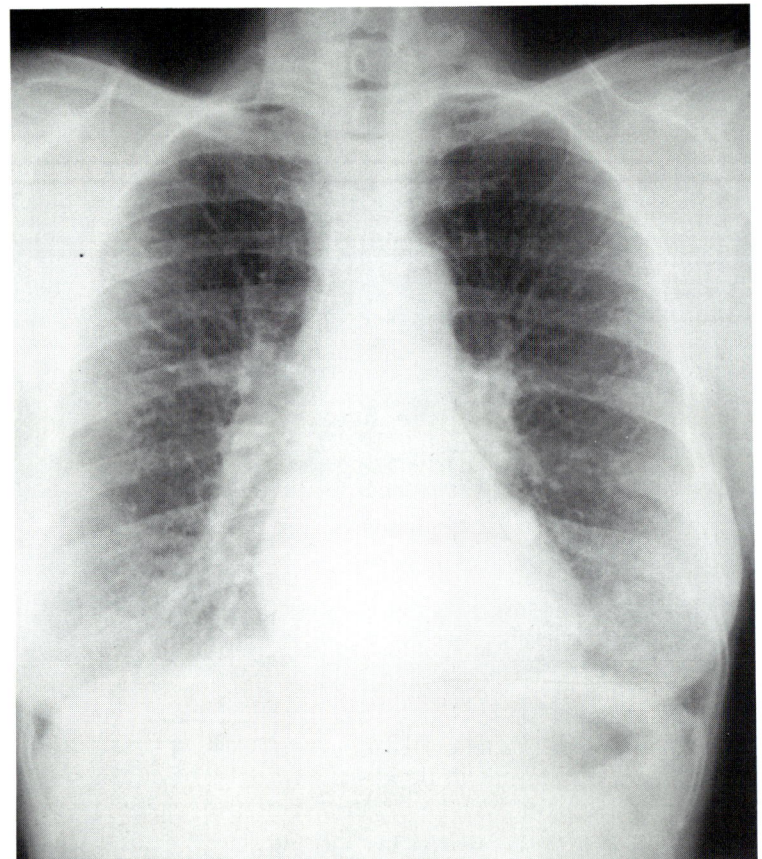

Figure 70

SECTION II—EXERCISES

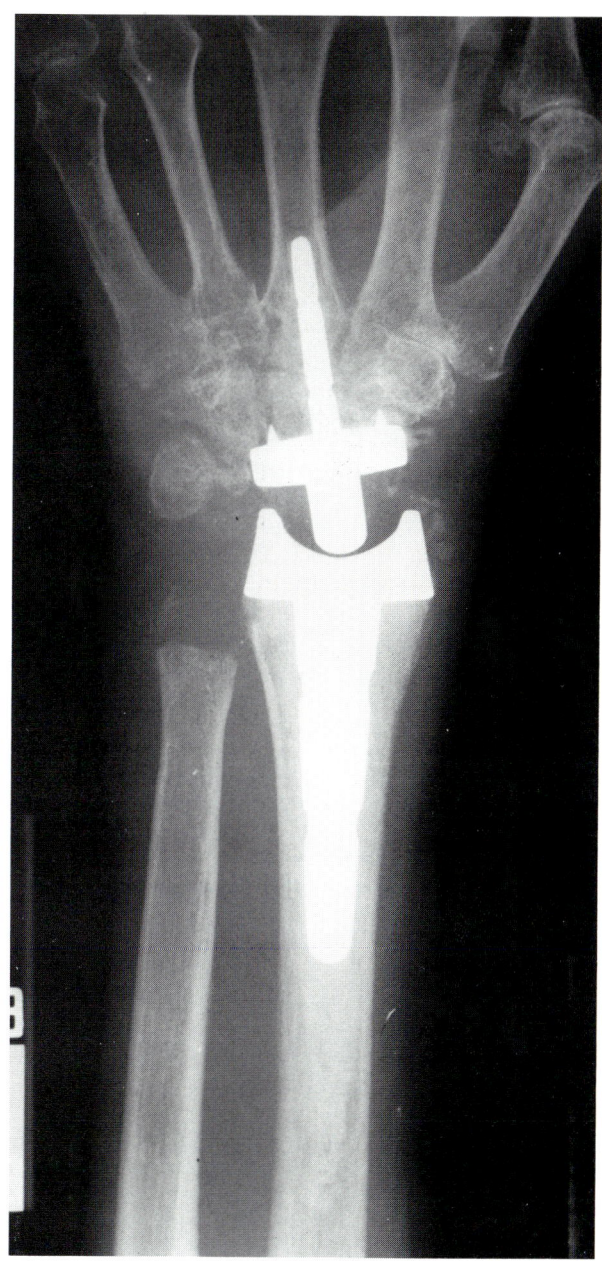

Figure 71

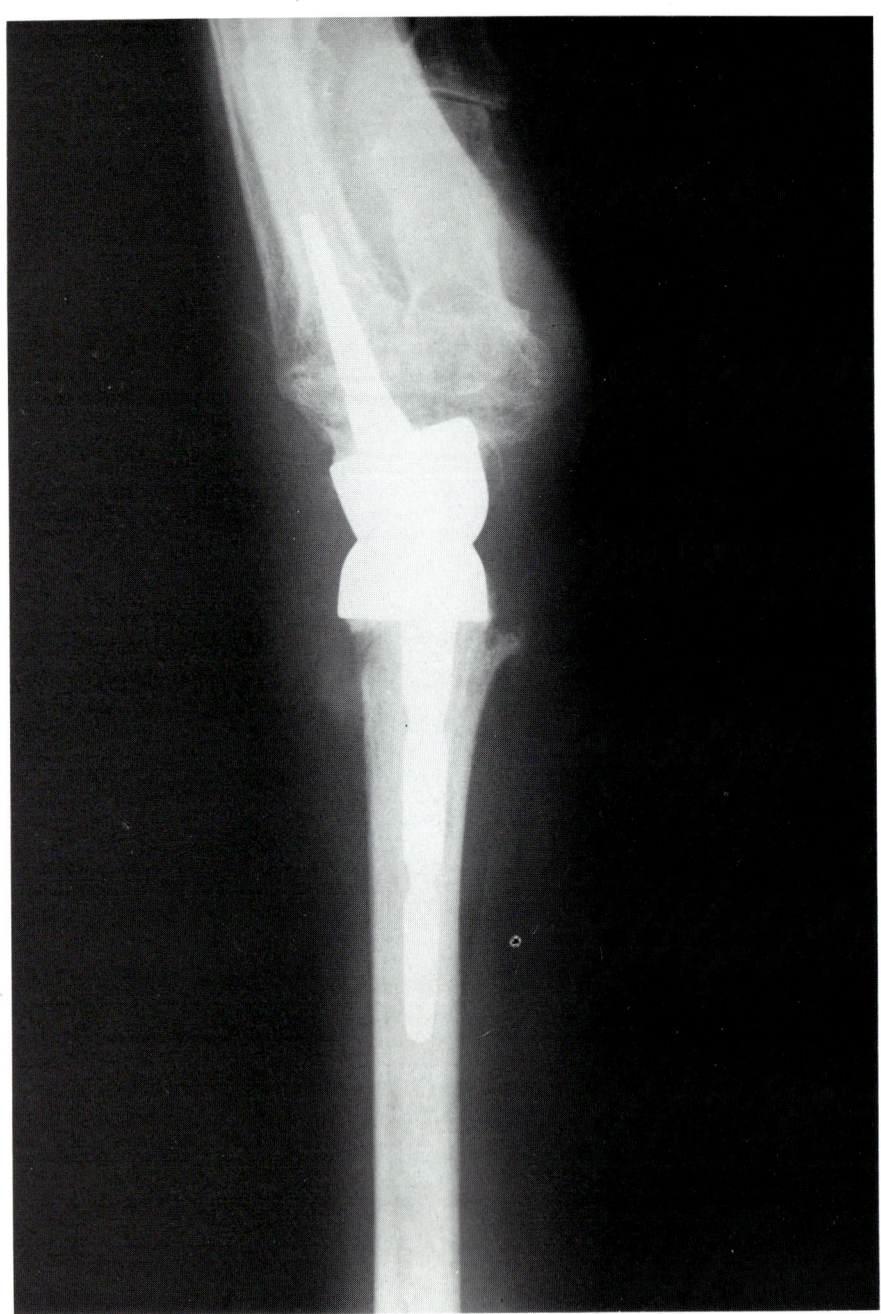

Figure 72

SECTION II—EXERCISES

Knees and Hips

Exercise 11

Sarah, 72 years old, has had increasing knee pain over the last several years and has noticed herself becoming increasingly bowlegged over that period. Recently, her symptoms have worsened a great deal. Look at her radiograph (Fig. 73) and decide what the cause of her knee pain is.

The radiograph shows that the bowlegged (varus) deformity is caused by bilateral medial cartilage narrowing associated with some sclerosis and osteophyte formation. This is typical OA. Compare this radiograph with that of the next case.

Exercise 12

You are reading bone films this week and are shown this pair of knee radiographs by the technician (Fig. 74). The intern forgot to write a history along with the radiograph request. Interpret the films and dictate a report.

You should have noted that there is uniform involvement of the

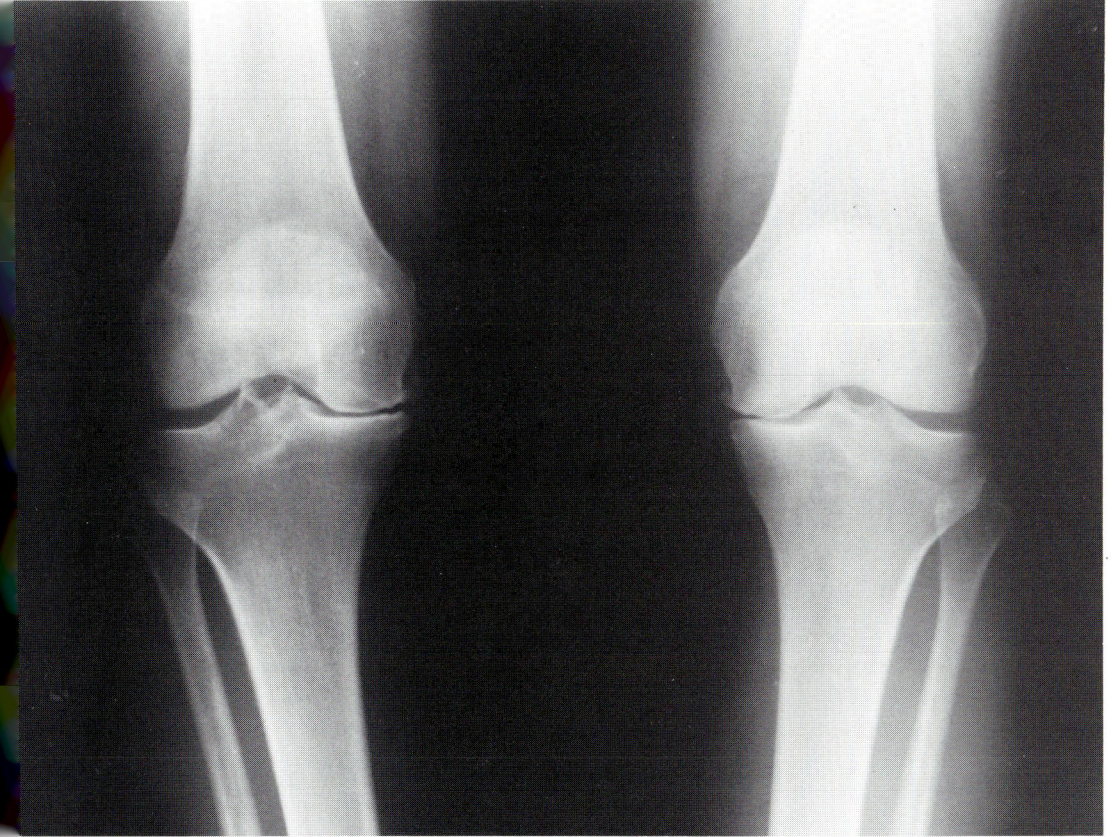

Figure 73

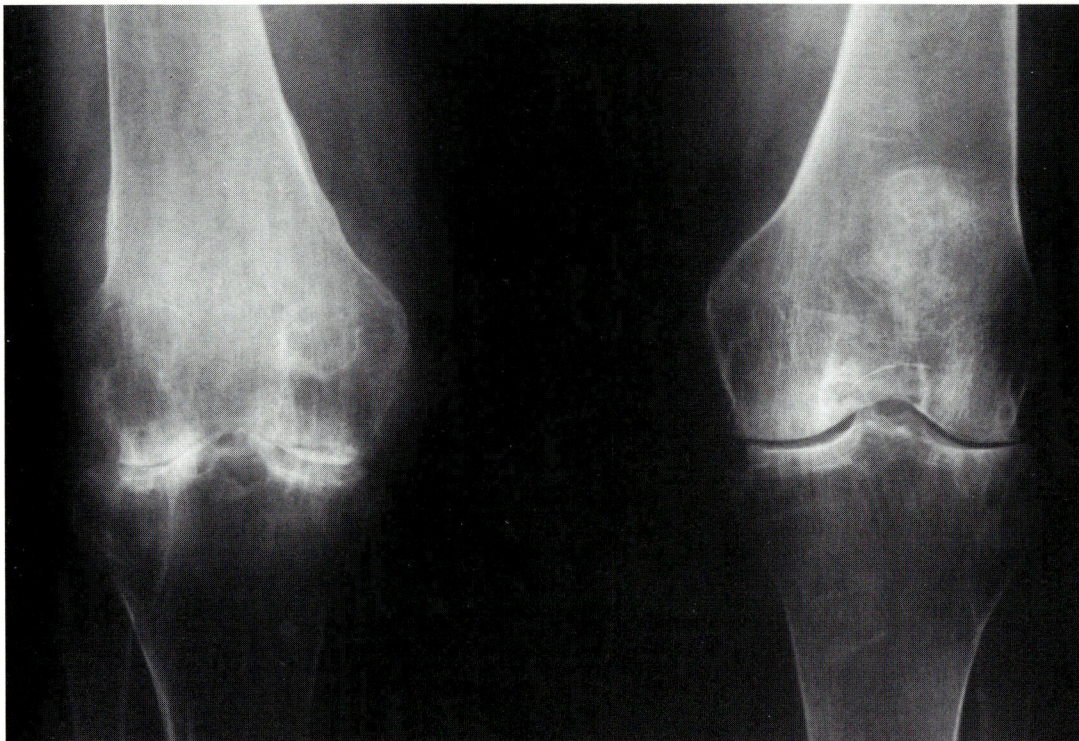

Figure 74

medial and lateral compartments of each knee. The joint spaces are narrowed. On the left, erosions are present on the nonweight-bearing areas of the femoral condyles and tibial plateaus as well as in the intracondylar notch. On the right, the changes are more extensive. The erosions have extended onto the weight-bearing areas and there is marked joint space narrowing. The absence of osteophytes indicates that this is an inflammatory disorder, probably RA because of the symmetric involvement. The minimal subchondral sclerosis is from mild secondary degenerative changes on top of a primary inflammatory illness. The intern later confirms your clinical impression.

Exercise 13

Joseph, 65 years old, shows you two radiographs (Figs. 75 and 76) of his painful hip, taken 5 years apart. He wants to know what you think he has and what he should do for it. What do you advise him to do?

The first radiograph shows narrowing superiorly between the head of the femur and the acetabulum, with mild sclerosis and no osteophytes bilaterally. Five years later the left hip has not changed. The right hip, however, has now completely abutted against the acetabulum, with increased sclerosis and large marginal osteophytes, especially inferiorly. This is the typical picture and time course of OA. Since conservative therapy has failed, Joseph requires a total hip replacement, which is what you recommend.

SECTION II—EXERCISES

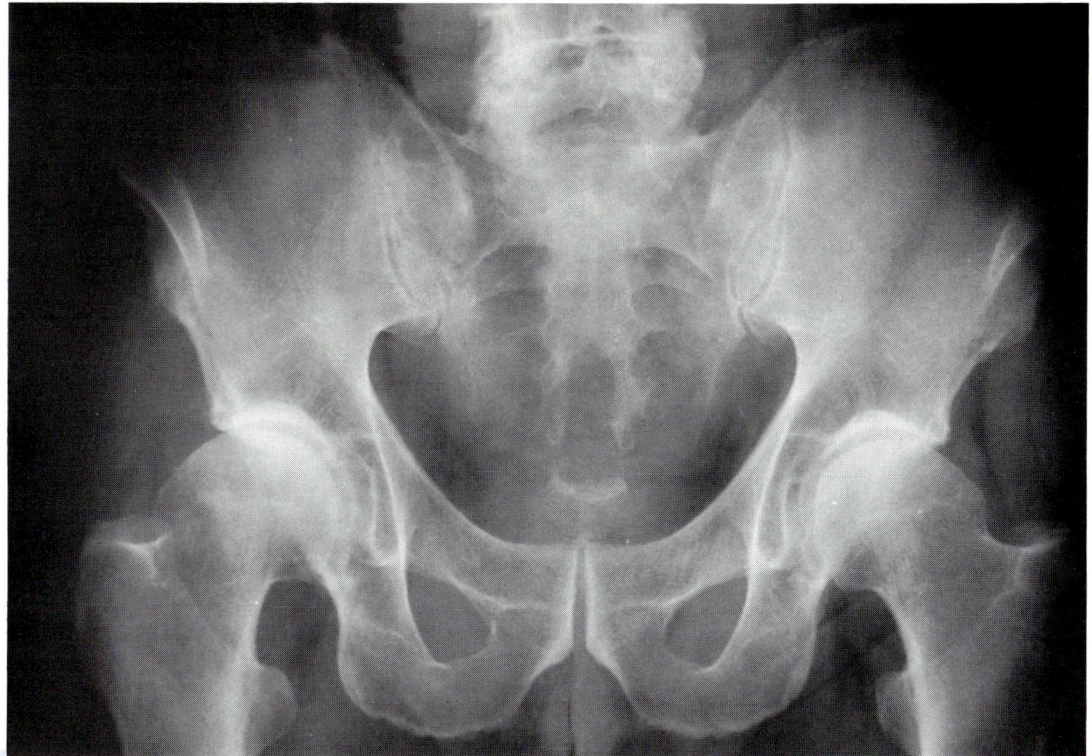

Figure 75

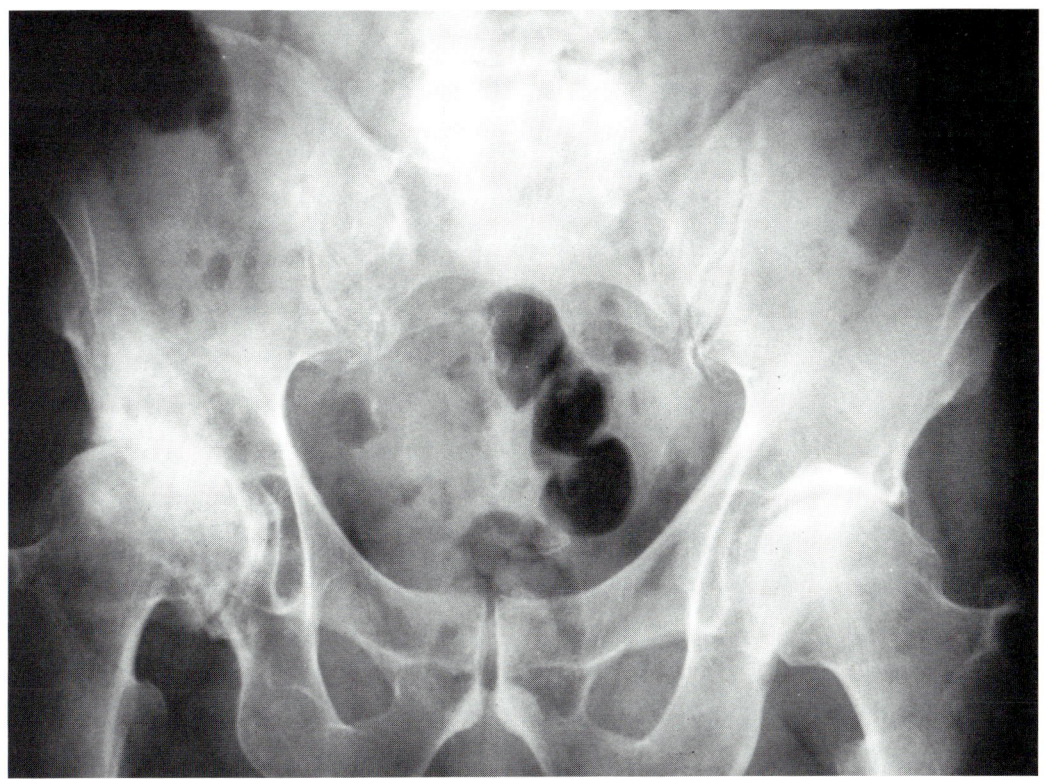

Figure 76

SECTION II—EXERCISES

Exercise 14

You are the orthopedic resident on call. The medical intern brings you a film (Fig. 77) on a patient he had admitted who has a polyarthritis and bilateral hip pain. He wonders if the radiograph suggests this patient has a congenital hip disease in addition to her other joint problems. What do you think?

The femoral heads are osteoporotic and deformed, and the joint space is evenly narrowed, suggesting an inflammatory disease. With the polyarthritis described in other joints, this is probably RA. The most striking abnormality, however, is the acetabulum, which is migrating into the pelvis. This is called protrusio acetabuli and is noted often in rheumatoid arthritis (compare with Figure 56).

Exercise 15

Laura Rose, 63 years old, awoke last night with severe pain in her right knee. When you examine the knee it is warm and very swollen. What does her radiograph (Fig. 78) tell you about the possible cause of her arthritis?

You should observe fine linear calcifications in both the medial and lateral menisci, which is consistent with chondrocalcinosis. The likely cause of Laura's knee swelling is an acute pseudogout attack. When fluid was aspirated from her knee, it revealed positively birefringent rhomboid-shaped crystals of CPPD, confirming the diagnosis.

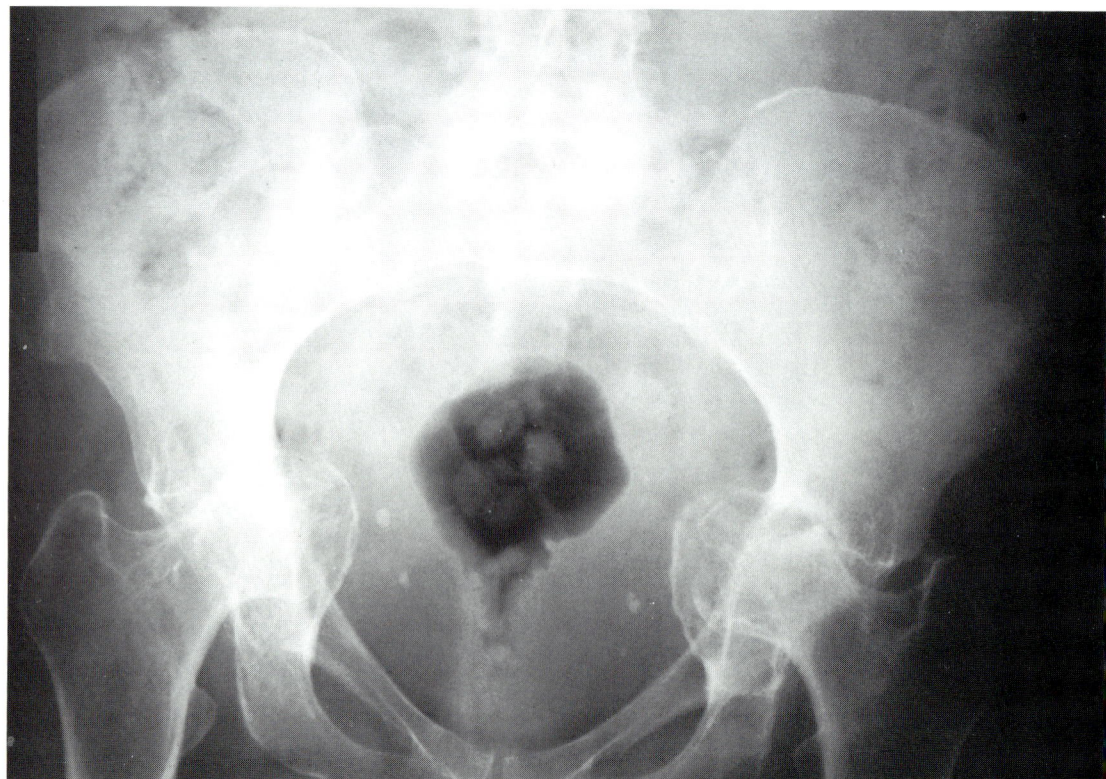

Figure 77

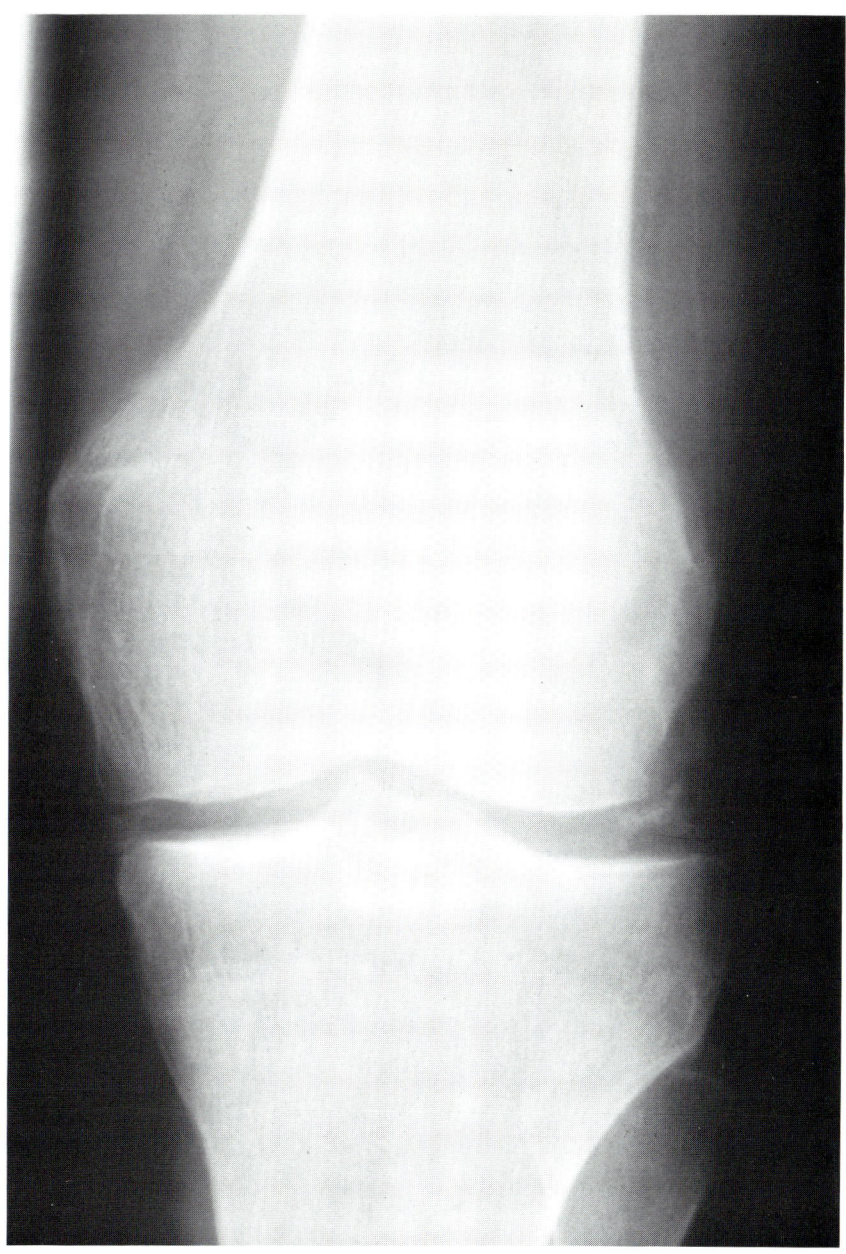

Figure 78

Exercise 16

Katie, 27 years old, had a history of arthritis in the knees and wrists as a young teenager, which had been diagnosed as rheumatic fever and subsequently improved with aspirin over a 2 year period. Since that time she has noted restricted range of motion of her affected joints. She comes to you now to clarify the original diagnosis and to seek advice on what to do next. On examination you notice no evidence of active arthritis and confirm her limitation of motion. Look at her radiographs (Figs. 79 and 80) and answer her question.

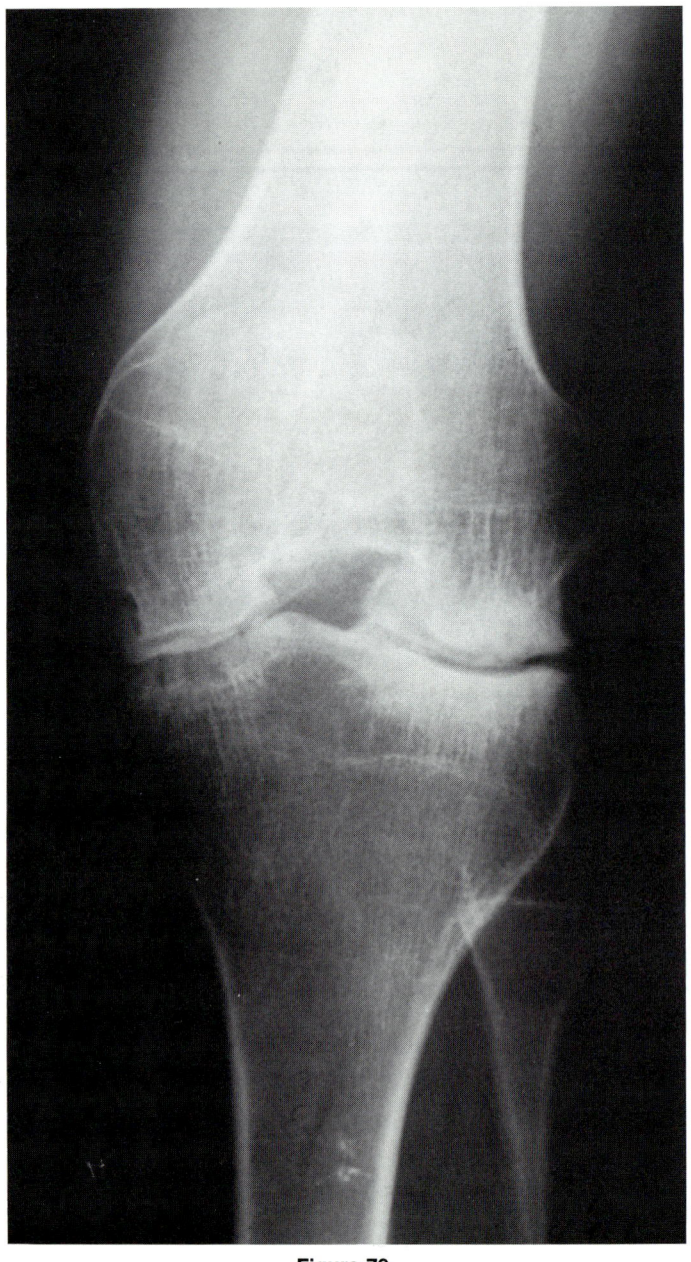

Figure 79

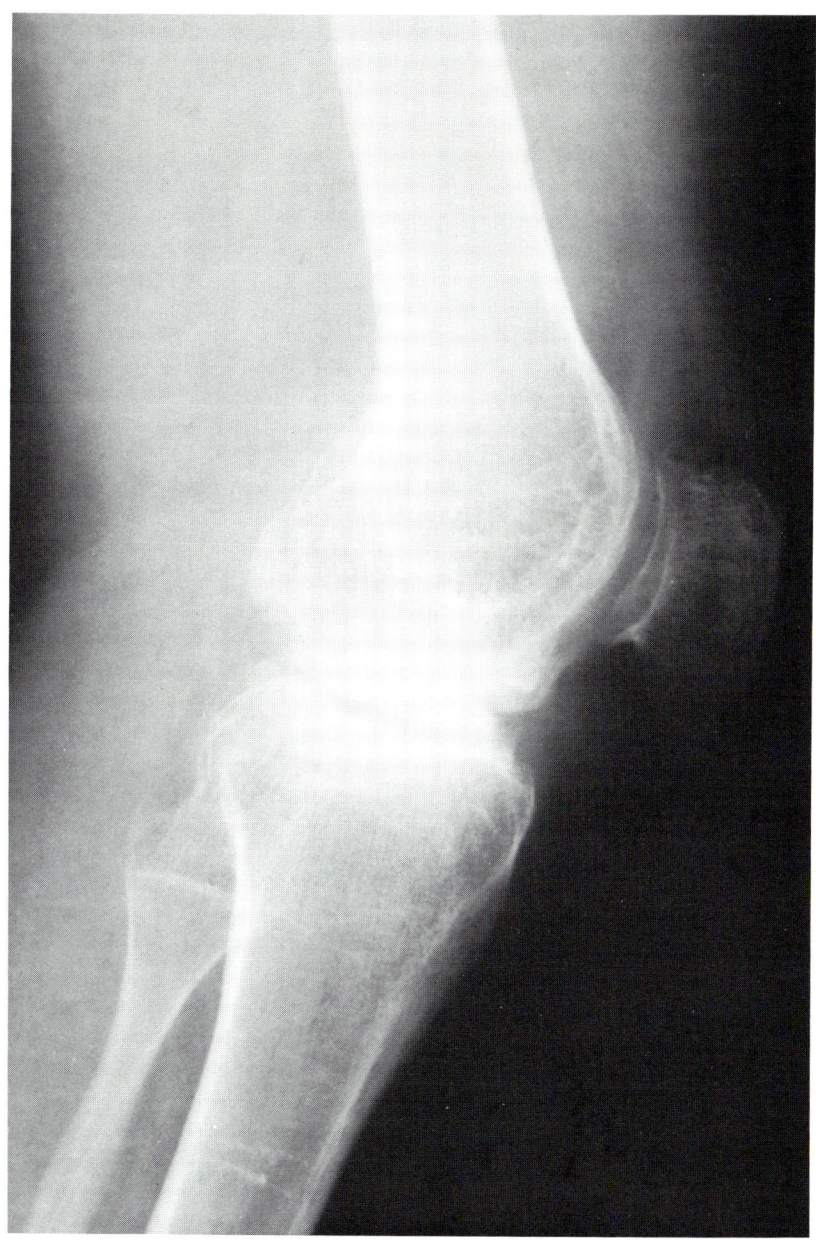

Figure 80

Katie's radiographs reveal osteopenia and uniform joint space narrowing of the right knee, which is consistent with an inflammatory arthritis. Her other knee and wrists also show this. She most likely has juvenile chronic polyarthritis (JCP), as rheumatic fever is not a destructive arthropathy. Notice, however, the subchondral sclerosis and beginnings of osteophytes at the margins; she is developing secondary degenerative changes in the knees. You have judged that she has no clinical evidence of inflammation, and with continuing pain despite good conservative therapy she requires a total knee replacement (Fig. 81).

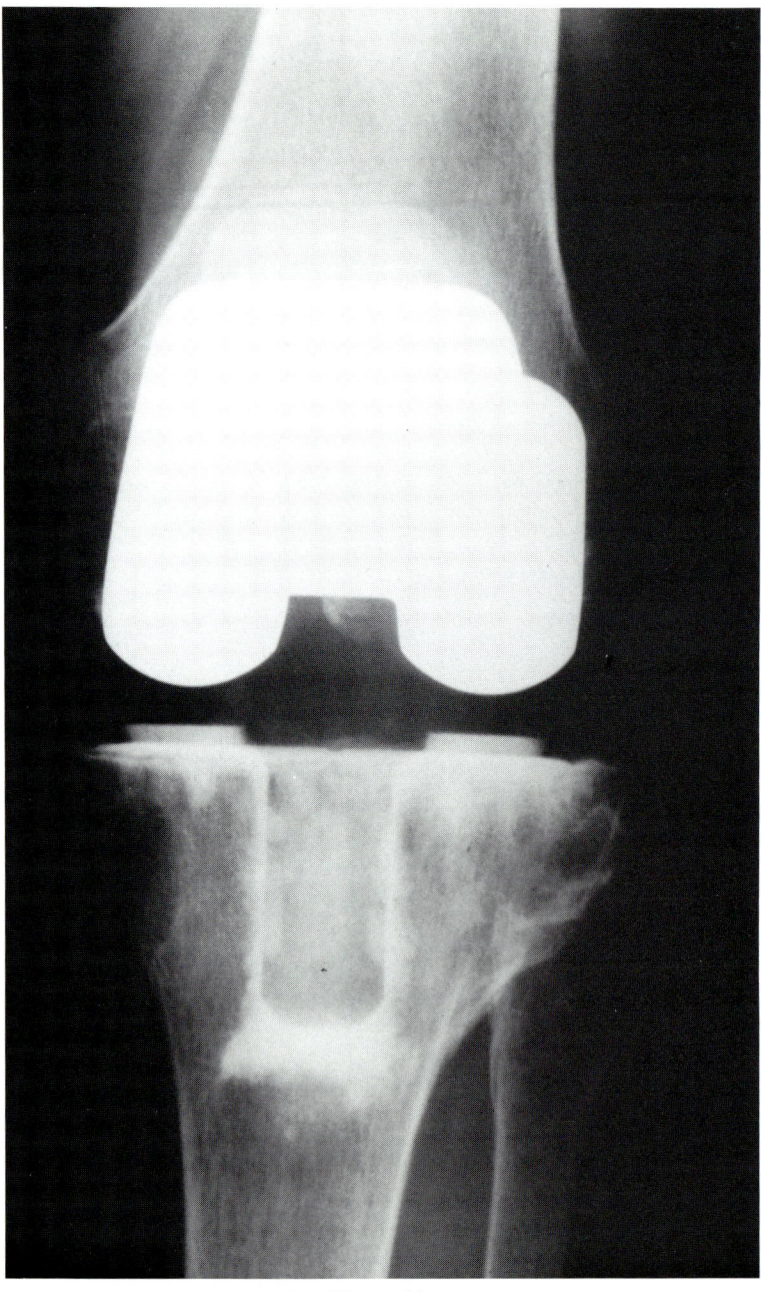

Figure 81

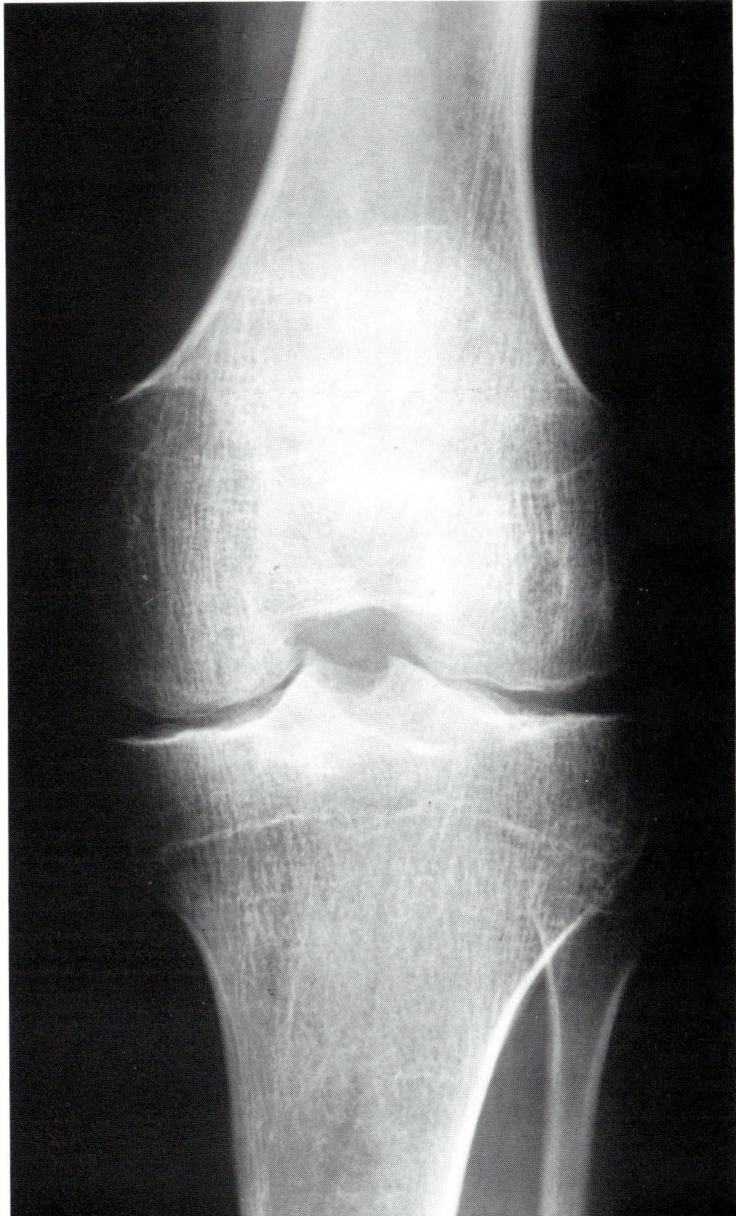

Figure 82

In view of Katie's diagnosis, look at the knee films of this 18 year old in Figures 82 and 83 and make a diagnosis.

The radiographs show symmetric narrowing and mild osteopenia consistent with an inflammatory arthritis. This is not JCP, however, but rather hemophilia arthropathy. This young man has had multiple episodes of hemarthrosis, which leads to a chronic inflammatory synovitis. The two are indistinguishable on radiographs. This patient also underwent a total knee replacement after factor VIII replacement without complication.

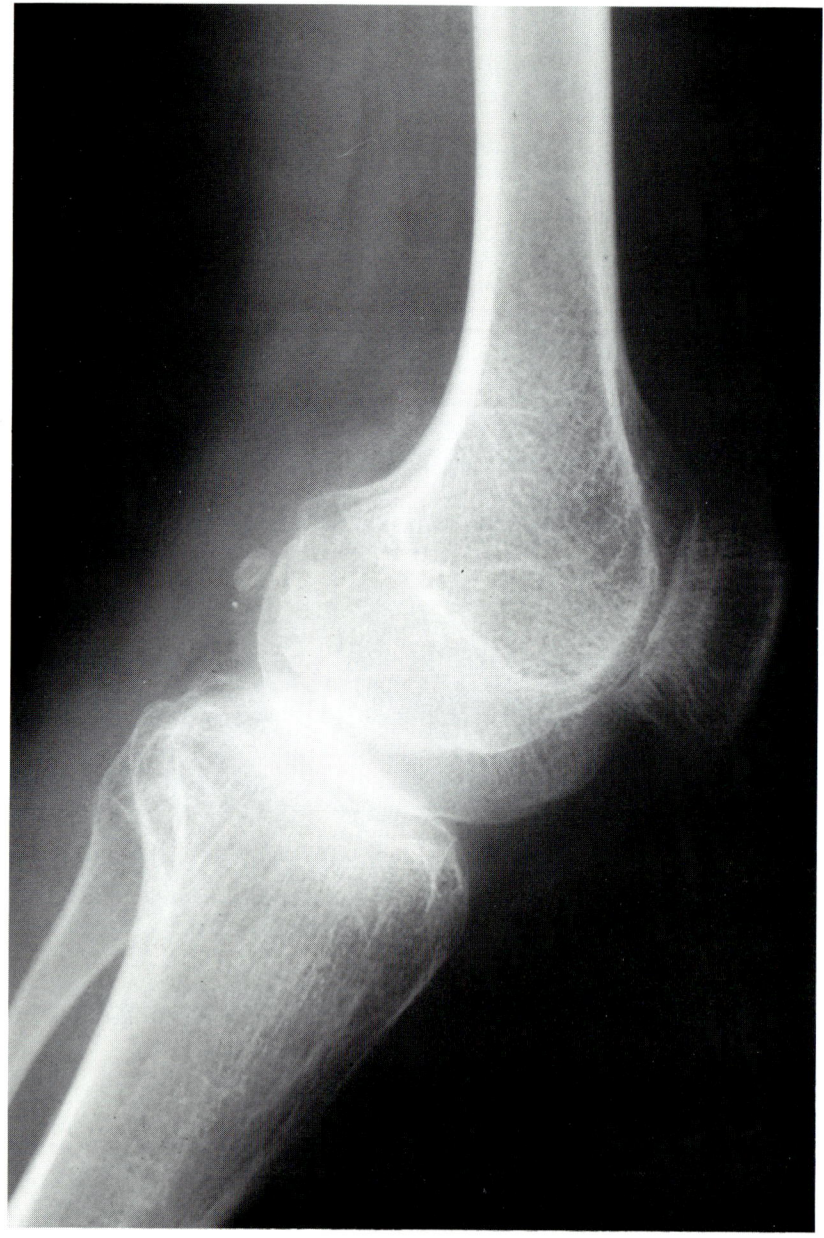

Figure 83

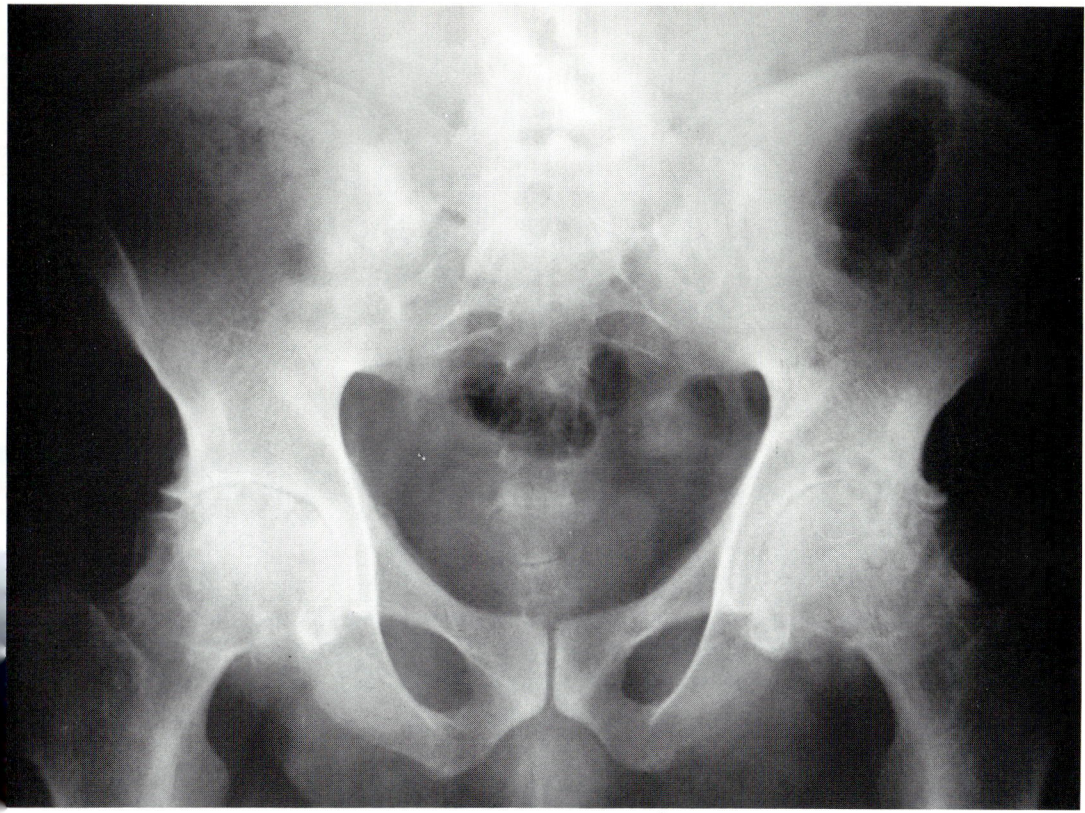

Figure 84

Exercise 17

This 32 year old man has bilateral hip disease and needs total knee replacements. Look at Figure 84 and decide on a diagnosis.

The radiograph demonstrates uniform narrowing of both hip joints. There are subchondral cysts around the right hip. There is no subchondral sclerosis, but there are small marginal osteophytes around both the femoral and acetabular components. Notice the sacroiliac joints, which are completely fused. This is ankylosing spondylitis. The hip changes are due to inflammatory destruction with minimal secondary degenerative changes.

Exercise 18

Tom, 55 years old and a deep sea diver, has been known to "put away" a few beers after a long day hunting for doubloons. About 4 months ago he noted some right hip pain, which has persisted and worsened as time has progressed. Look at his radiograph (Fig. 85) and make a diagnosis. Would you do any other radiographic studies on him?

The radiograph reveals a "crescent sign," or pseudofracture line, just under the rim of the femoral head (Fig. 86). This is best seen on the frog leg view and is pathognomonic for avascular necrosis. This is a condition in which a piece of subchondral bone has suffered some

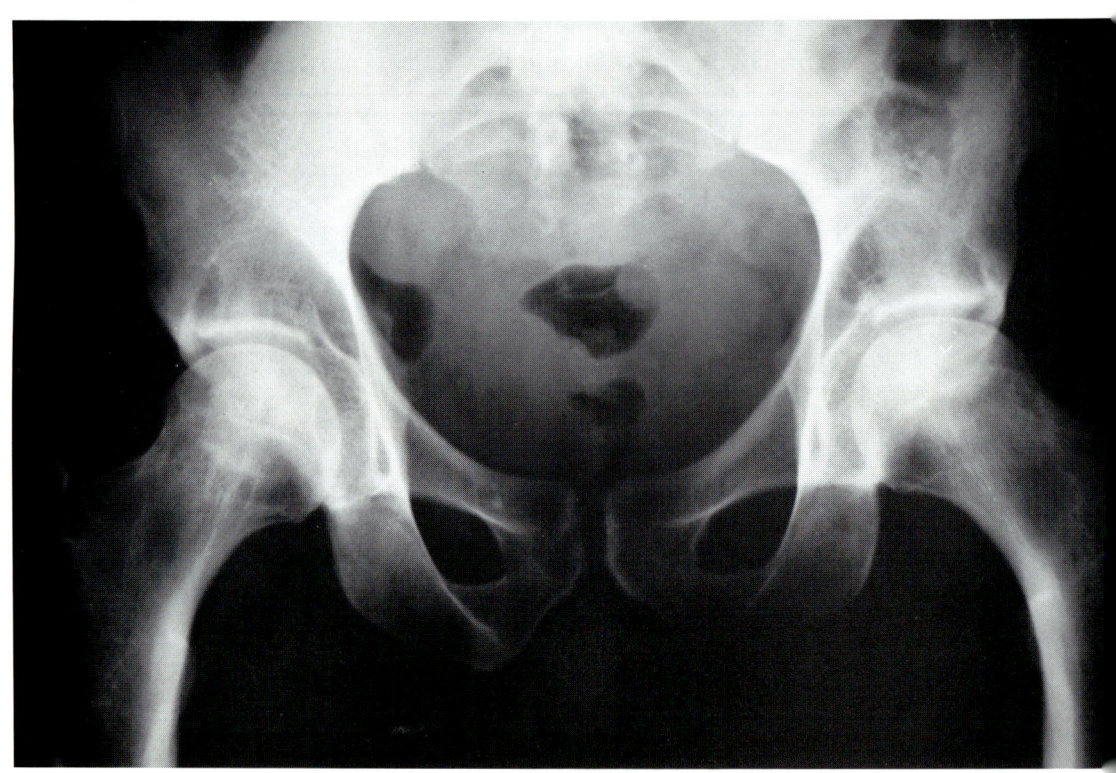

Figure 85

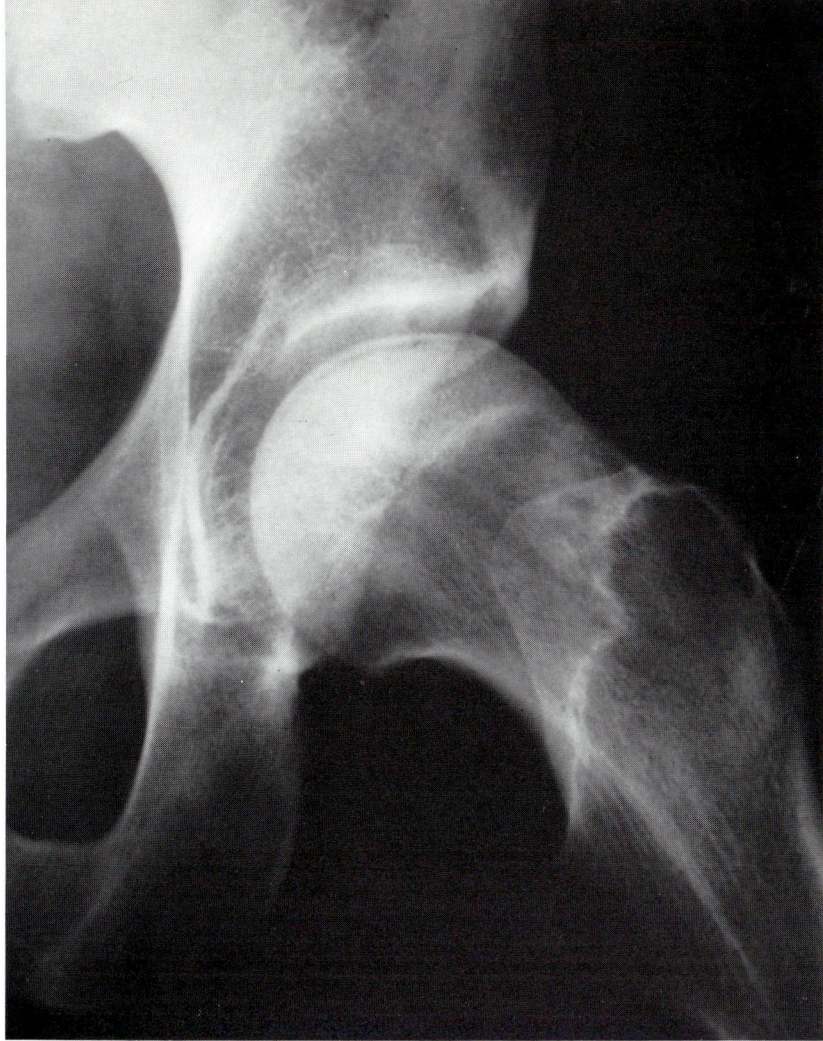

Figure 86

vascular insult and is no longer viable. The "crescent sign" represents an unossified space demarcating the area of dead bone. There are multiple causes of this condition, including steroid therapy, SLE, femoral neck fracture and intracapsular hip infection. There are two other potential causes: alcohol abuse and nitrogen toxicity. Unfortunately for him, the end result of this illness is usually a collapsed femoral head requiring a total joint replacement.

Another type of avascular necrosis is osteochondritis dessicans, demonstrated in the knee in Figures 87 and 88. Notice the lucent defect in the medial femoral condyle (arrow). Such areas may detach from the condyle, forming loose bodies called "joint mice."

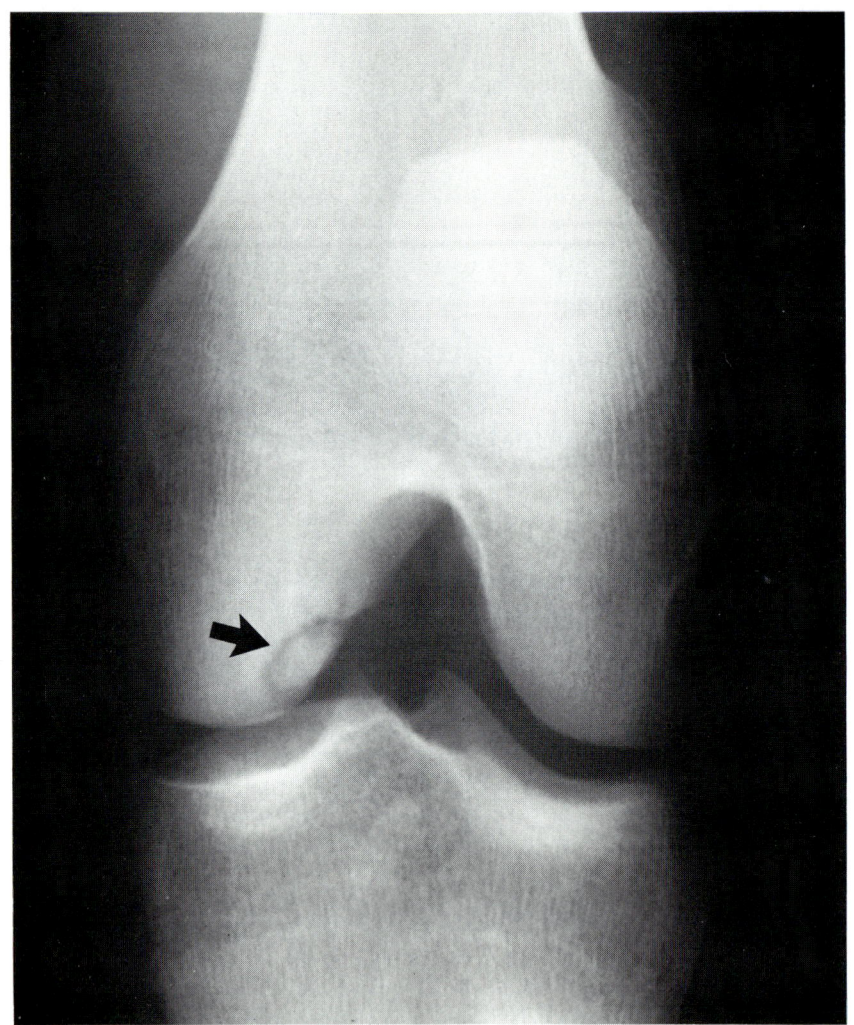

Figure 87

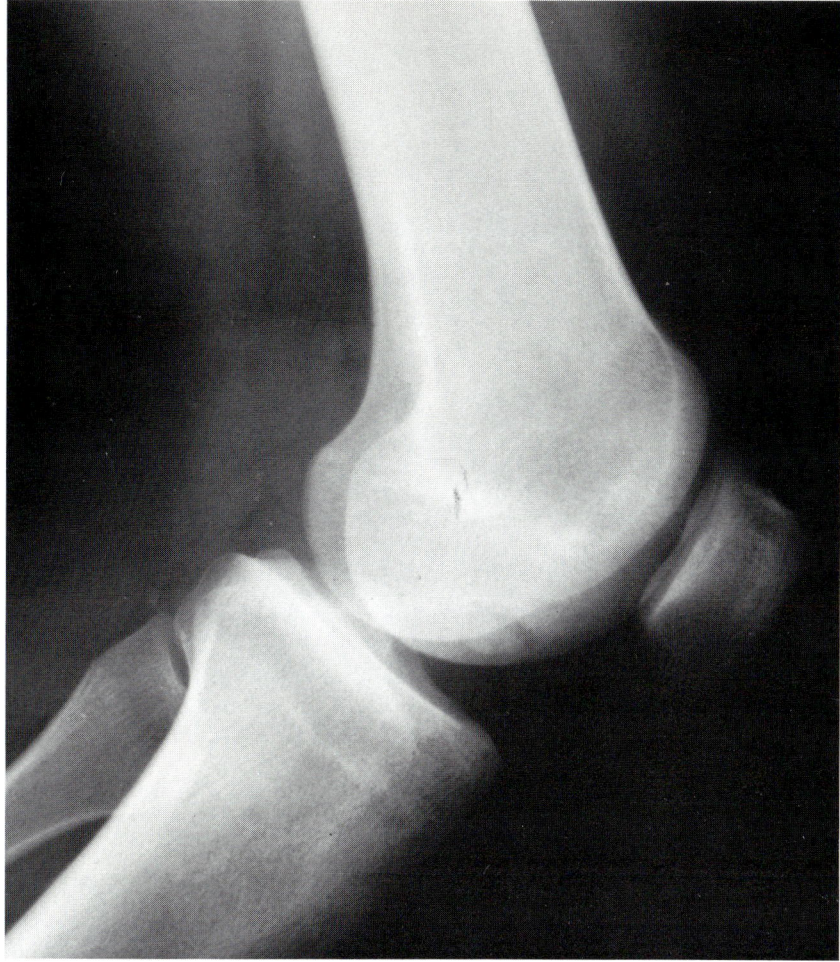

Figure 88

Exercise 19

Look at the radiographs of these two hips (Figs. 89 and 90) and decide which is inflammatory and which is degenerative arthritis.

The first radiograph (Fig. 89) shows uniform narrowing of the left hip. Although the bone looks sclerotic, closer attention reveals that this is the acetabulum seen though the femoral head. In fact, there is little if any new bone growth. Look at the right hip. The narrowing is more difficult to see here, but did you notice the erosion laterally at the base of the femoral head? This is RA. Look at Figure 91, which is another rheumatoid hip that again demonstrates the erosions in the femoral head and neck (arrow). In contrast, Figure 90 demonstrates much more marginal osteophyte growth with sclerosis. This is OA. Did you notice the calcification unattached to the bone, near the lateral femoral head, which was thus not an osteophyte? Figure 92 shows a closeup of this condition. This is probably chondrocalcinosis. Look at the pubis closely to see the thin line of calcification there. This patient

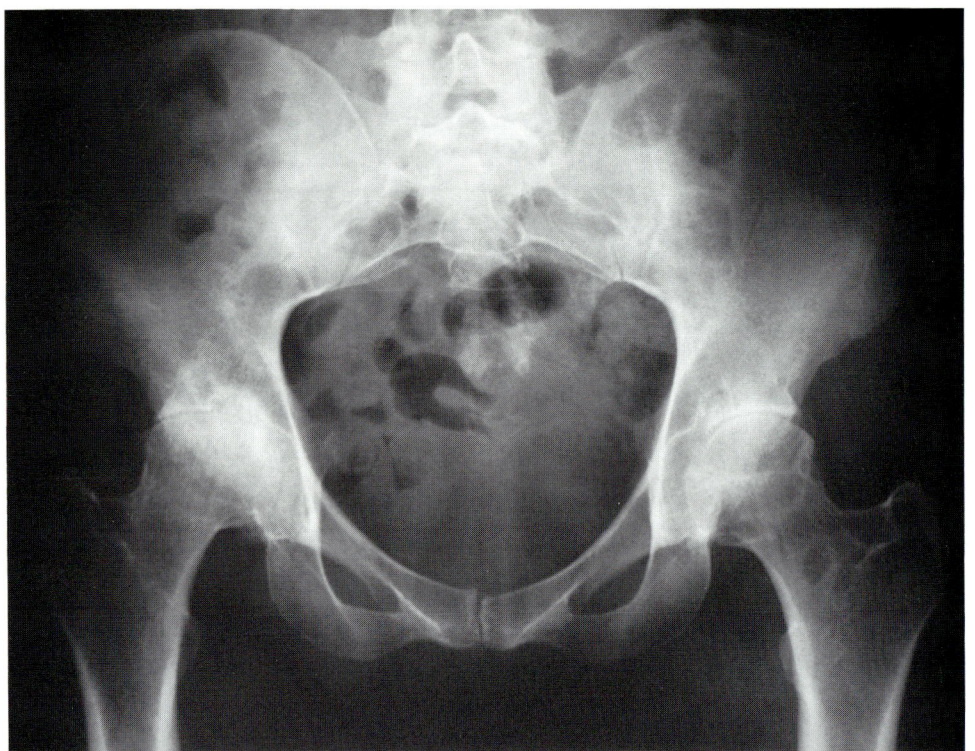

Figure 89

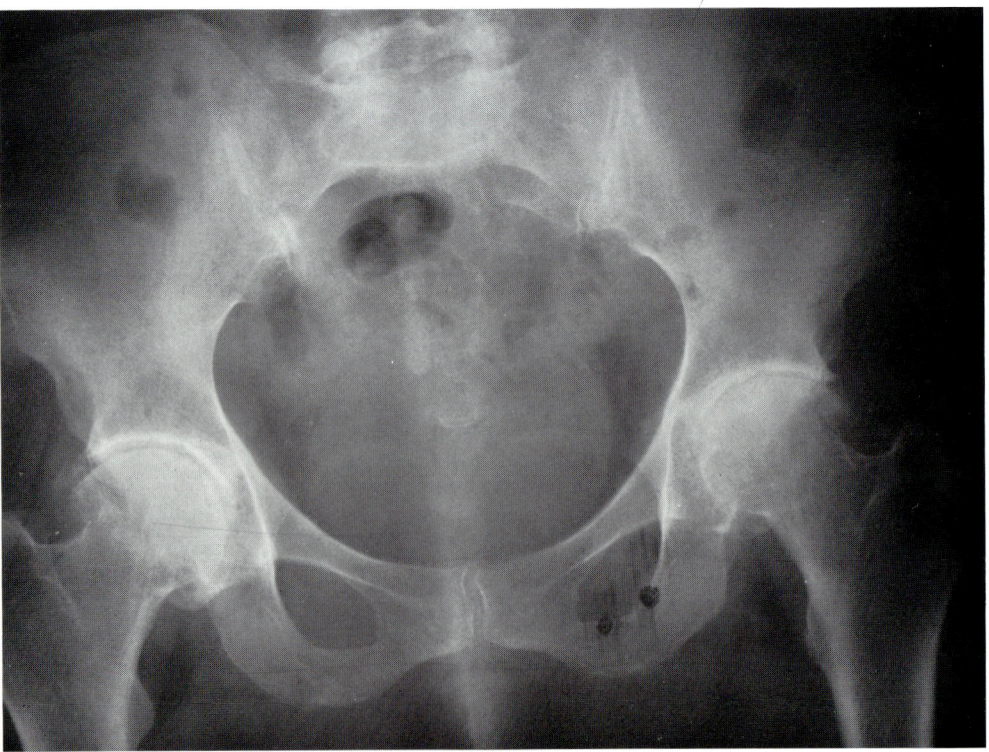

Figure 90

SECTION II—EXERCISES

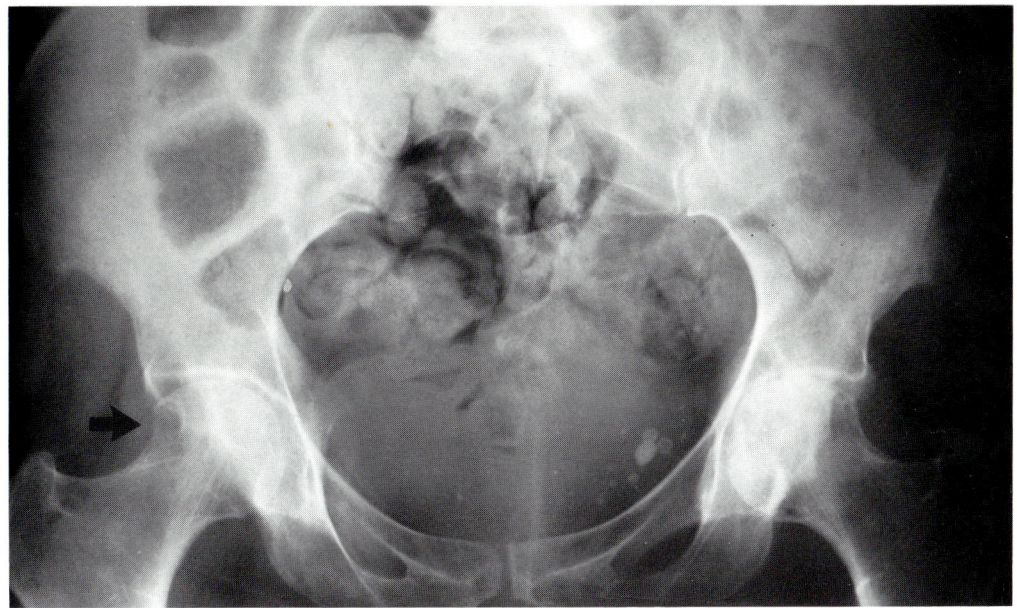

Figure 91

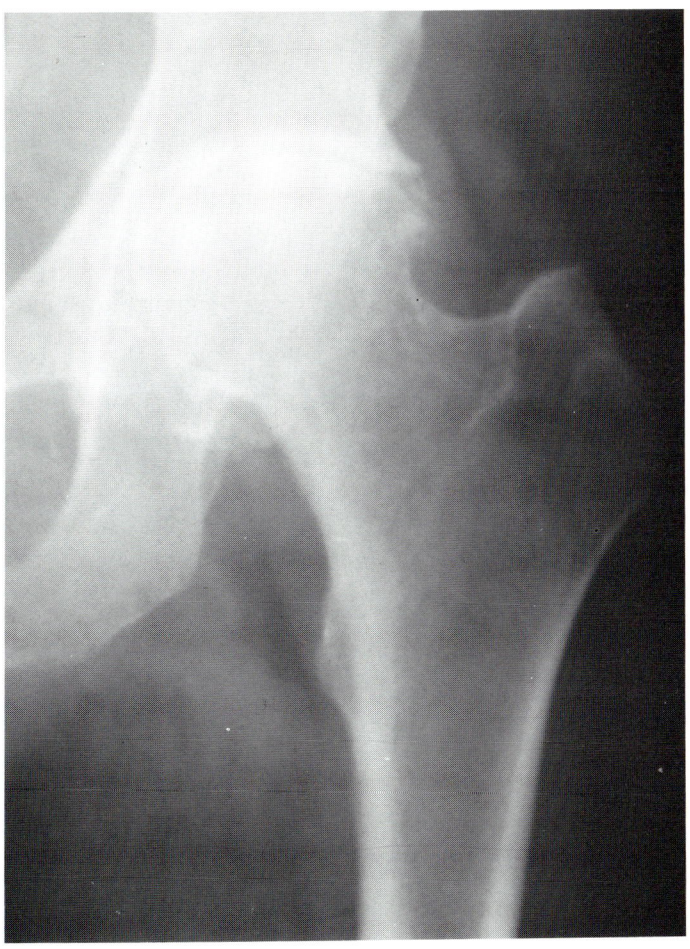

Figure 92

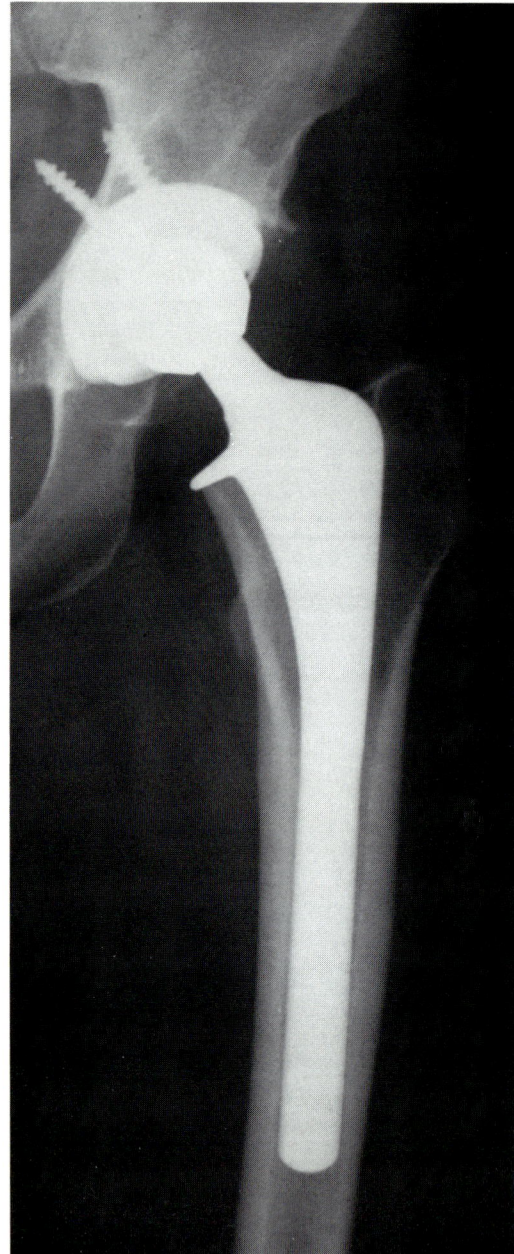

Figure 93

had suffered several bouts of pseudogout in the past. Look at Figure 93, which is a cementless hip prosthesis that was placed in this patient, and compare it to the cemented prosthesis of the knee shown previously in Figure 81.

Exercise 20

Harold comes to you with pain in his right hip of 1 month's duration following a bout of rather severe diarrhea. On examination, limitation of motion on movement and pain of the right hip are obvious. Look at his radiograph (Fig. 94) and decide your next move.

You should be able to determine that Figure 94 is a radiograph of a normal hip. If you still suspect articular disease despite a normal radiograph, a bone scan may help to confirm your impression. Look at Figure 95, which is a bone scan of Harold's hip, demonstrating intense uptake of radionuclide around the right hip. This is highly suggestive of an inflammatory arthritis. Figure 96 is a radiograph taken of Harold's hip 4 weeks later. There is diffuse osteopenia and loss of subarticular cortex in both the acetabulum and the femoral head. An irregular erosion is present in the femoral neck. These rapid changes suggest an infectious process. An aspiration of the hip revealed cloudy fluid that grew *Salmonella* on culture. Figure 97, a hip radiograph done 6 months later, demonstrates further destruction of the femoral head and joint space narrowing despite adequate antibiotic therapy.

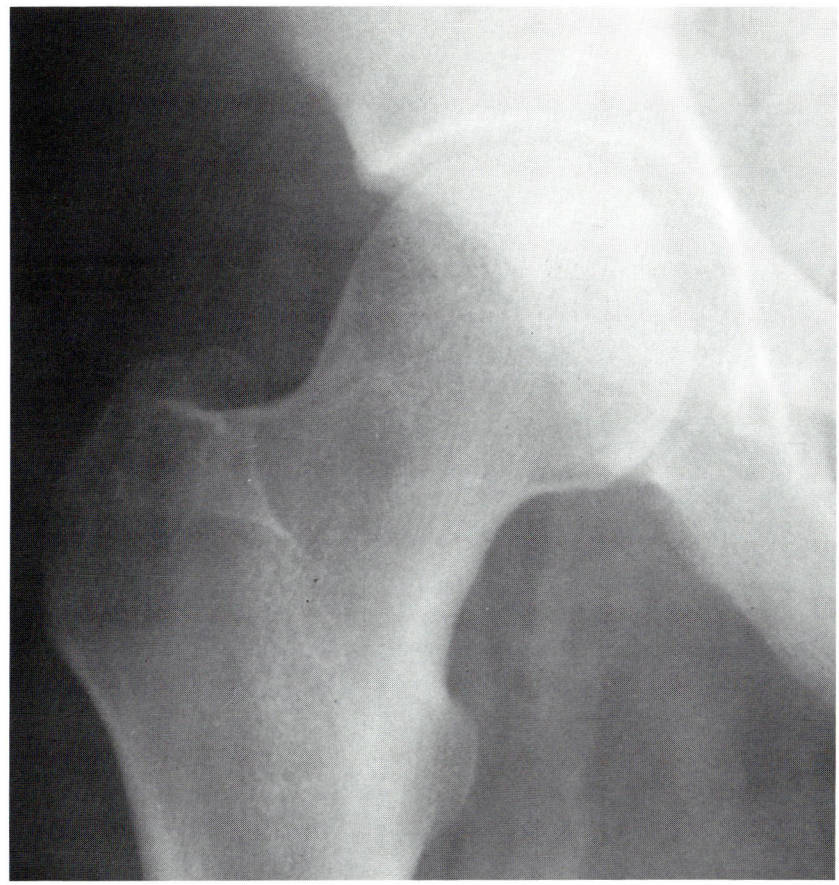

Figure 94

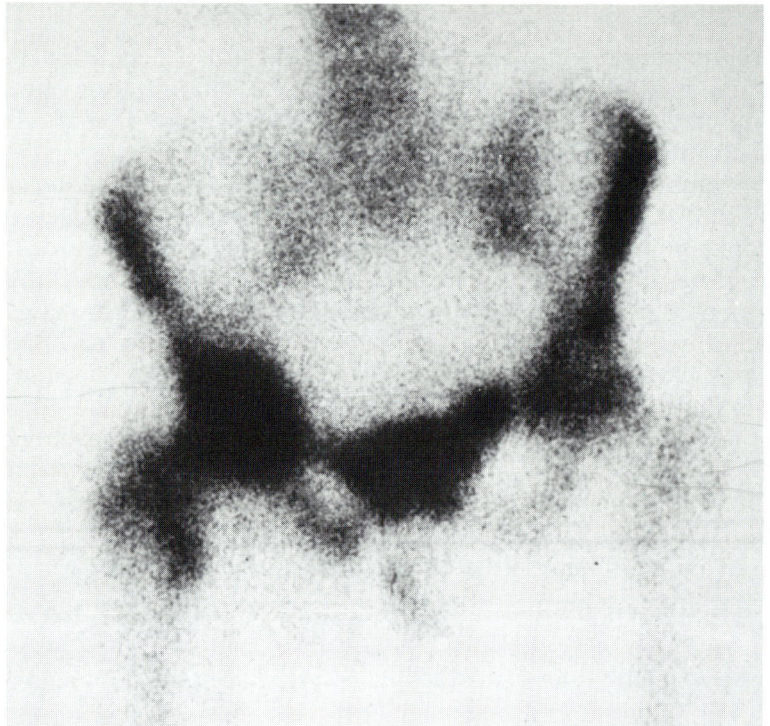

Figure 95

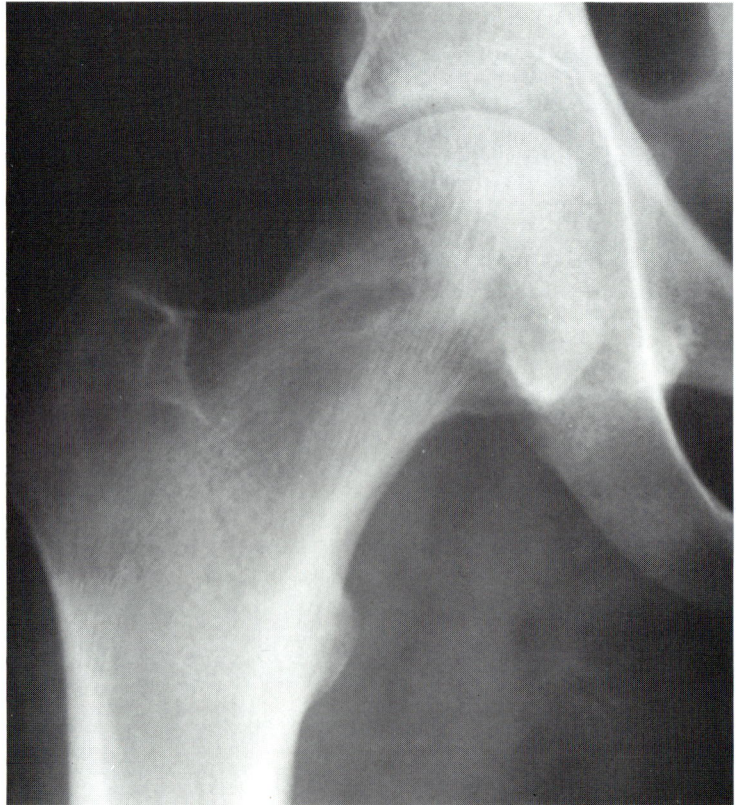

Figure 96

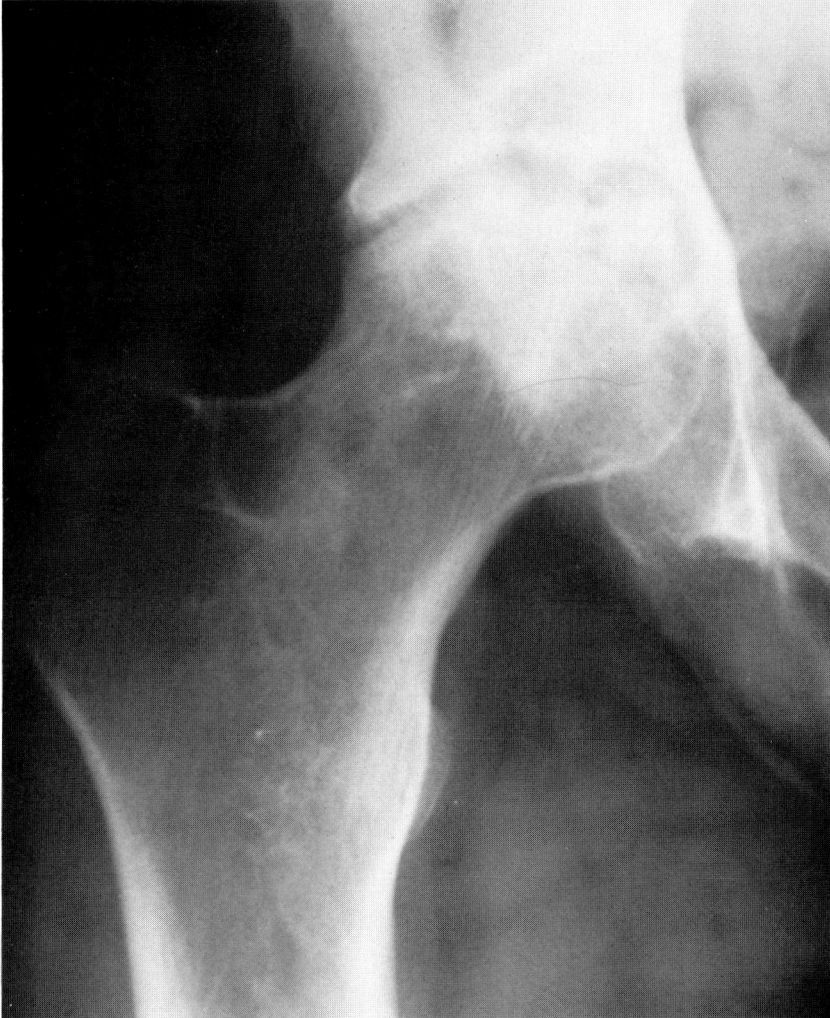

Figure 97

Exercise 21

Look at Victoria's hip radiograph (Fig. 98) and attempt to deduce the illness from your interpretation.

There are diffuse osteopenia, uniform joint space narrowing and several small subchondral cysts. In addition, a large erosion is noted laterally at the base of the femoral head. There is no new bone formation in the form of osteophytes and there is only slight subchondral sclerosis. This is clearly an inflammatory arthritis. In fact, the patient has RA. The large femoral neck erosion is characteristic of a synovial proliferative disease and is seen quite frequently in RA. Look at her hand and foot films next (Figs. 99 and 100).

Her hand radiograph (Fig. 99) shows extensive destruction involving the carpus, the distal radius and the ulnar styloid, with associated soft tissue swelling, particularly over the ulnar styloid regions. The intercarpal and radiocarpal joints are narrowed and there are erosions at the radioulnar joint. All these changes are consistent with the diagnosis of

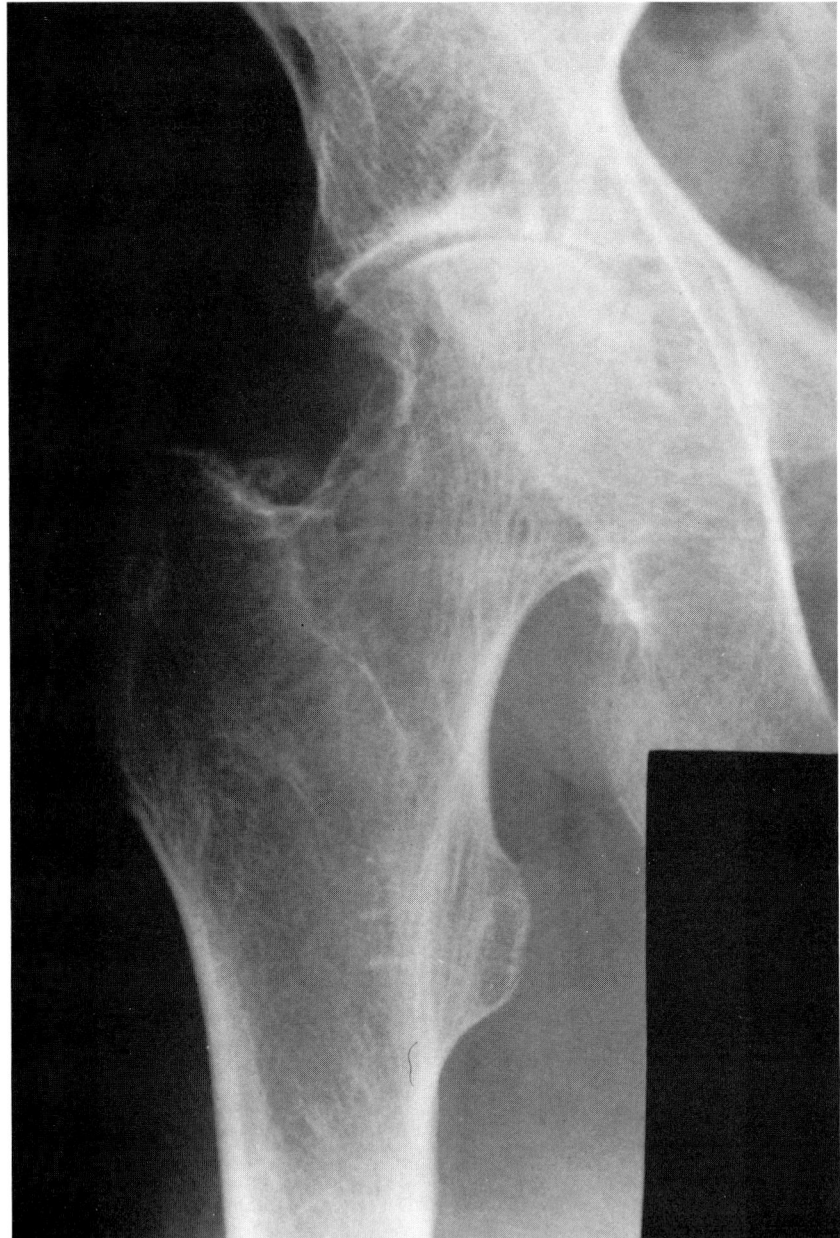

Figure 98

RA. Now look at her foot films (Fig. 100). The oblique radiograph demonstrates erosions in all of the distal metatarsal heads. There is subluxation of the proximal phalanges of the second through the fourth MIP joints. There is a "pencil and cup" lesion at the fifth MIP joint. Although this is more typical for psoriatic arthritis, it is not specific and can be seen in other inflammatory arthritides, as this radiograph demonstrates.

SECTION II—EXERCISES

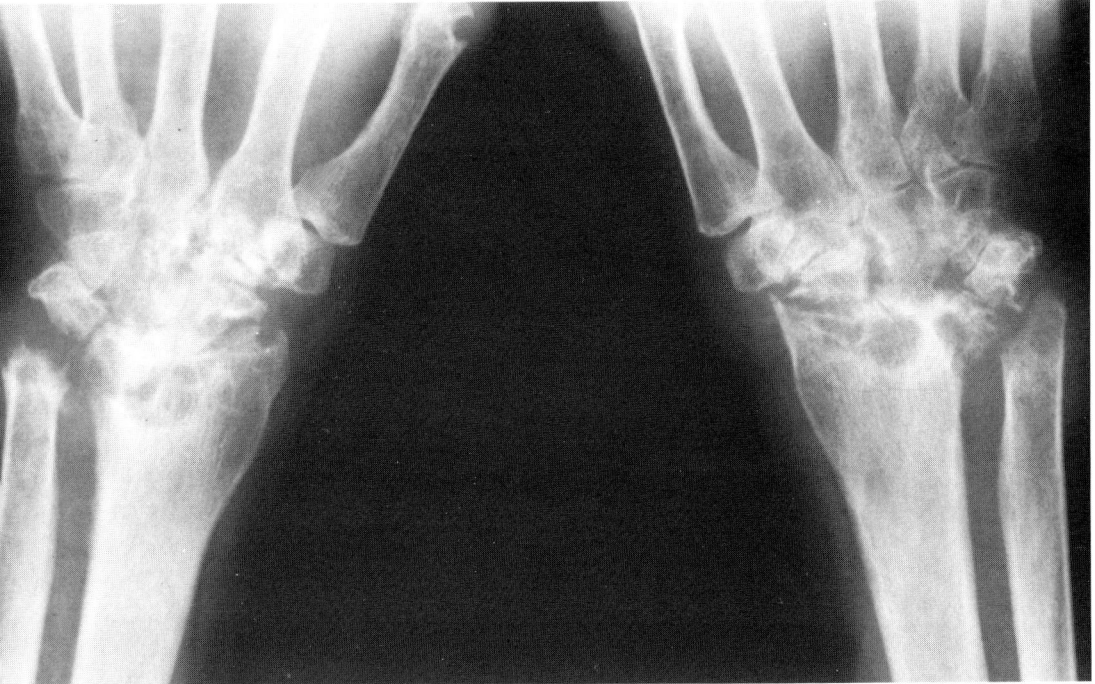

Figure 99

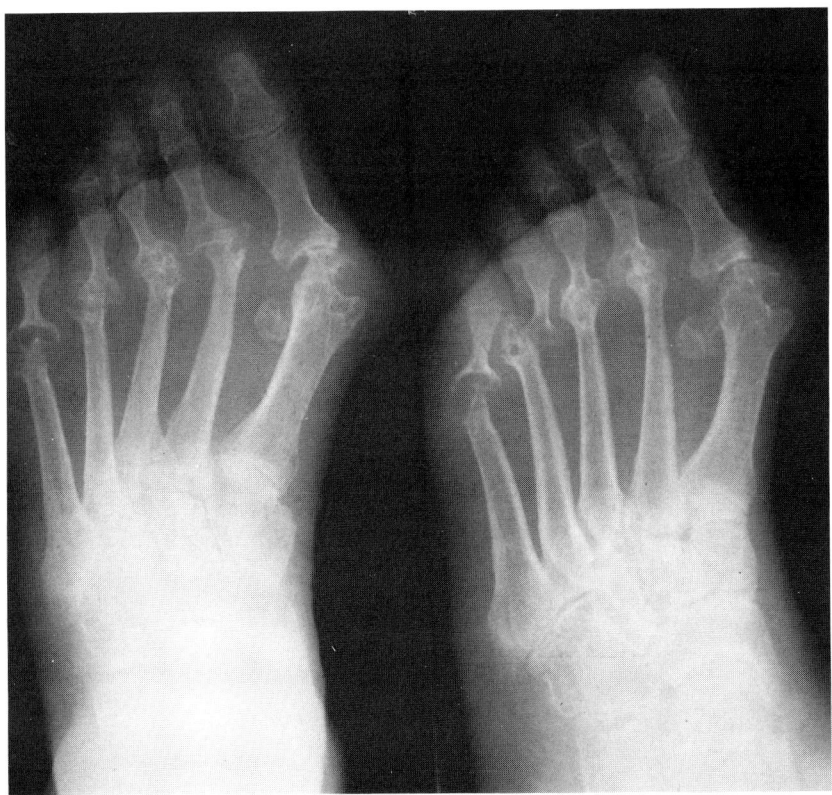

Figure 100

Exercise 22

Jessie, 55 years old, has had progressive pain in her right hip for the last 3 years, and her ambulation is getting worse. She wonders if she should have her hip replaced and asks your advice. She shows you two radiographs (Figs. 101 and 102) taken 3 years apart. What do you think?

The first radiograph shows severe narrowing with sclerosis superiorly. Also noted is fragmentation and cyst formation of the femoral head. Although no osteophytes are present, the findings suggest a severe

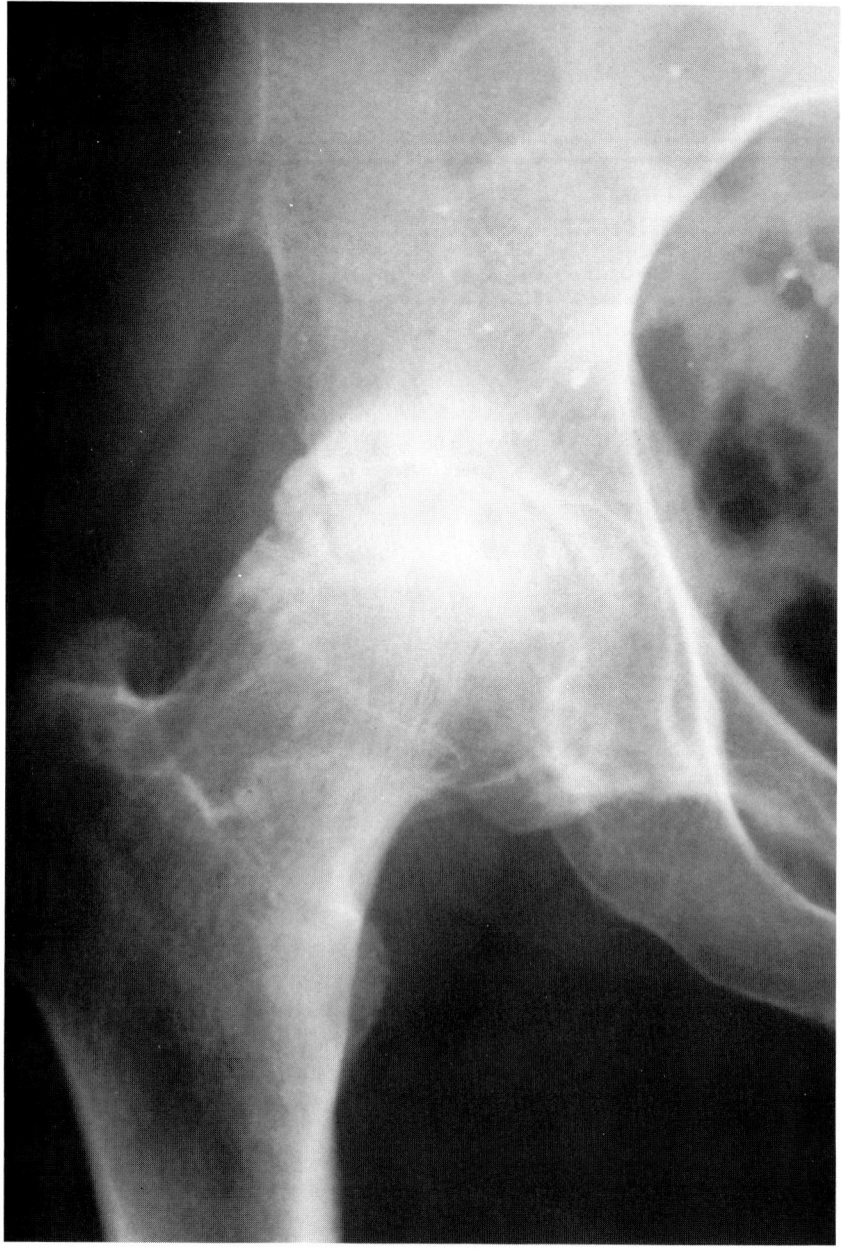

Figure 101

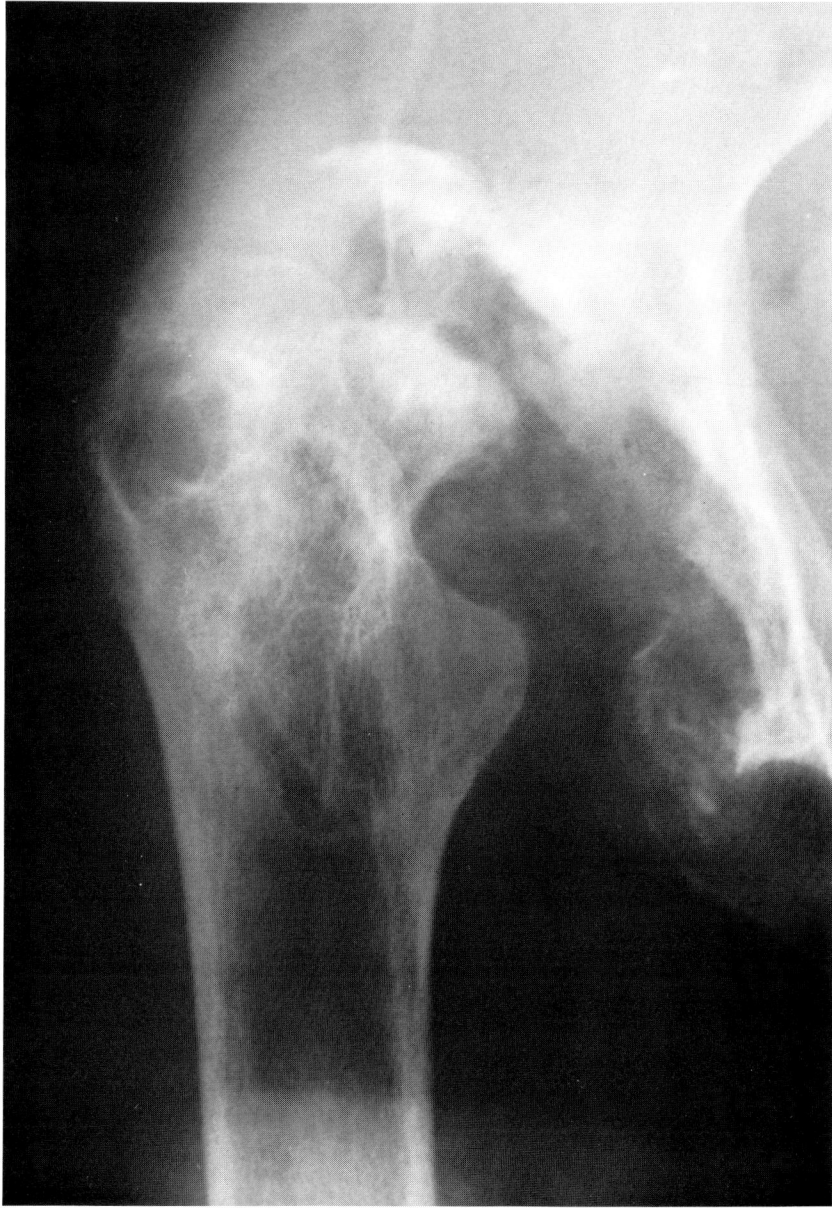

Figure 102

degenerative and destructive process. The second radiograph, taken 3 years later, demonstrates progression with severe bone resorption and destruction. This is a Charcot, or neuropathic, arthropathy. Such a joint develops when there is a loss of proprioception or pain sensation in the articular structures, leading to increased stress and accelerated destruction. Diabetes is a common cause of this disease, especially when it occurs around the foot and ankle. In Jessie's case, it is tabes dorsalis. Look at her knee radiographs, which show changes similar to her hip radiograph (Fig. 103). Jessie should not have a total hip replacement because they do not hold well in Charcot bone.

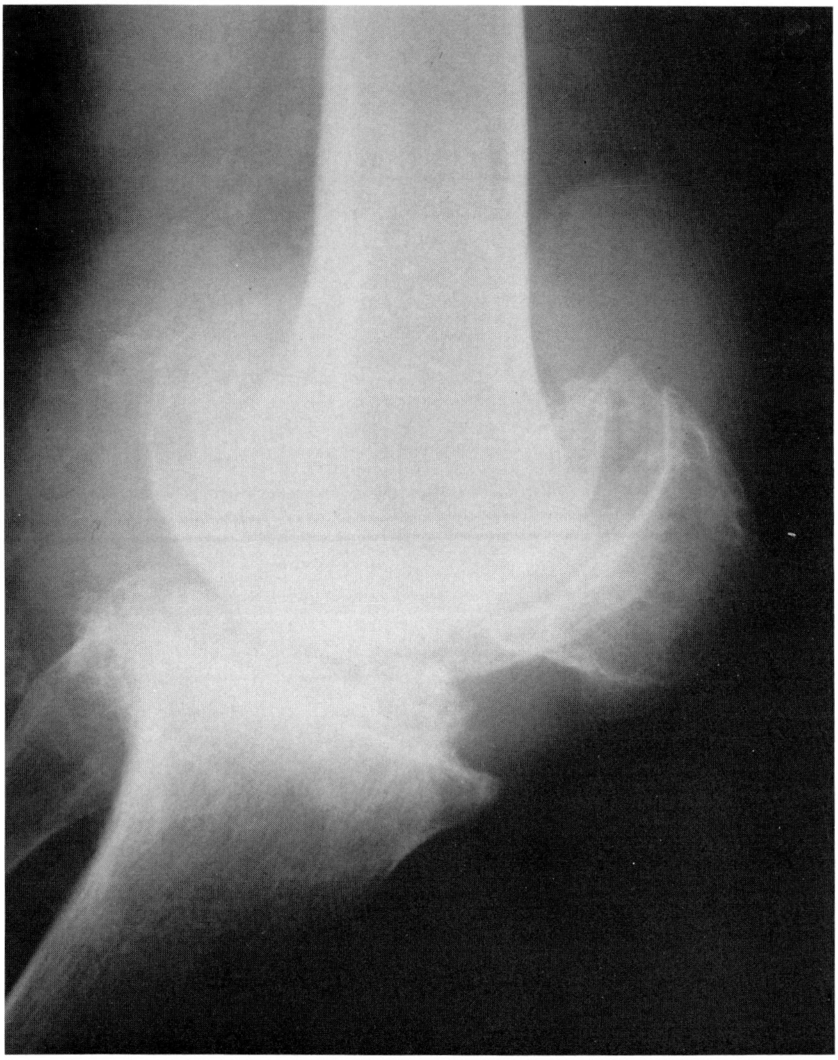

Figure 103

Exercise 23

Joan is a 48 year old waitress with a longstanding polyarthritis involving the upper and lower extremity large and small joints symmetrically. Her hand radiograph is shown in Figure 104. Recently, her knees have been particularly bad, making her sit more often in the restaurant. Two days ago, she developed a sudden onset of calf pain and pitting edema in the left leg. A radiograph of her knees is shown (Fig. 105). Which radiographic procedure would you like performed next?

Joan has periarticular osteopenia, joint space narrowing and erosions around the PIP and MCP joints, the carpal bones and the ulnar styloid, suggesting RA. Her knee films reveal uniform narrowing without osteophytes or subchondral sclerosis, and an effusion, which is also consistent with RA. Joan had a rupture of a Baker's cyst, a herniation of the posterior joint capsule dissecting through the popliteal space and

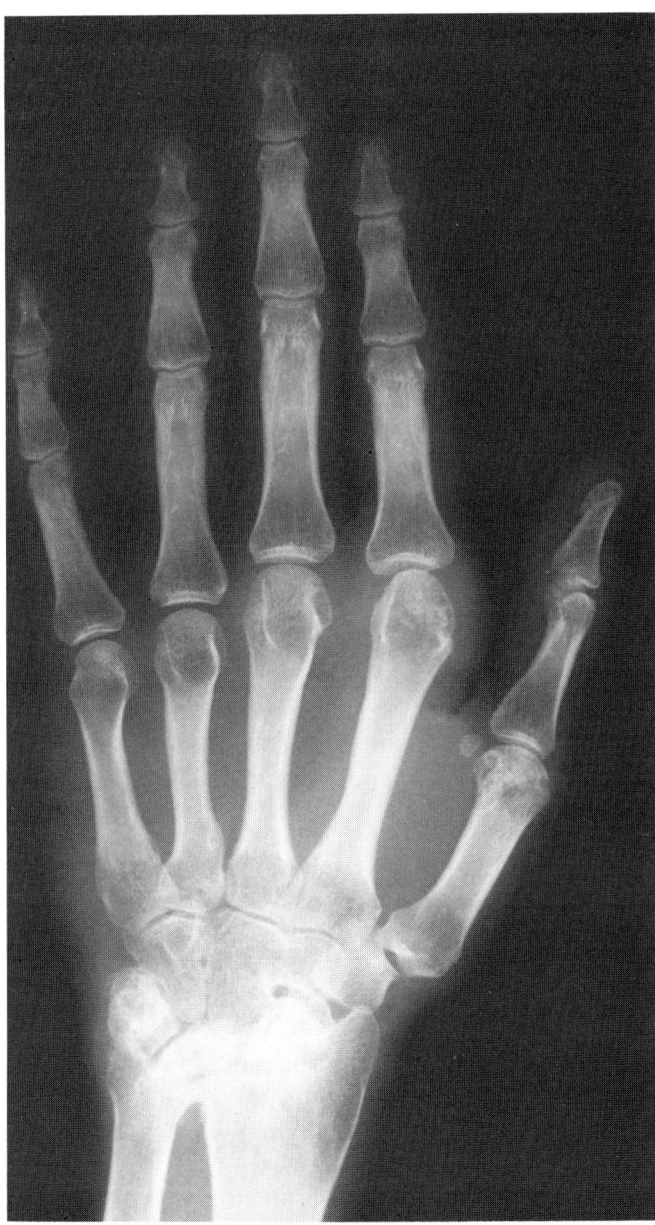

Figure 104

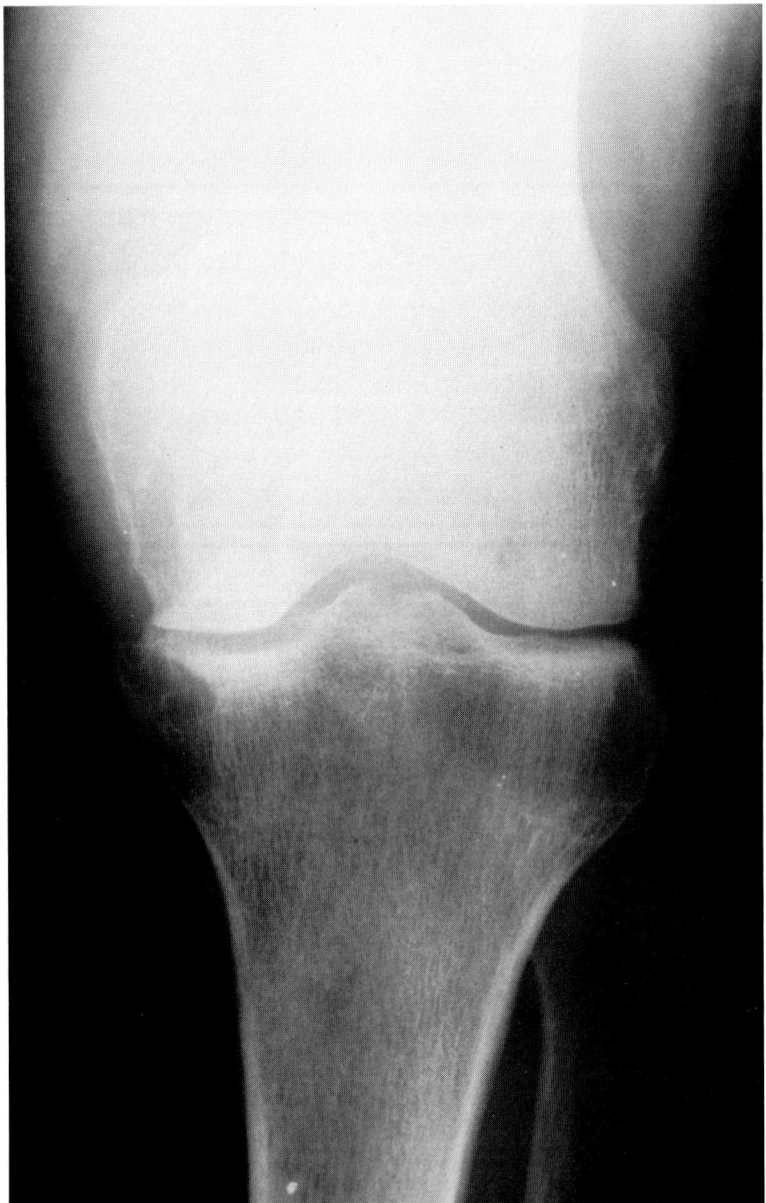

Figure 105

down into the calf muscles, which caused her sudden calf pain and swelling. This is demonstrated most easily by ultrasound, but shown here instead is an arthrogram (Fig. 106). This clearly demonstrates that contrast medium injected into the knee joint leaks out posteriorly and fills a cyst in the calf. If you thought she had a deep venous thrombosis and ordered a venogram, you were "taken in" by the similar clinical presentation of the two illnesses. This similarity has earned the ruptured Baker's cyst the name "pseudothrombophlebitis."

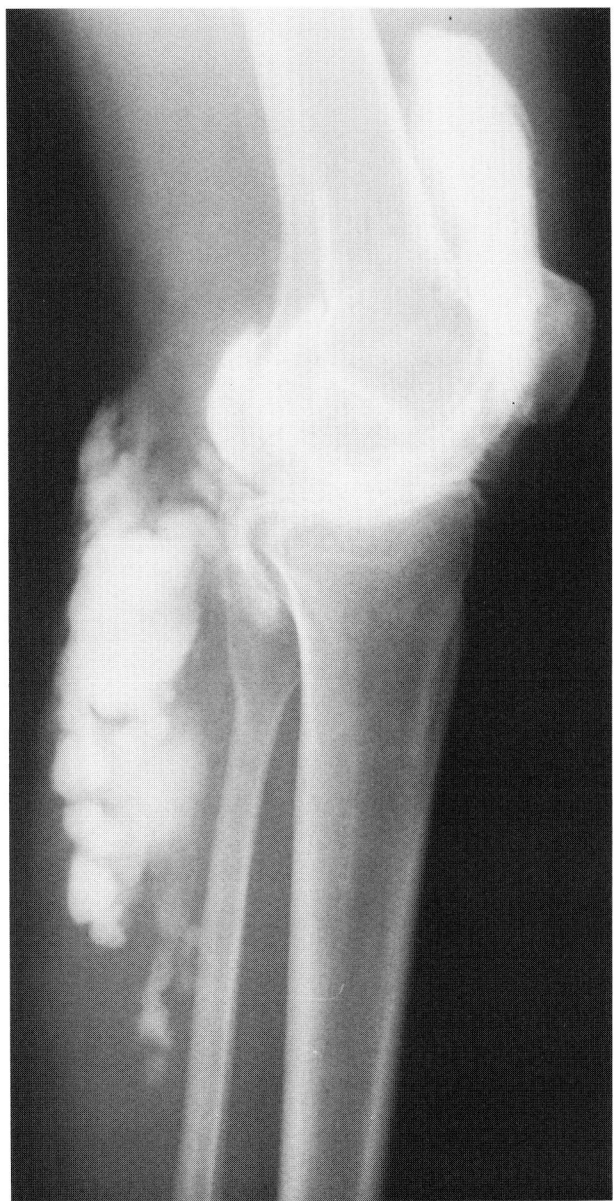

Figure 106

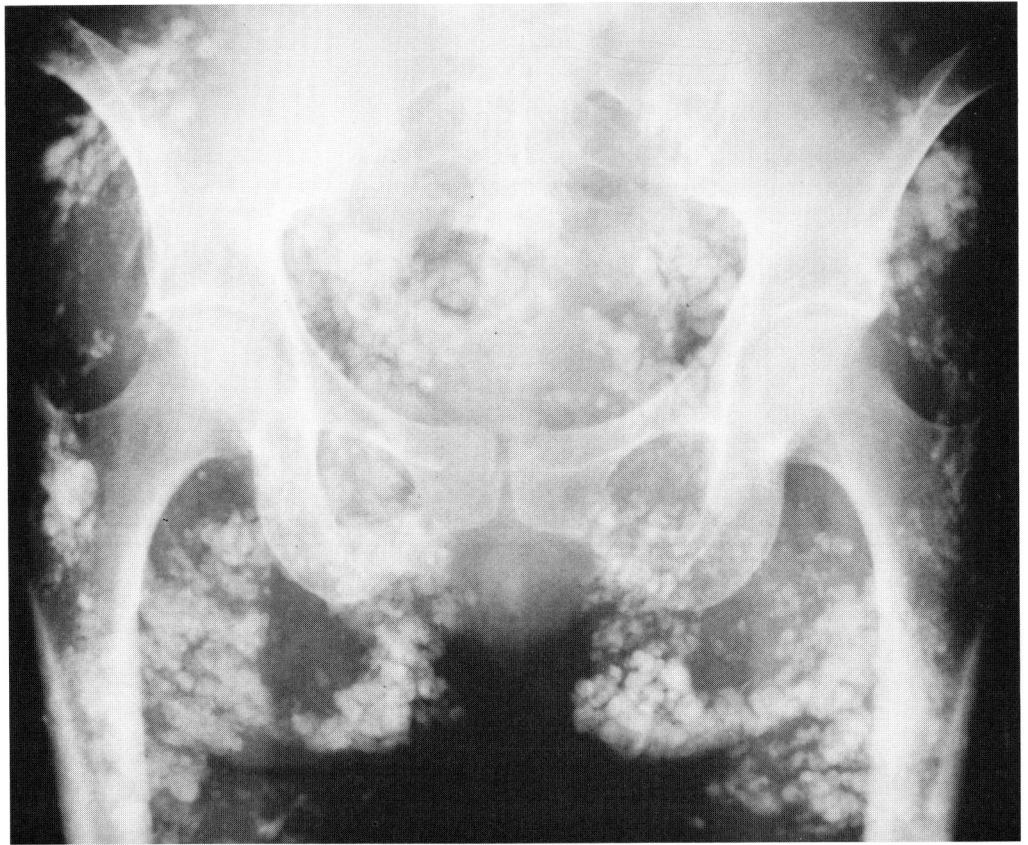

Figure 107

Exercise 24

Edna, 46 years old, complains of two months worth of difficulty rising from a chair or combing her hair. Although some pain is involved, the predominant features are stiffness and weakness and a periorbital rash. You obtain a radiograph of her hips. Look at the radiograph (Fig. 107) and diagnose her condition.

Edna has diffuse soft tissue calcification. Although this can be seen in the scleroderma, CREST syndrome, myositis ossificans or the hypercalcemia of renal failure, her clinical story makes the likely cause of her calcification dermatomyositis. In fact, her creatine phosphokinase (CPK) level was elevated, and an electromyogram and a muscle biopsy were consistent with this diagnosis.

Exercise 25

Ronald, 41 years old, has complained of pain in his hip for the last 6 months. He has no history of trauma to this joint. On examination you note that there is limitation of motion and that he has a noticeable limp. Look at his radiograph (Fig. 108) and tell him what he has.

Ronald's radiograph shows a normal joint space, normal bone density and alignment and no osteophytes. The obvious abnormality is the diffuse soft tissue nodular calcification. A CAT scan (Fig. 109)

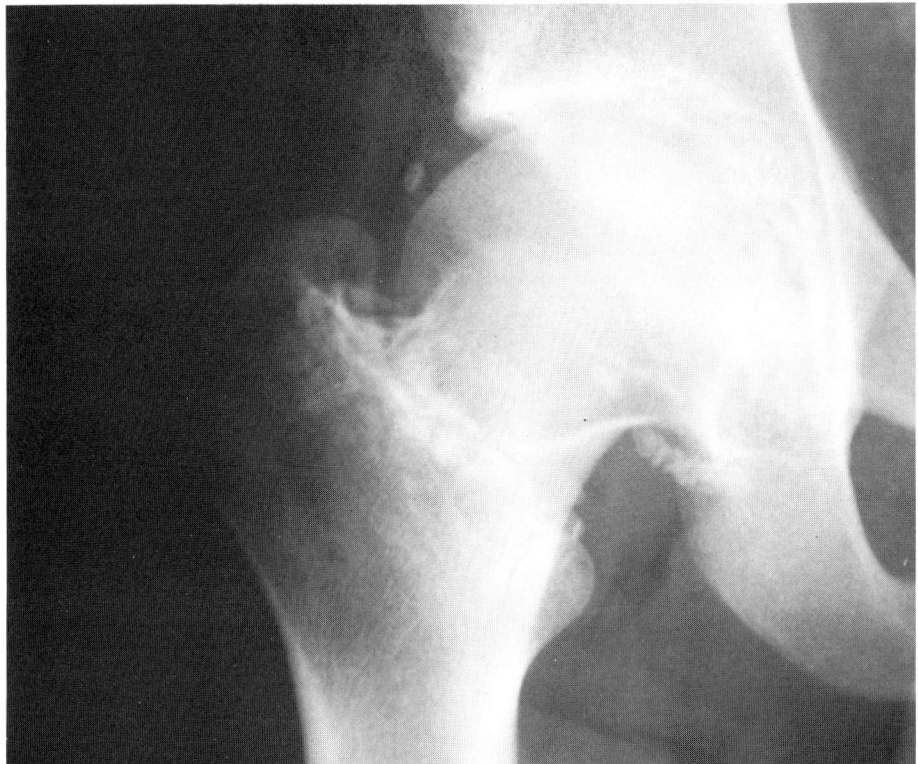

Figure 108

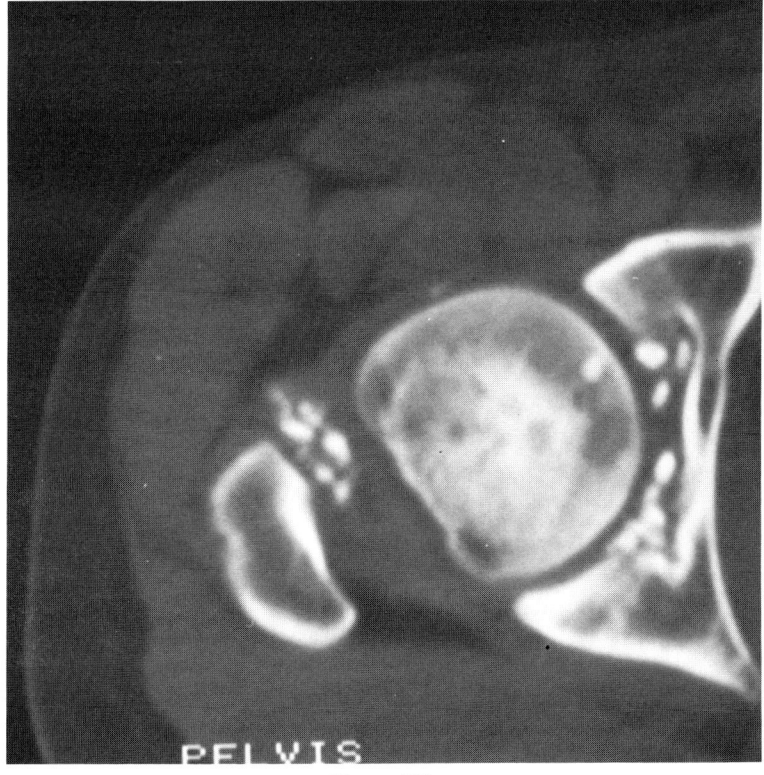

Figure 109

confirms the intra-articular location of the calcium deposits. This suggests a diagnosis of synovial chondromatosis, a condition in which multiple foci of cartilage metaplasia occur in synovium, often undergoing ossification. This leads to pain and stiffness of the affected joint. Synovectomy is usually curative, which is what you recommend to Ronald. Figures 110 to 112 demonstrate similar changes in the knee and ankle of two other patients.

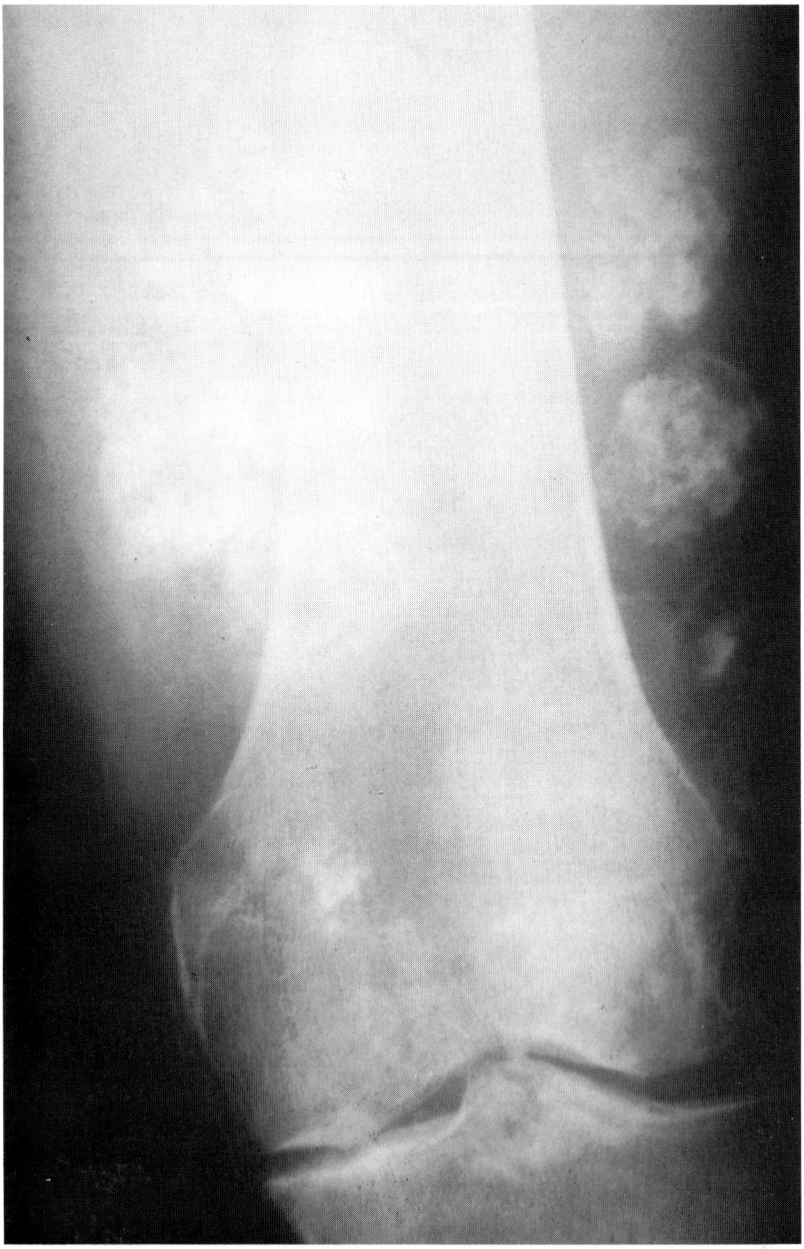

Figure 110

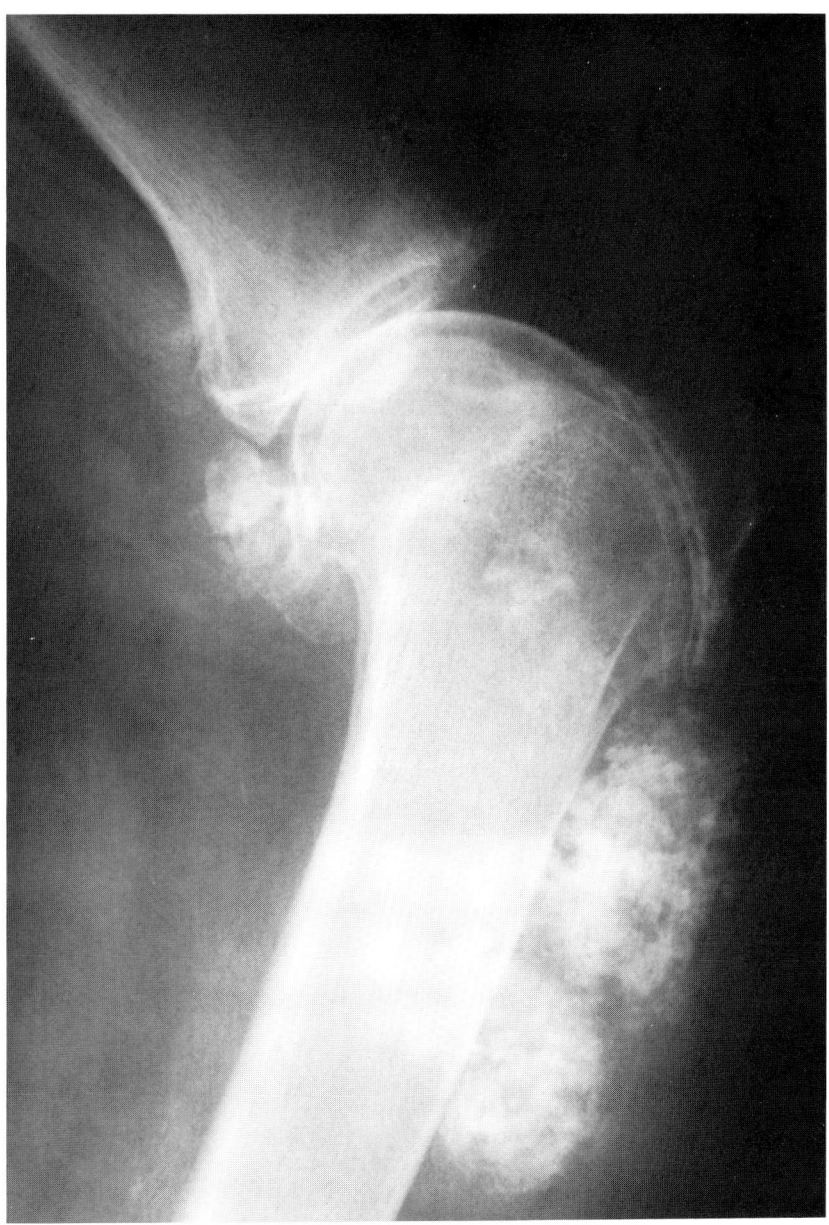

Figure 111

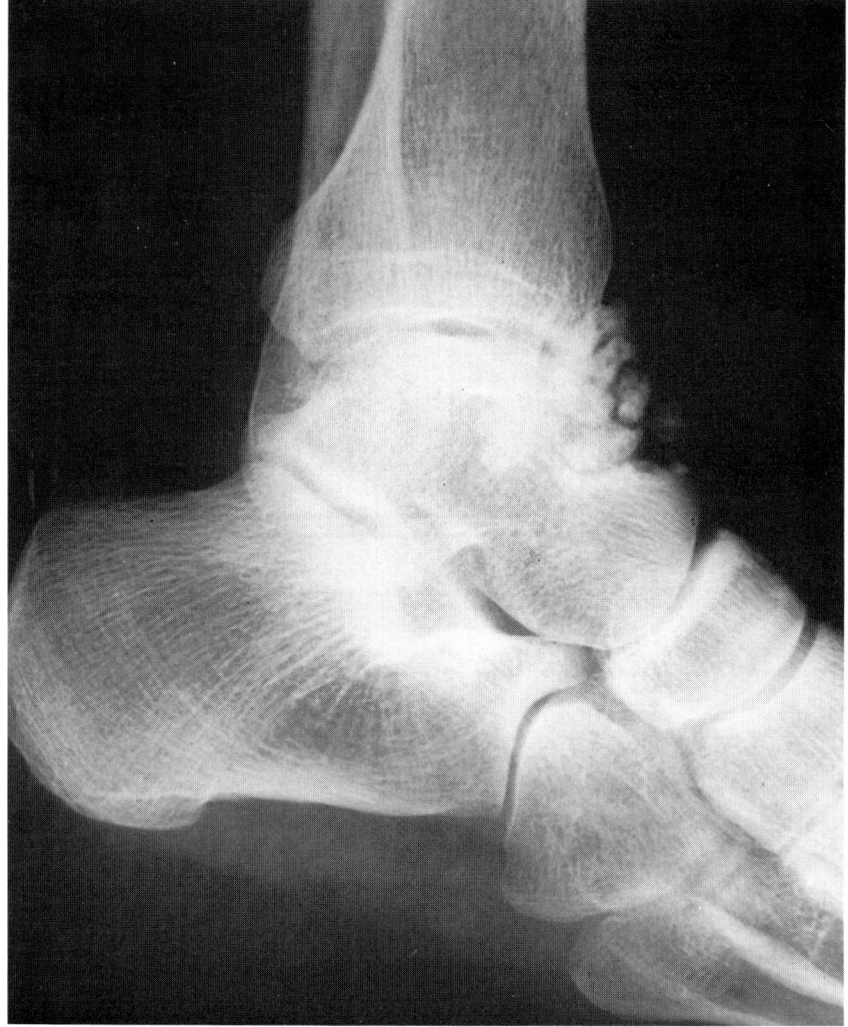

Figure 112

Foot and Ankle

Exercise 26

Your associate shows you a set of radiographs of the foot and ankle (Figs. 113 and 114). Based on your interpretation of the films, tell him what the likely cause of this person's ankle pain is and how you might treat it.

The radiographs reveal narrowing of the tibiotalar and intertarsal joint spaces. Note the erosive disease in the subtalar joint (arrow) as well as at the point of insertion of the Achilles tendon in the os calcis. The narrowed and eroded joint spaces in the absence of reactive bone changes are characteristic of an inflammatory arthritis such as RA. A procedure that is done to relieve pain from such destruction is a triple arthrodesis, which fuses several of the subtalar joints. This procedure

SECTION II—EXERCISES

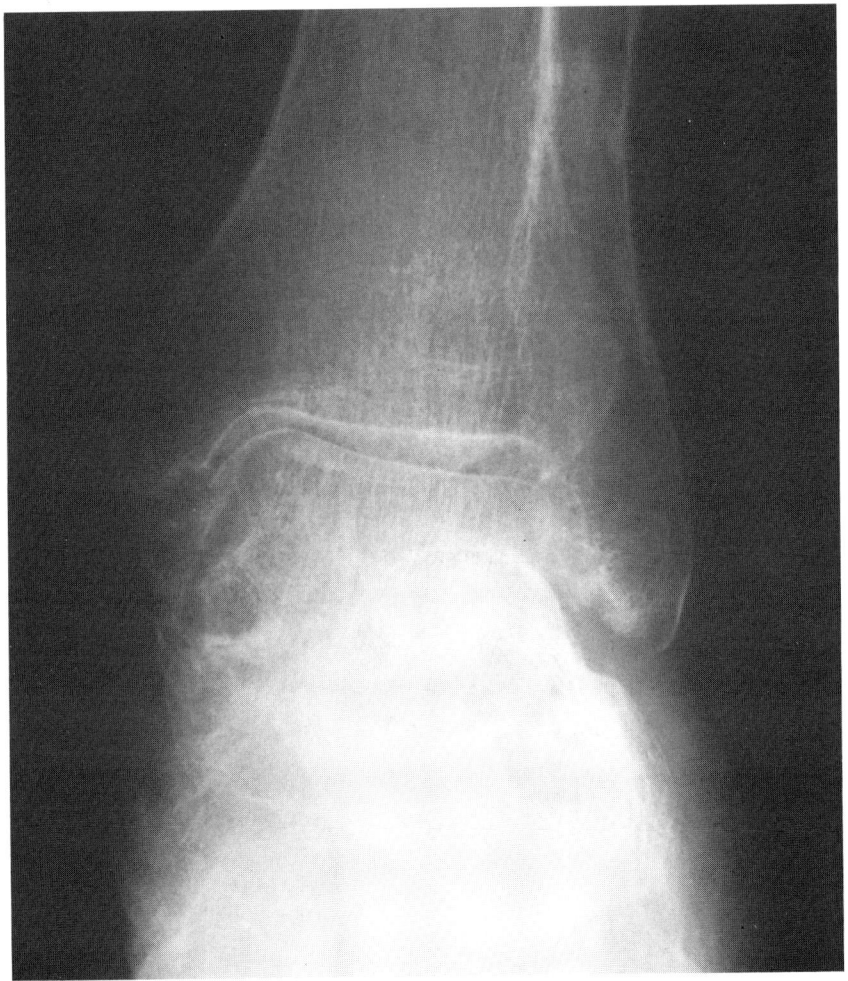

Figure 113

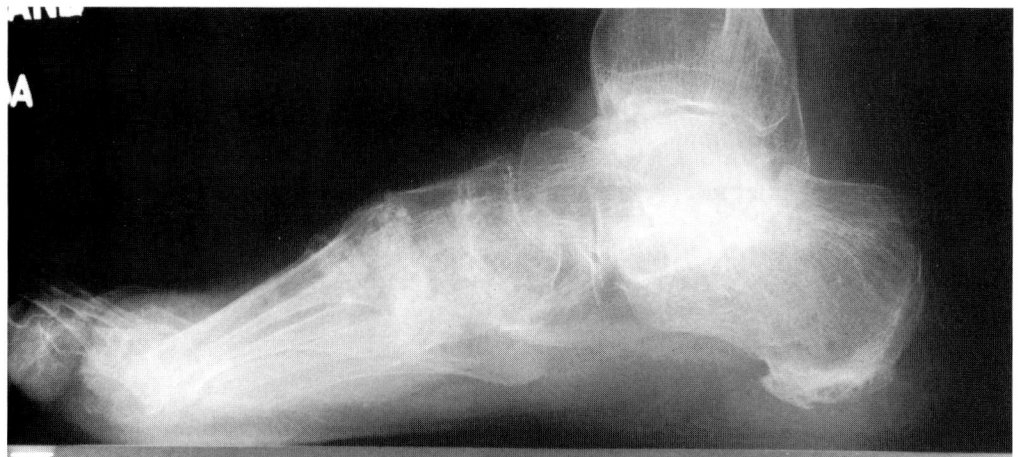

Figure 114

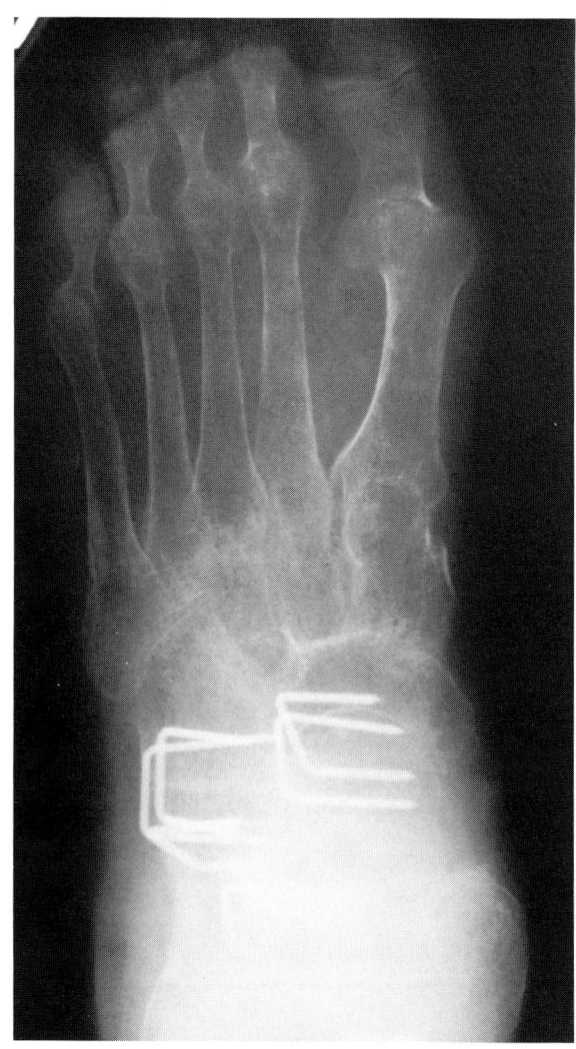

Figure 115

is demonstrated in the patient in Figure 115. Note again on this radiograph the marked inflammatory changes in the intertarsal and metatarsal joints.

Exercise 27

Donald, 35 years old, is an ex-soccer player who is having considerable pain in his big toe. Look at his radiographs (Figs. 116 and 117) and tell him the cause of his pain.

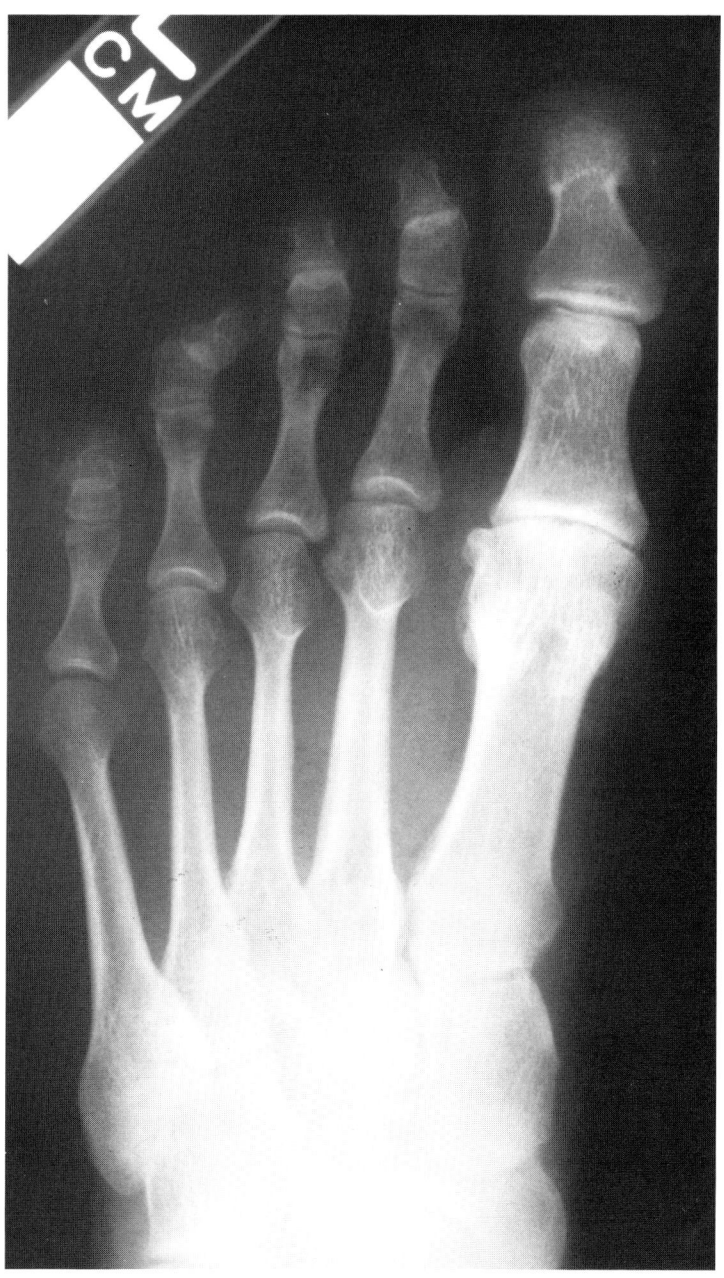

Figure 116

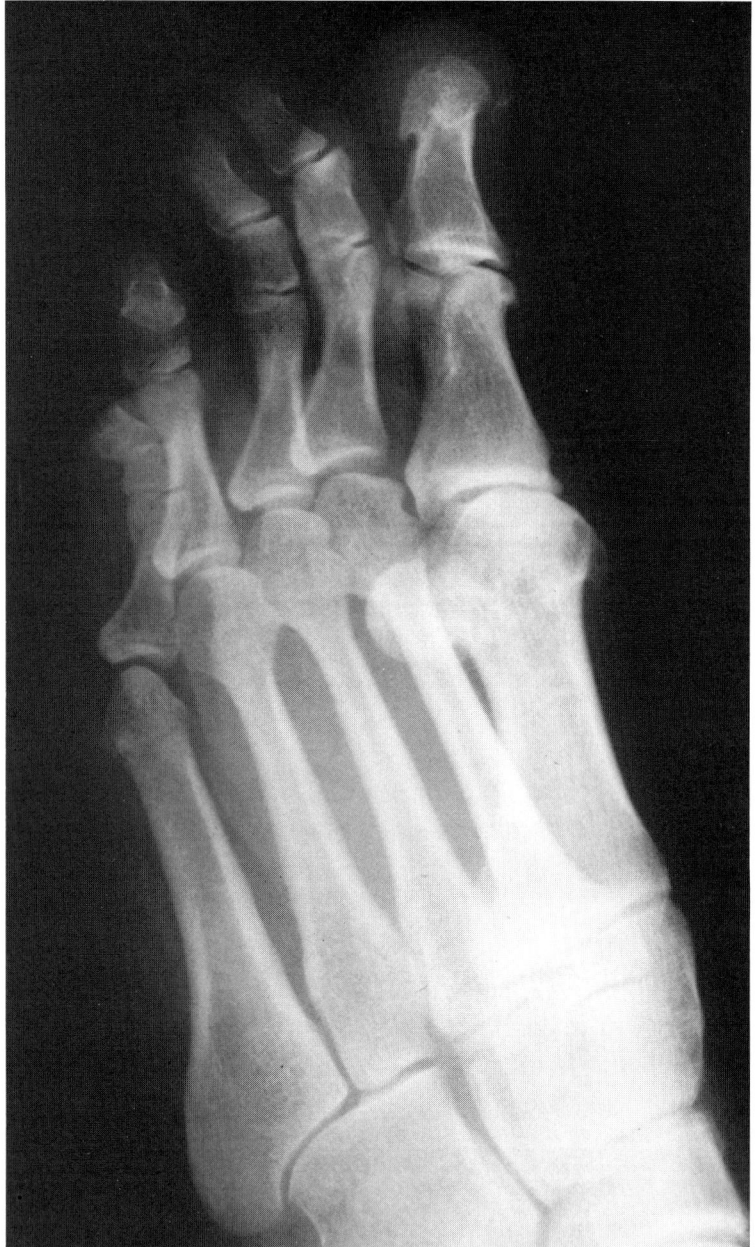

Figure 117

Donald's radiographs reveal that the first MTP joint has joint space narrowing with sclerosis and osteophyte formation. This is consistent with degenerative arthritis, presumably secondary to the repeated trauma his sport is associated with. Note the absence of malalignment of the first MIP joint. Frequently such degeneration is associated with a valgus deformity at the MTP joint and formation of a medial osteophyte with an overlying swollen bursa, often called a bunion.

Exercise 28

Two sets of hand and foot films are shown (Figs. 118–119 and Figs. 120–122). Describe each and decide what the patient has based on your radiographic interpretation. The key to interpretation of these radiographs is the asymmetric distribution of the joint involvement.

Figure 118 shows soft tissue swelling around the fourth DIP and third PIP joints. The third PIP joint has accompanying joint space narrowing and erosions; the fourth DIP joint has joint space narrowing and what looks like marginal new bone growth. Both the DIP and MCP joints of the thumb are swollen, with erosions and narrowing. The foot (Fig. 119) shows erosion at the first, fourth and fifth DIP joints, as well

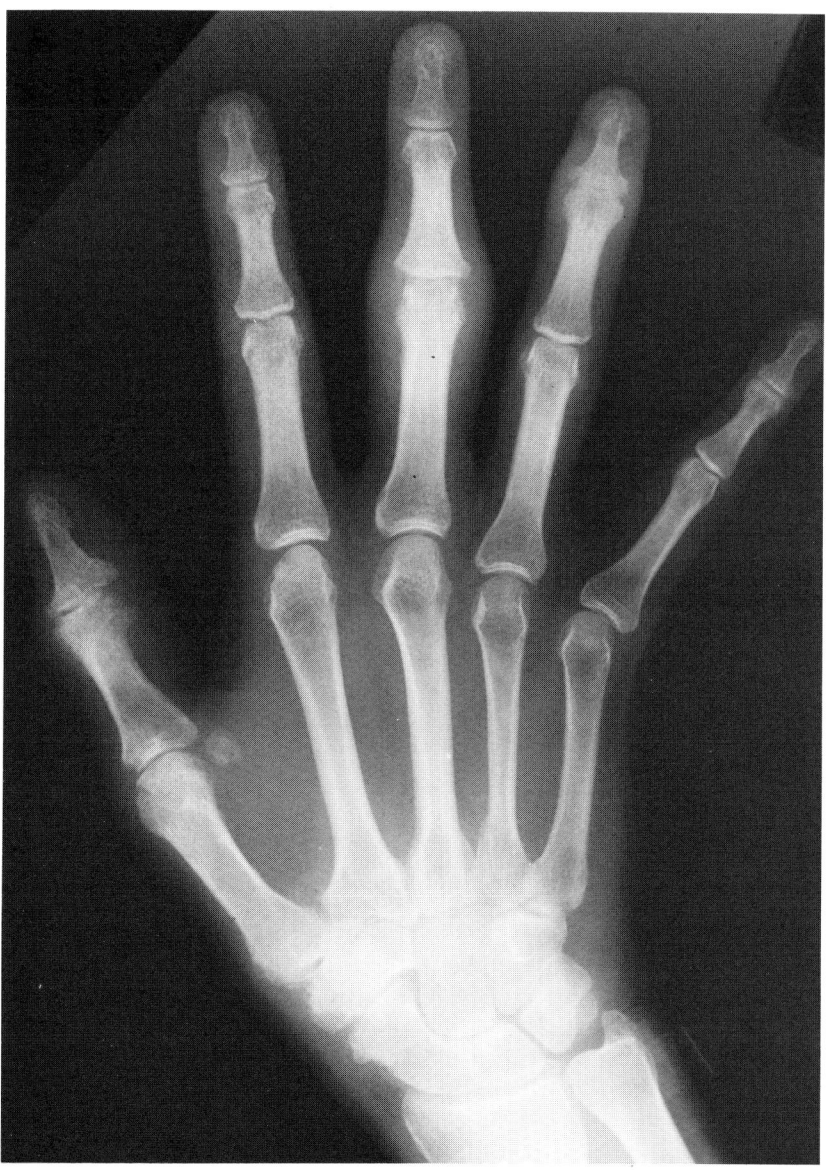

Figure 118

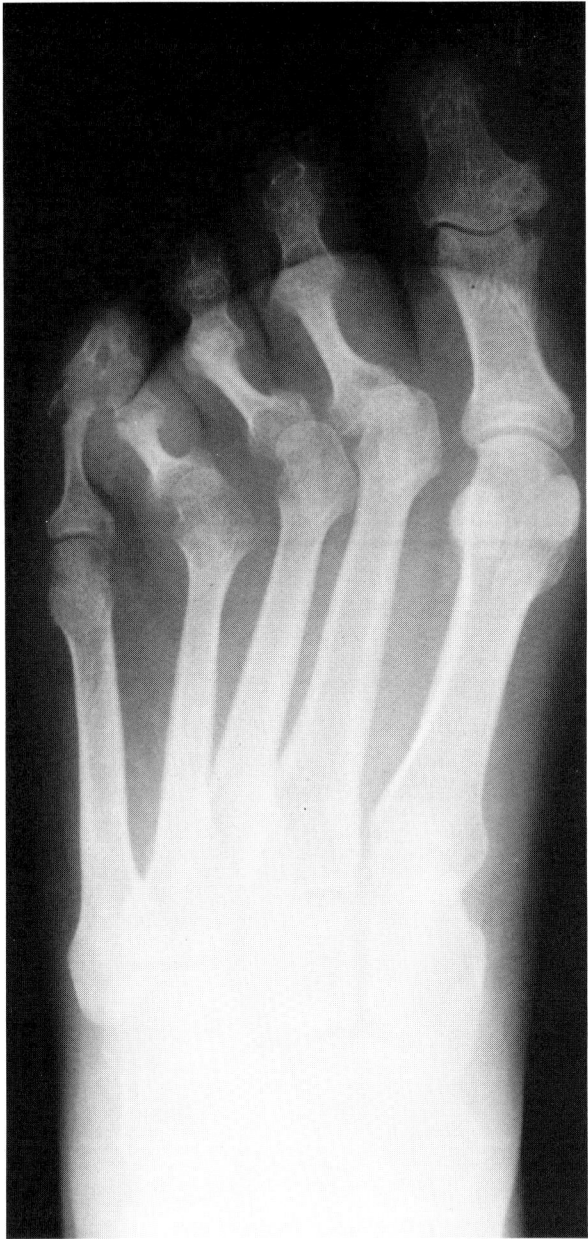

Figure 119

as at the fifth MIP joint. The second, third and fourth MIP joints are subluxed, forming hammer toes. The uniform narrowing of the joints, along with erosions and absence of sclerosis or osteophyte formation, suggests an inflammatory illness. The asymmetry of the distribution demonstrated in these radiographs favors psoriatic arthritis as the type of inflammatory illness.

Figure 120 shows destruction and erosion in the right fifth MCP, PIP and DIP joints, with widening of the joint spaces. The rest of the hand is normal. The foot (Figs. 121 and 122) shows the first and fifth MTP and DIP joints to be involved with a destructive process, with

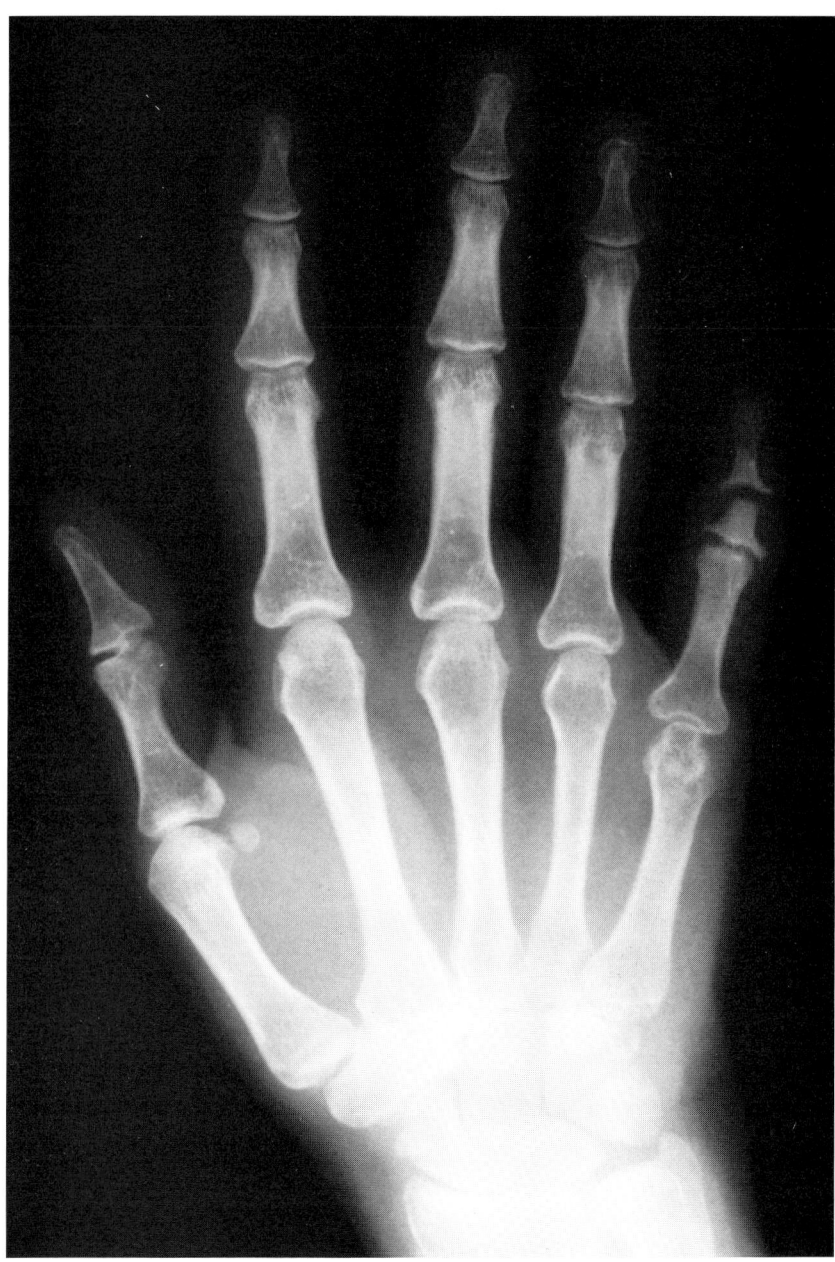

Figure 120

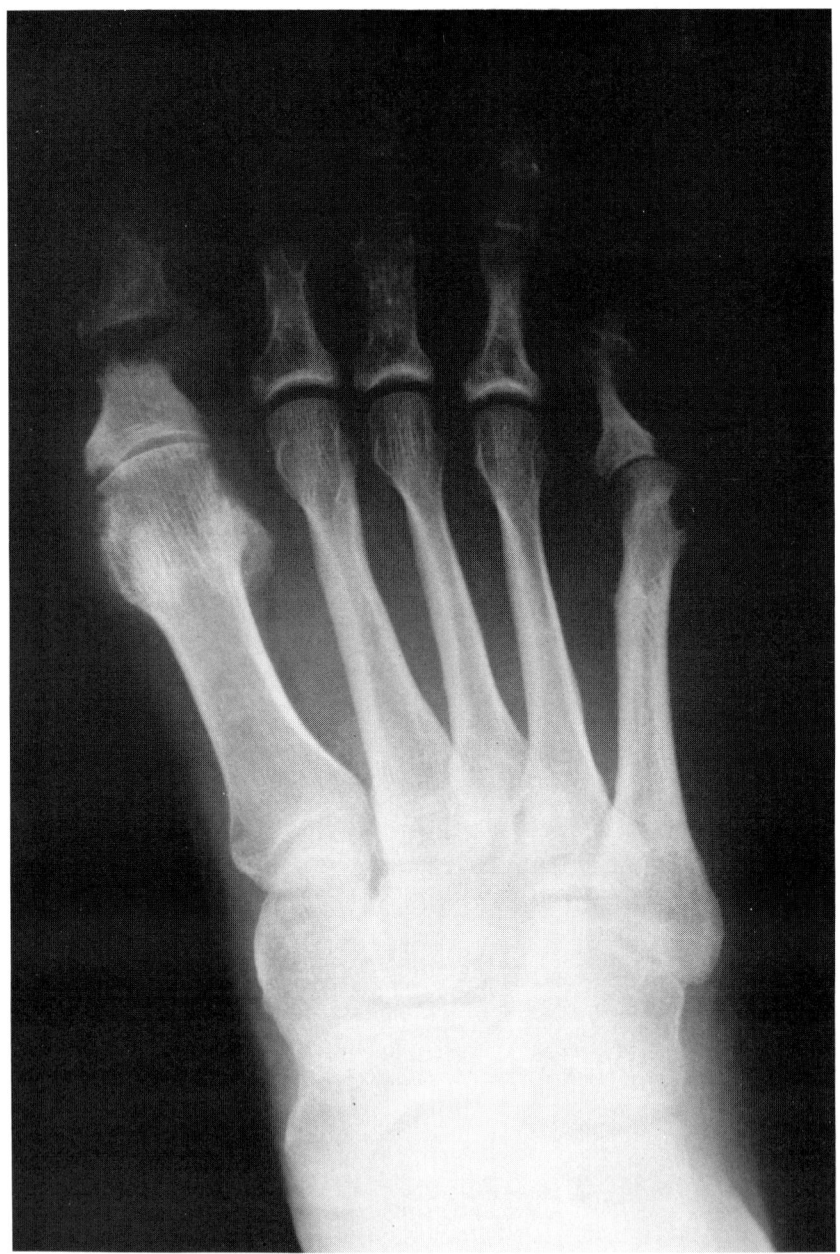

Figure 121

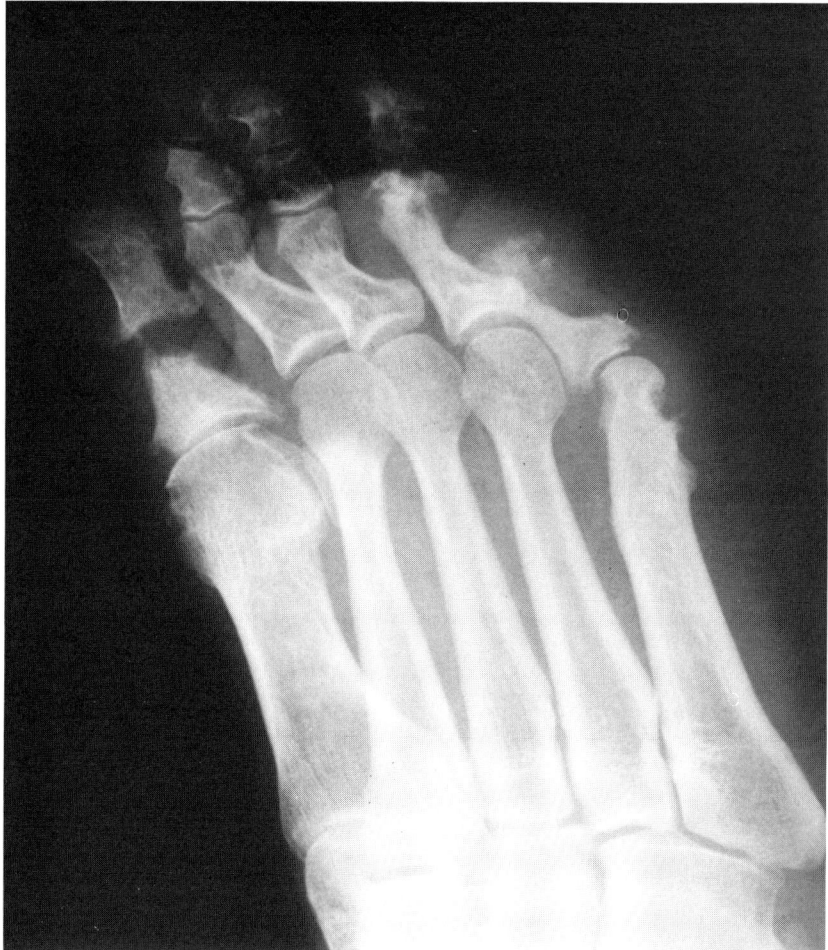

Figure 122

erosion and whittling of the bone. Again, this proved to be psoriatic illness.

Exercise 29

Barry has had recurrent attacks of acute arthritis for the last 5 years. He has recently noted nodule formation around his elbows and his big toes. Look at the radiograph of his foot (Fig. 123) and decide what he has.

There are cystic changes associated with destruction of cartilage at the first MTP joint. There is no subchondral sclerosis or osteophyte formation. This seems to be an inflammatory arthritis but in fact is tophaceous gout. The soft tissue calcification and overhanging lip typical of the radiographic changes of tophaceous gout are not seen in this case. Barry's serum uric acid level was elevated, and aspiration of the elbow nodule revealed urate crystals.

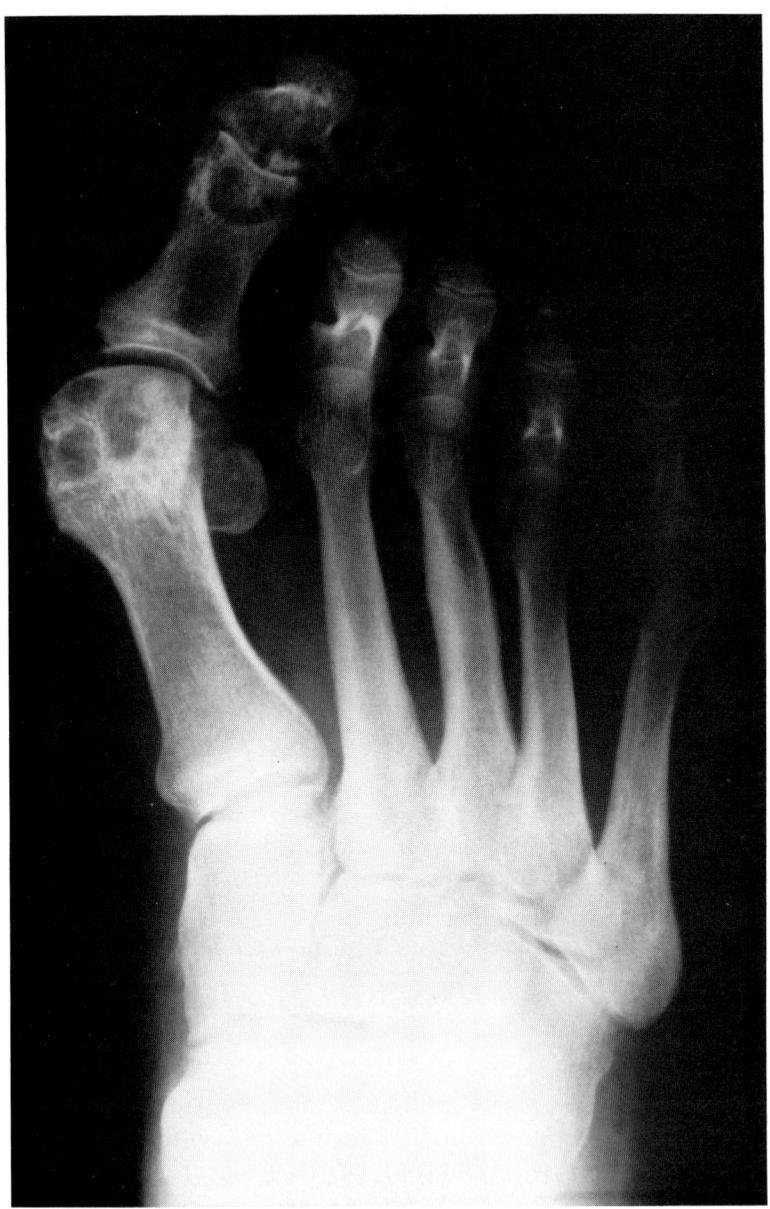

Figure 123

Exercise 30

Harvey, 26 years old, has just finished a 4 month bout of urethritis, conjunctivitis and knee and shoulder arthritis, which was treated with indomethacin. He now presents to you with heel pain. On examination you note tenderness under the calcaneus and around the Achilles tendon. Look at his radiograph (Fig. 124) and decide if the findings fit your diagnosis.

The constellation of symptoms Harvey noted suggests the Reiter's syndrome triad. Arthritis in Reiter's syndrome may be acute or chronic, and the joints tend to be affected asymmetrically. Reiter's syndrome may also involve the sacroiliac joints and spine in a pattern that is similar to other forms of spondylitis. Also involved are multiple entheses, or sites of tendon and ligamentous insertion, throughout the body. His persistent heel pain, in the Achilles tendon and the plantar fascia, is a common site for the enthesitis of Reiter's syndrome. His radiograph demonstrates reactive new bone formation on the posterosuperior margin of the os calcis at the point of attachment of the Achilles tendon and on the inferior surface at the plantar fascia insertion. These changes are typical for Reiter's syndrome. Restarting his indomethacin therapy made his symptoms abate.

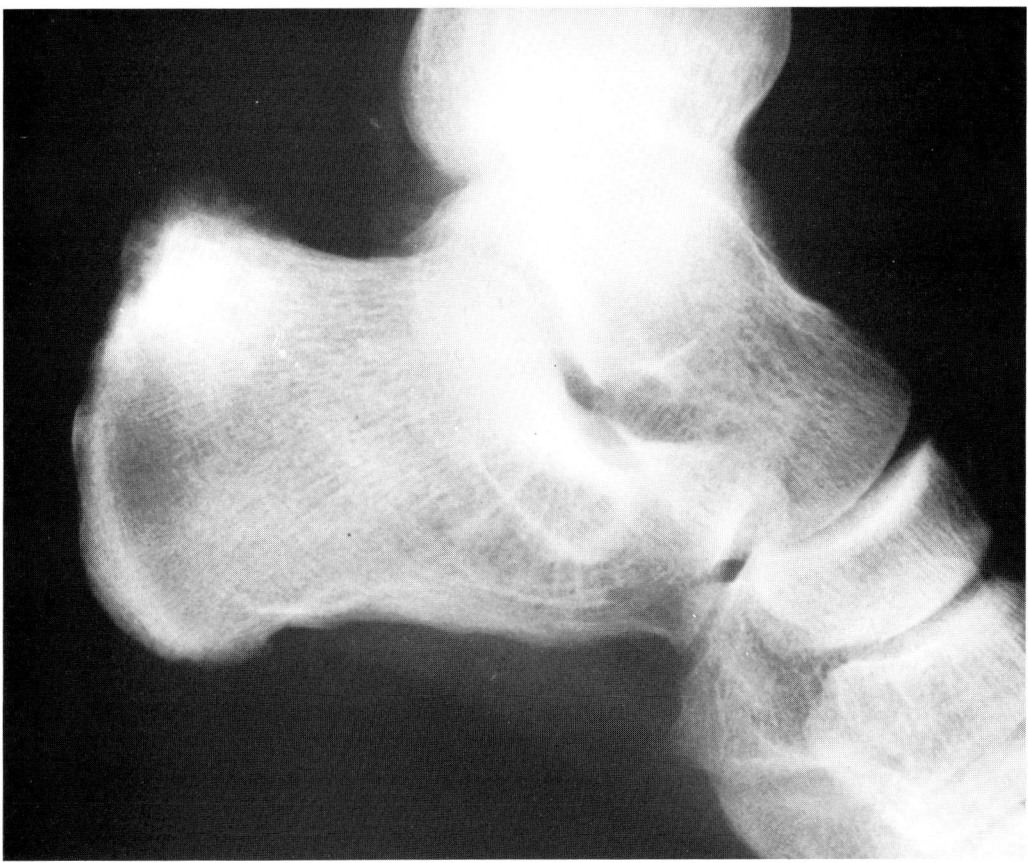

Figure 124

Exercise 31

Sally, 17 years old, has had hand and foot pain for 2 years. Her pediatrician has been giving her aspirin for presumed JCP, and this has allowed her to function reasonably well. Lately, however, she has noted an increase in her stiffness and more pain. Both her physician and her mother would like you to comment on how effective the aspirin has been. Look at her films (Figs. 125 and 126) and tell them.

The hand film (Fig. 125) shows soft tissue swelling around several PIP joints and osteopenia around the PIP and MCP joints and the wrist. Although the MCP joint surfaces appear all right, the second and fifth

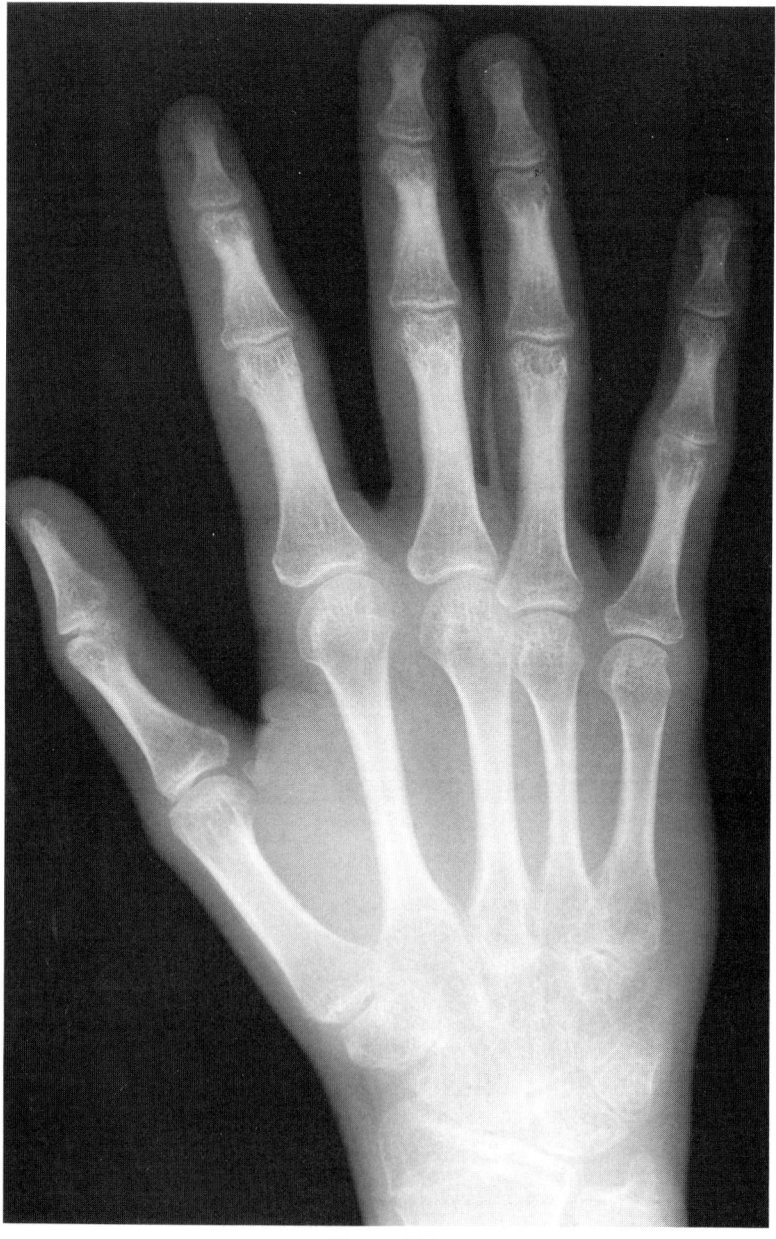

Figure 125

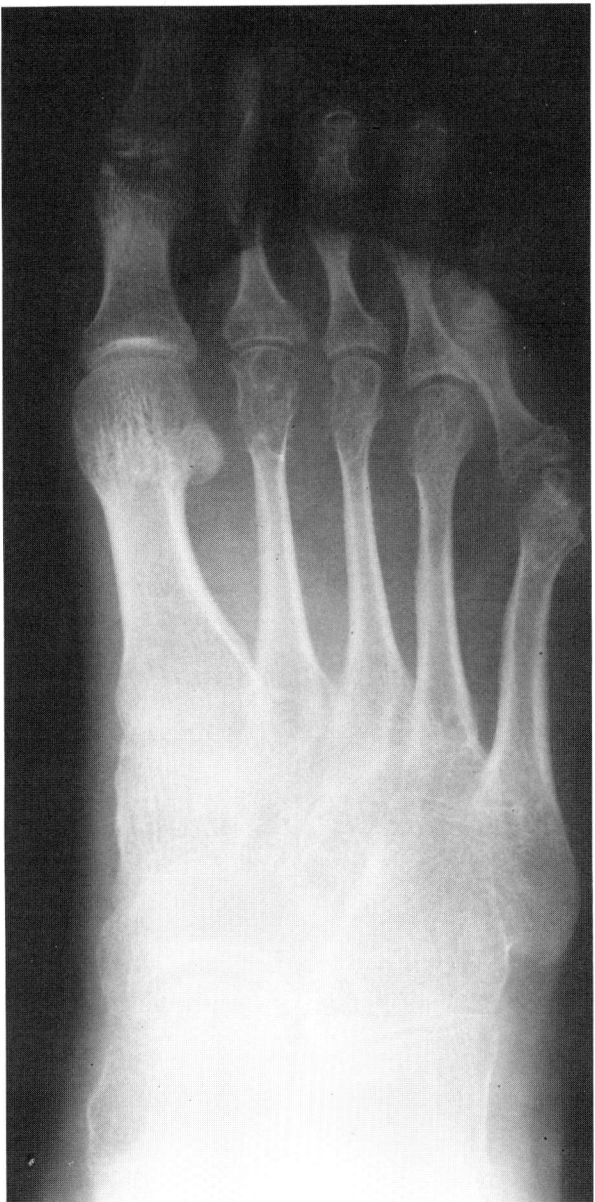

Figure 126

PIP joints are narrowed, as is the radiocarpal joint. Her feet reveal erosions at most of the MTP joints, especially the fifth (Fig. 126). Did you notice the erosions in the DIP joint of the great toe and the malalignment of the third and fifth toes? In view of the destructive nature of her arthropathy, you conclude that she has not responded well to the aspirin and recommend adding gold therapy.

Exercise 32

Geraldine, 43 years old, developed progressive pain and swelling in her foot following what seemed to be a minor trauma. Over the past month it has limited her ability to use the limb. You note that the foot is swollen, mottled and cool. You obtain a radiograph (Fig. 127). On the basis of these facts and the radiograph, what kind of treatment do you recommend?

Geraldine's radiograph shows osteoporosis and some subperiosteal bone resorption diffusely throughout the foot. In conjunction with her symptoms, this suggests a reflex sympathetic dystrophy. Other radiographic findings include a diffuse flush in the extremity on bone scan. Geraldine was helped by a lumbar sympathetic block, steroids and exercise.

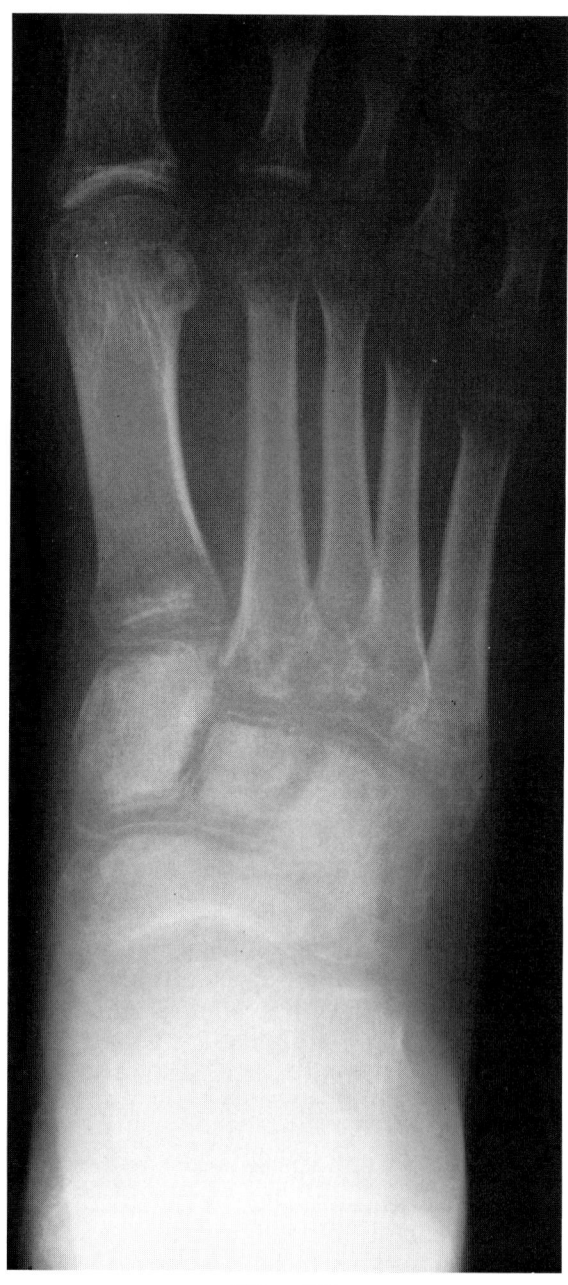

Figure 127

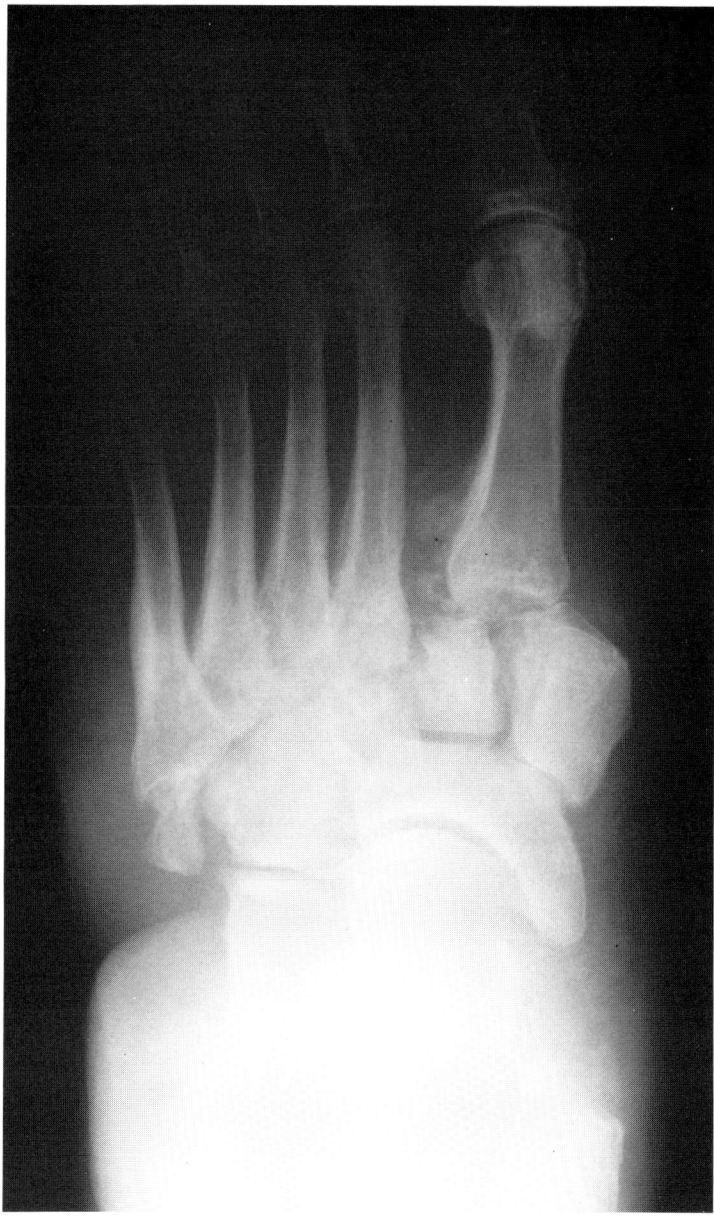

Figure 128

Exercise 33

Joan has had diabetes for 23 years. She comes to you with ankle pain of 2 months' duration. There is no history of trauma, but she has twisted her ankle several times lately while walking. On examination you notice decreased sensation to pinprick over her foot and a small pressure sore under her metatarsal bones. Her ankle is swollen with fluid and is somewhat hypermobile. Look at her radiographs (Figs. 128 and 129) and state your differential diagnosis.

AP and lateral radiographs of the foot demonstrate severe destruction and disruption of the normal relationship of the tarsal-metatarsal

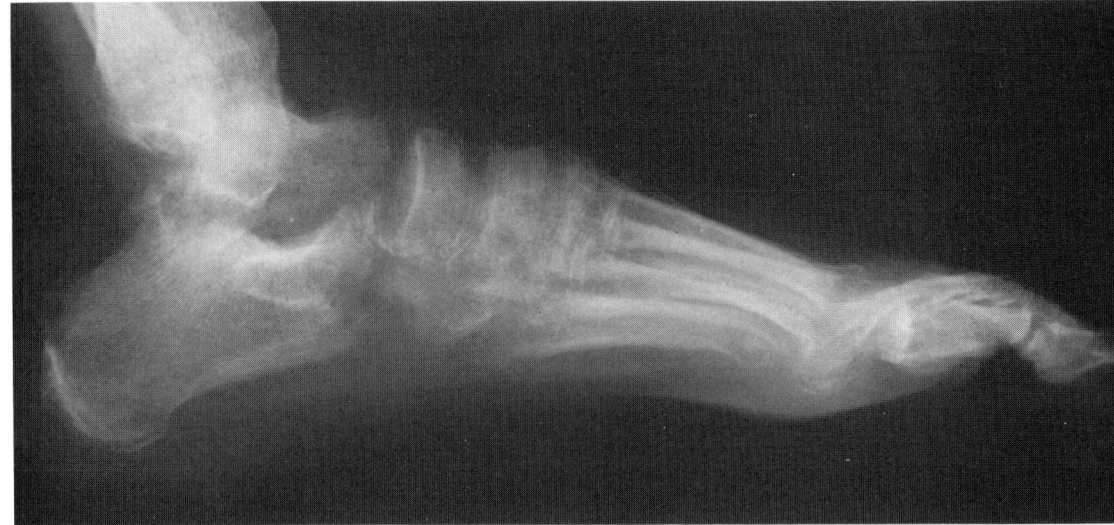

Figure 129

region. Soft tissue swelling and bony fragmentation are noted at the first tarsal-metatarsal joint and the proximal end of the fifth metatarsal bone. Note the absence of osteoporosis. This much destruction often represents a Charcot or neuropathic joint. Look at the lateral view of the foot in Figure 130, which shows the same changes. Compare this

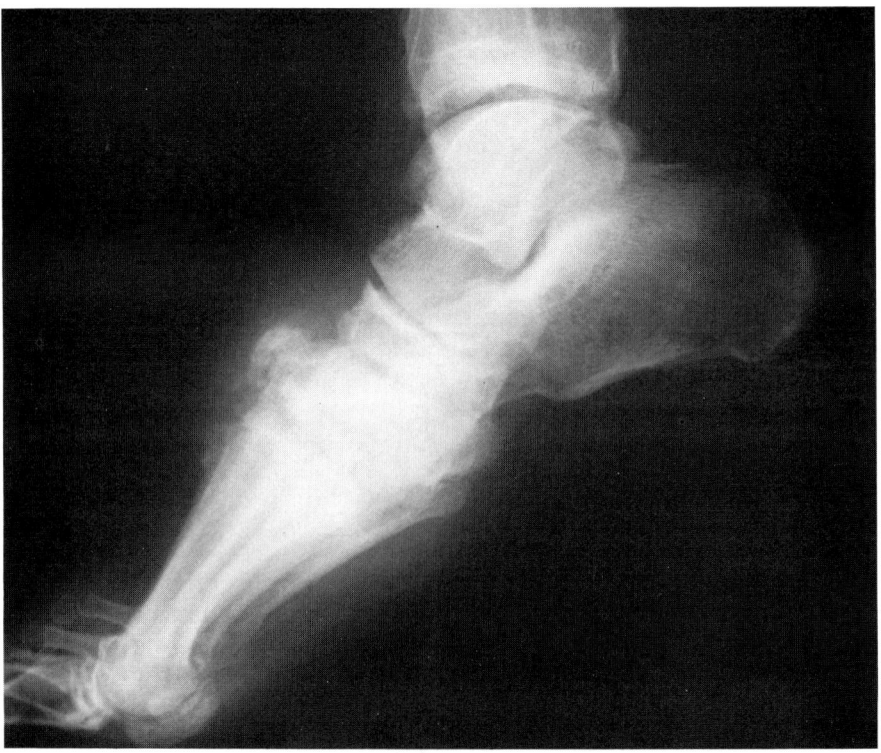

Figure 130

with the hip and knee radiographs shown in Exercise 22, p. 100. Again, Charcot joints occur in illnesses in which there is a loss of sensation, especially proprioception, and therefore there is increased trauma to the area. Pain may be a prominent feature despite the denervation, and it is generally associated with laxity of ligaments and effusion. Diabetic patients succumb to this in their lower extremities, especially around the ankle and foot. Tabes may cause Charcot changes in knees, hips or lumbosacral spine. Figures 131 and 132 show AP and lateral views of the knee with heterotopic new bone growth, exensive fragmentation and advanced degeneration consistent with Charcot joints in a patient with tabes. Syringomyelia may cause Charcot joints around the shoulder or elbow. Figure 133 is such an example. In the diabetic patient, be

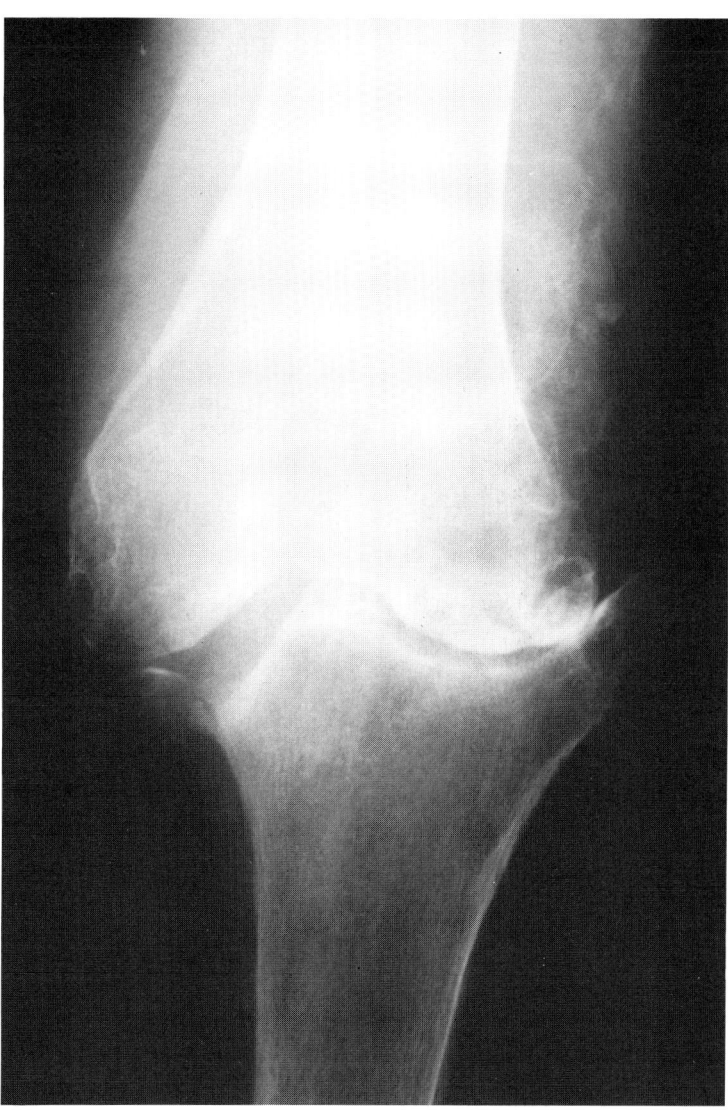

Figure 131

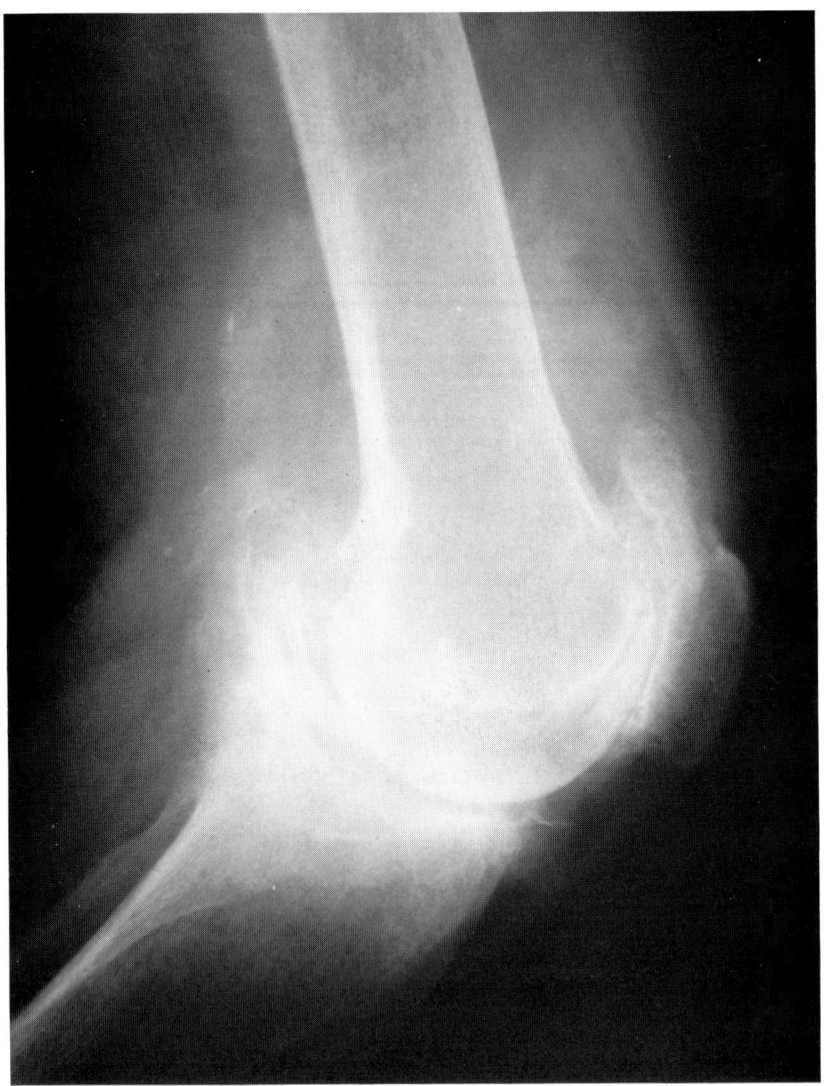

Figure 132

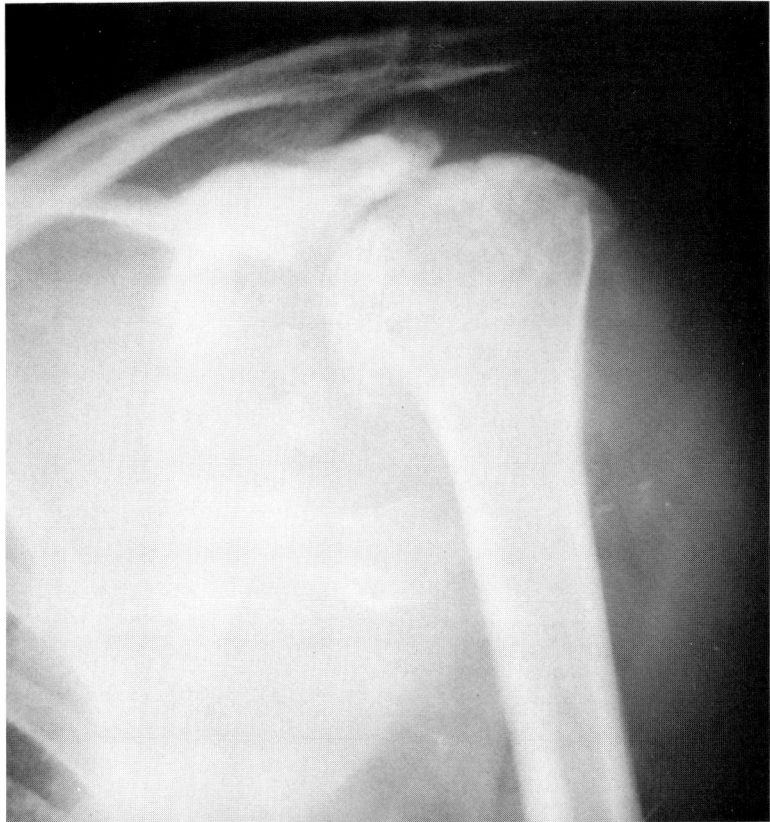

Figure 133

careful to rule out a septic joint or osteomyelitis, as the radiographic changes may be similar, and both are common in diabetes.

Exercise 34

Two heel radiographs are shown to you (Figs. 134 and 135). Decide what you think is abnormal about them and what the underlying disease process is.

Both have abnormalities at the point at which the plantar fascia inserts on the calcaneus. Figure 134 shows an erosion, whereas Figure 135 shows some calcification. Both represent an enthesitis, or inflammation at tendinous or ligamentous insertions. Such inflammation may cause erosive damage, or upon healing may undergo ossification, sometimes called "lover's heel." Although seen in all inflammatory arthritides, they are most common in the HLA-B27-related illnesses, especially Reiter's syndrome. Look at the pelvis film (Fig. 136) of the patient shown in Figure 134. This radiograph demonstrates asymmetric narrowing of the sacroiliac joints with an irregular contour to the joints, especially on the left. This patient has Reiter's syndrome. Calcification of the plantar fascia may also occur in noninflammatory conditions, such as aging, or in the DISH syndrome (see Exercise 45). In fact, the patient depicted in Figure 135 is an elderly woman who presented with calcaneal bursitis.

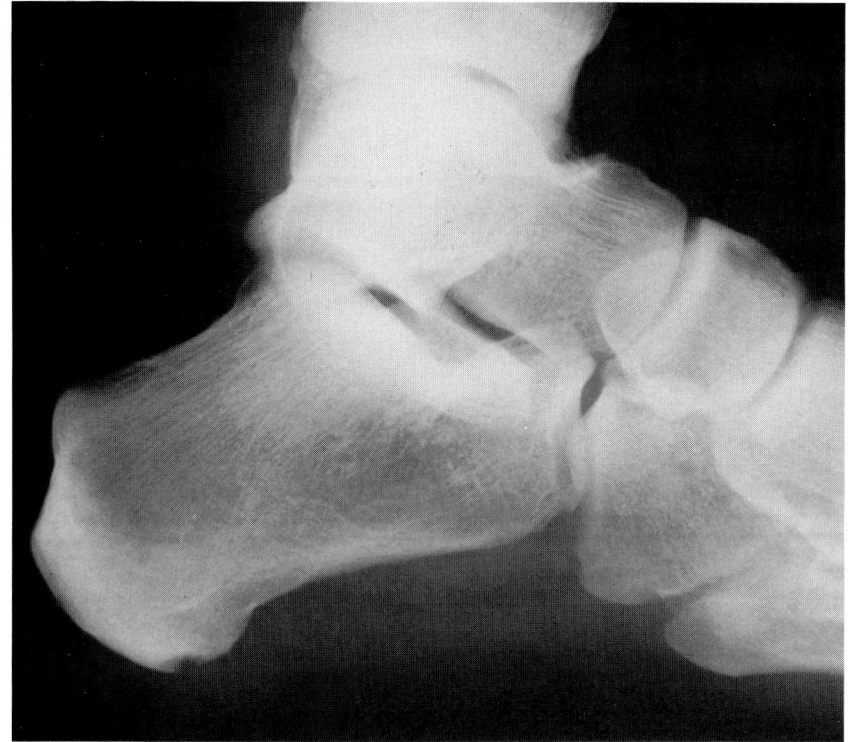

Figure 134

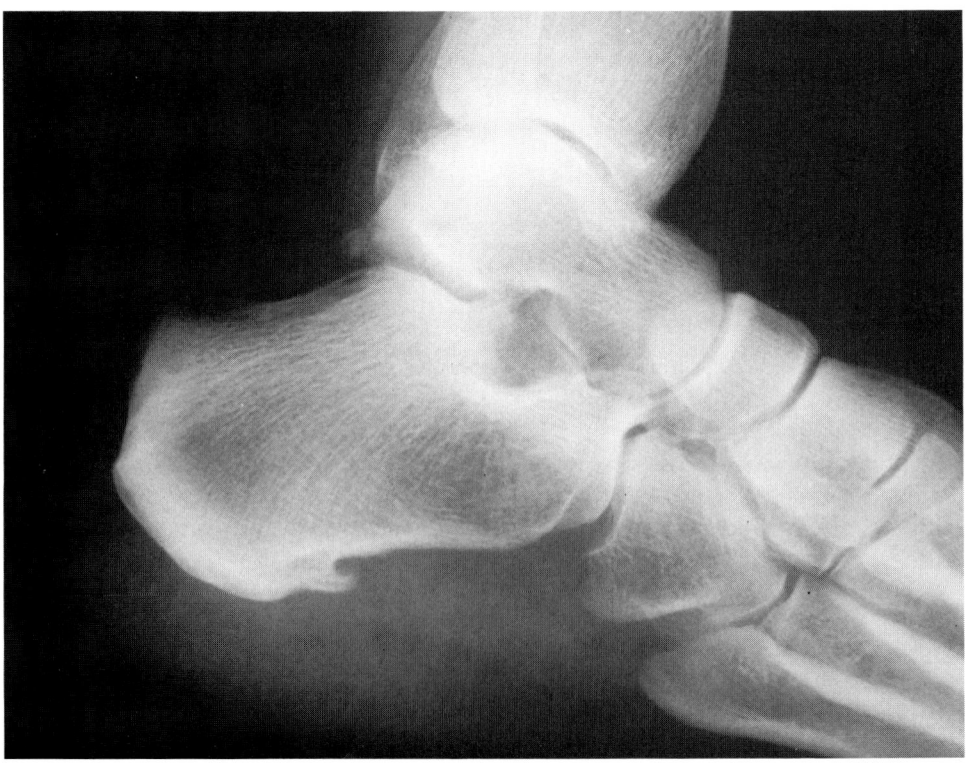

Figure 135

SECTION II—EXERCISES

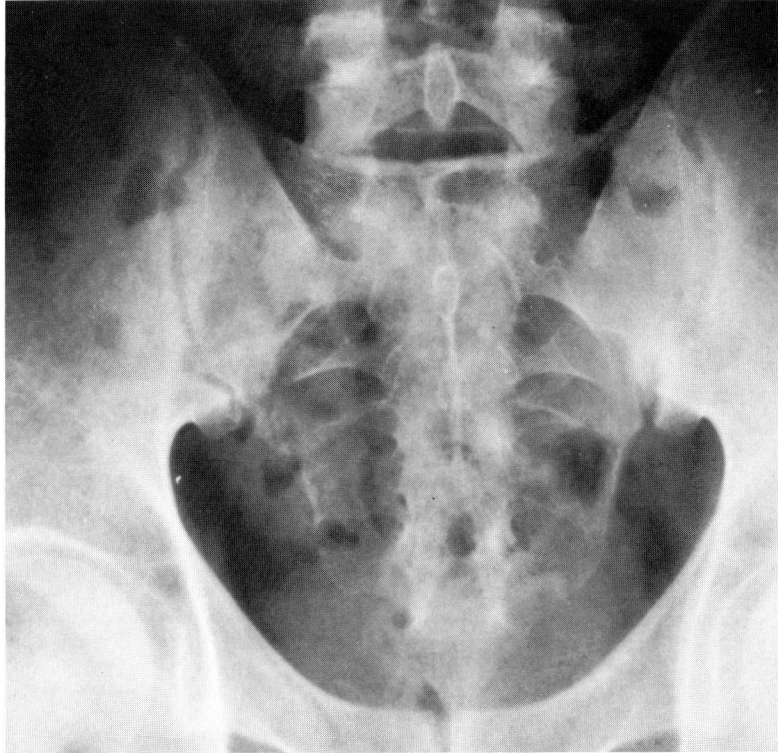

Figure 136

Shoulder

Exercise 35

Sally developed pneumonia and you hospitalized her immediately. One day after admission her right shoulder becomes painful and swells up. Aspiration reveals cloudy fluid with the viscosity of water. Analysis of the fluid reveals 85,000 white blood cells with 90 per cent granulocytes, no crystals and a negative Gram stain. Look at her radiograph (Fig. 137) and decide what you think she has.

Sally's first radiograph is normal. However, this should not deter you from diagnosing a septic arthritis. Radiographic changes lag 7 to 14 days or more in pyogenic arthritis and even more in nonpyogenic infections. *Streptococcus pneumoniae* was cultured from her joint fluid 2 days later, and she responded well to therapy with penicillin. Look at the radiograph 3 weeks later (Fig. 138), which demonstrates an erosion on the superior aspect of the greater tuberosity (arrow).

Exercise 36

Nancy is a 66 year old woman with bilateral shoulder pain. She also notes pain in her wrists, knees, ankles and the small joints of the hands. Her illness has been present now for 3 years but is getting worse. Her only therapy has been aspirin. You note synovial proliferation at her wrists and fingers, with effusion in her knees. Her shoulder radiograph is shown (Fig. 139). Do you think age plays a role in this illness?

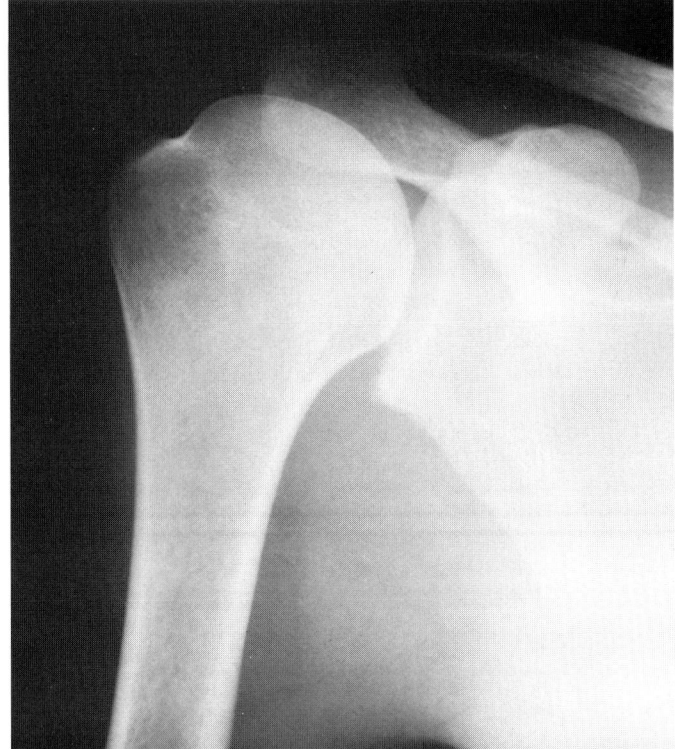

Figure 137

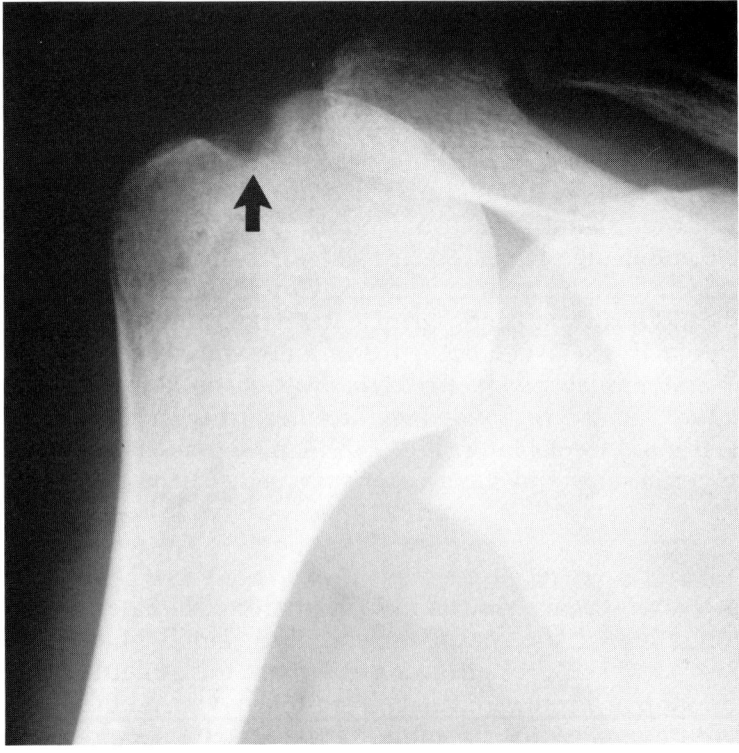

Figure 138

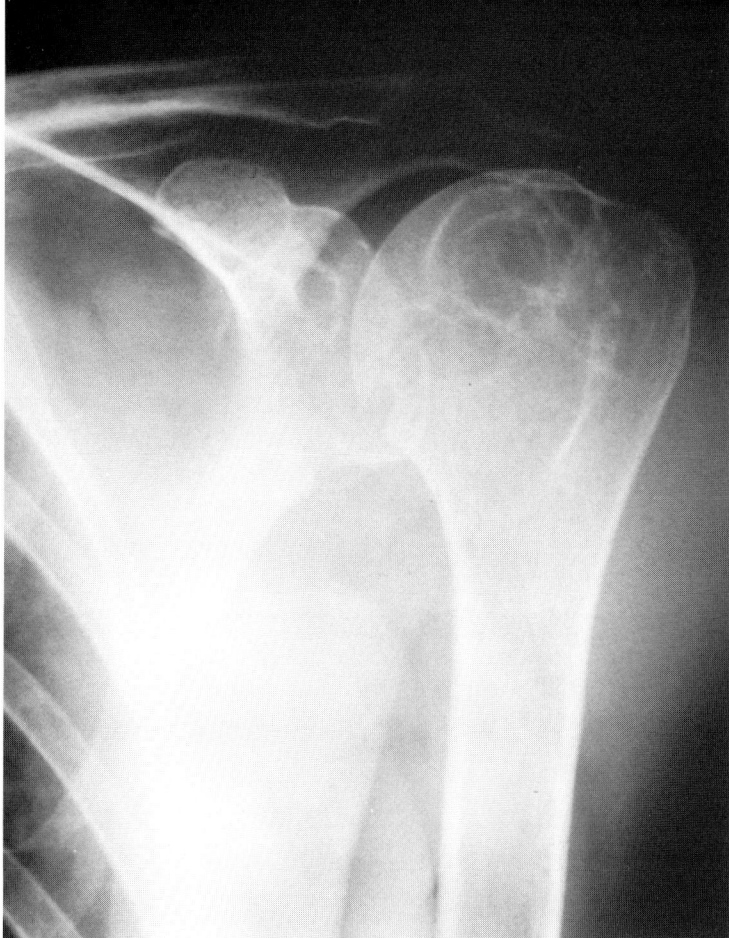

Figure 139

Nancy's radiograph shows uniform narrowing of the glenohumeral joint, periarticular osteopenia and multiple erosions of the humeral head and the glenoid fossa. There is a lack of osteophytes and reactive subchondral sclerosis. These changes are characteristic of an inflammatory arthritis. Does it surprise you to learn that her rheumatoid factor is positive? Nancy has RA. This illness can occur at any age.

Exercise 37

Norman, 56 years old, recently developed pain in his right shoulder, especially when lying on his right side at night or on abducting his arm. On examination he has limited range of motion of his shoulder and tenderness to palpation over the subdeltoid area. Look at his radiograph (Fig. 140) and decide on a course of therapy.

Norman's radiograph shows a deposit of amorphous calcium adjacent to his humeral head in the area of clinical tenderness. He has a calcific bursitis caused by a deposit of CHO. A local injection of cortisone into the area around his subdeltoid bursa soon relieved his symptoms.

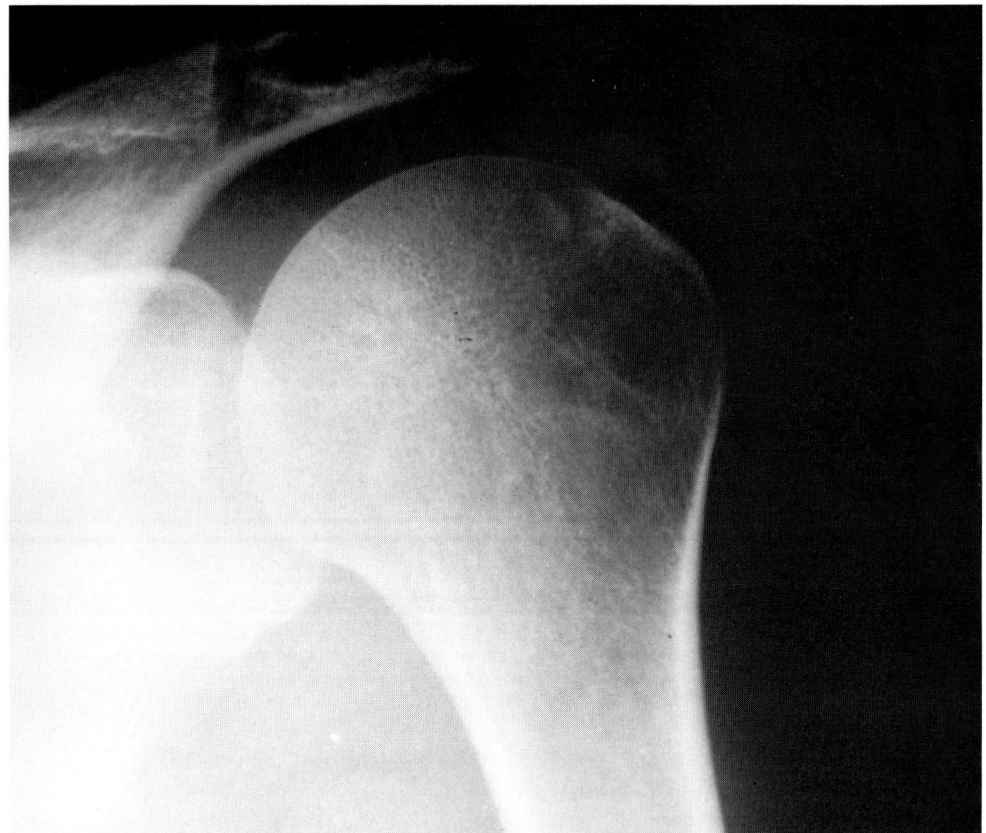

Figure 140

Exercise 38

Todd has chronic active hepatitis and has been on prednisone therapy for the last 18 months. For the last 10 months he has noted pain in his left shoulder. You note that he can abduct his arm 90 degrees but that internal and external rotation are limited and painful. Look at his shoulder radiograph (Fig. 141) and suggest a diagnosis.

Todd's radiograph shows sclerosis of the humeral head with a pseudofracture line similar to that seen in Figure 85. He also has partial collapse of the humeral head with some secondary degenerative changes. He has developed avascular necrosis of the humeral head secondary to his steroid use. Because of severe pain he underwent a total shoulder replacement (shown in Fig. 142) with complete relief of symptoms and good return of function.

Exercise 39

Sam, 54 years old, slipped on a grease spot at the warehouse and caught himself on his outstretched arm. He has since lost the ability to lift his arm over his head. A radiograph taken at a local hospital (Fig. 143) is read as normal. He comes to see you 3 months later. On examination, he is unable to abduct his shoulder more than 60 degrees,

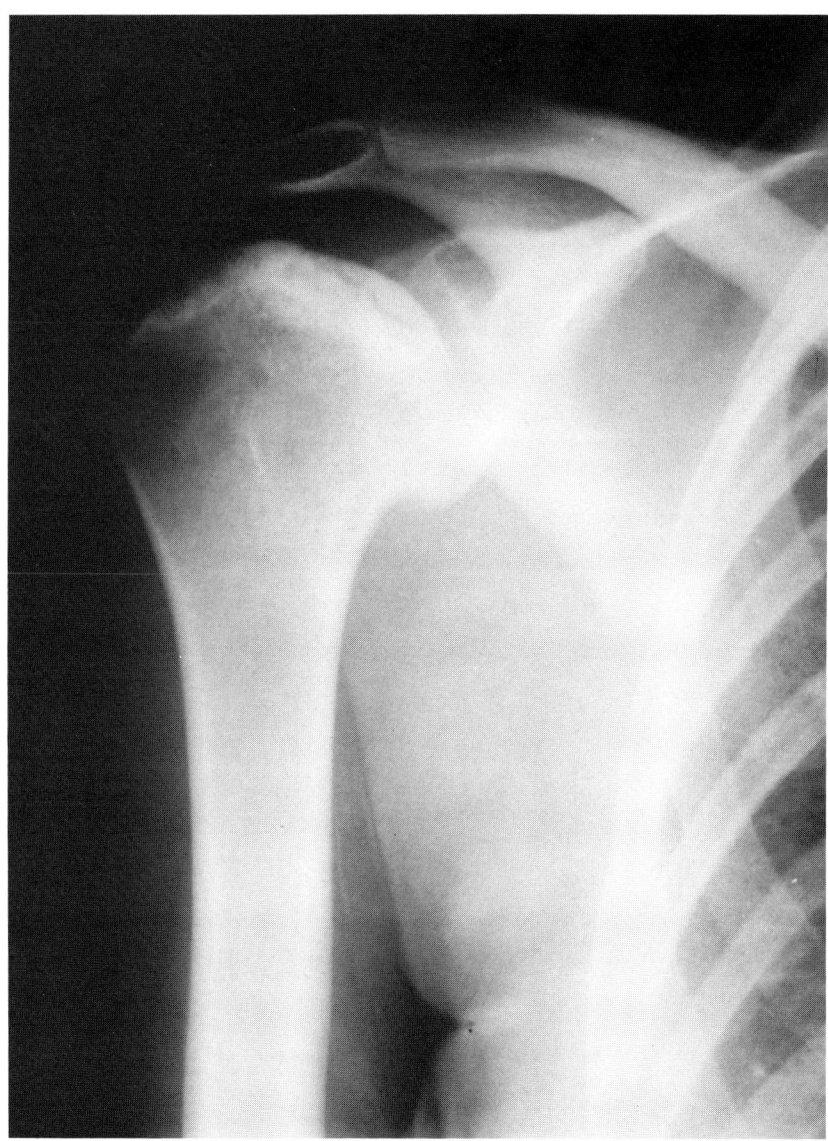

Figure 141

136 SECTION II—EXERCISES

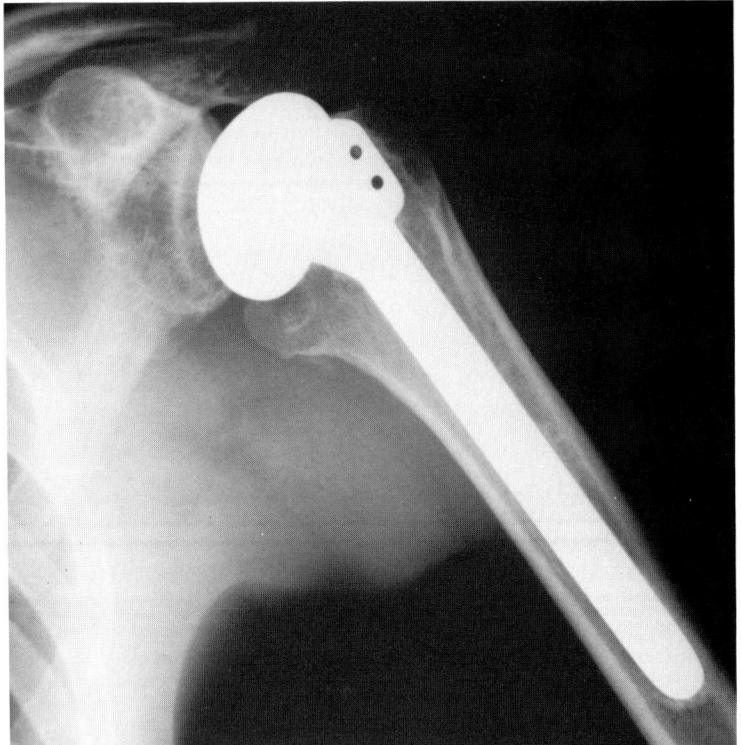

Figure 142

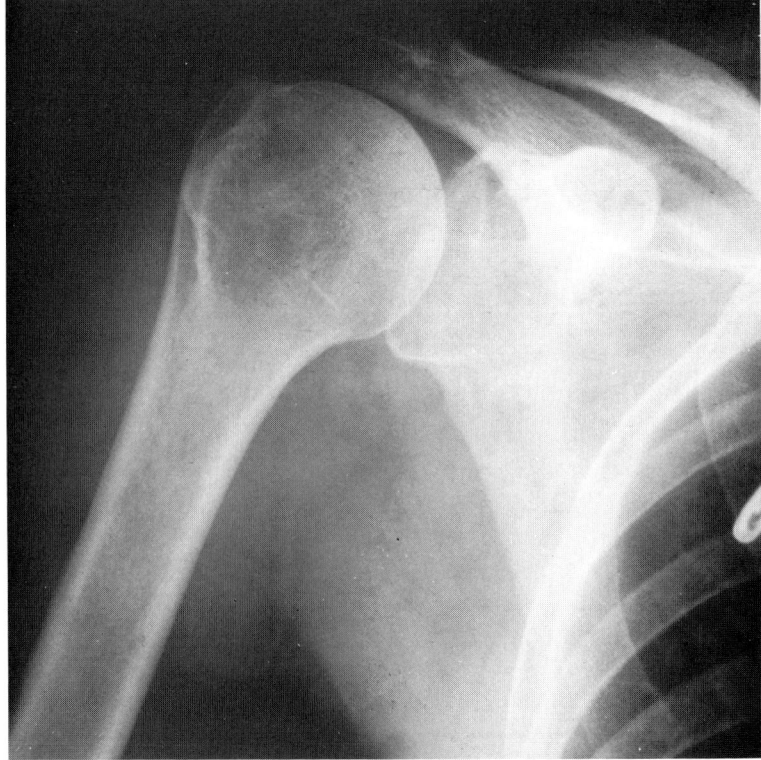

Figure 143

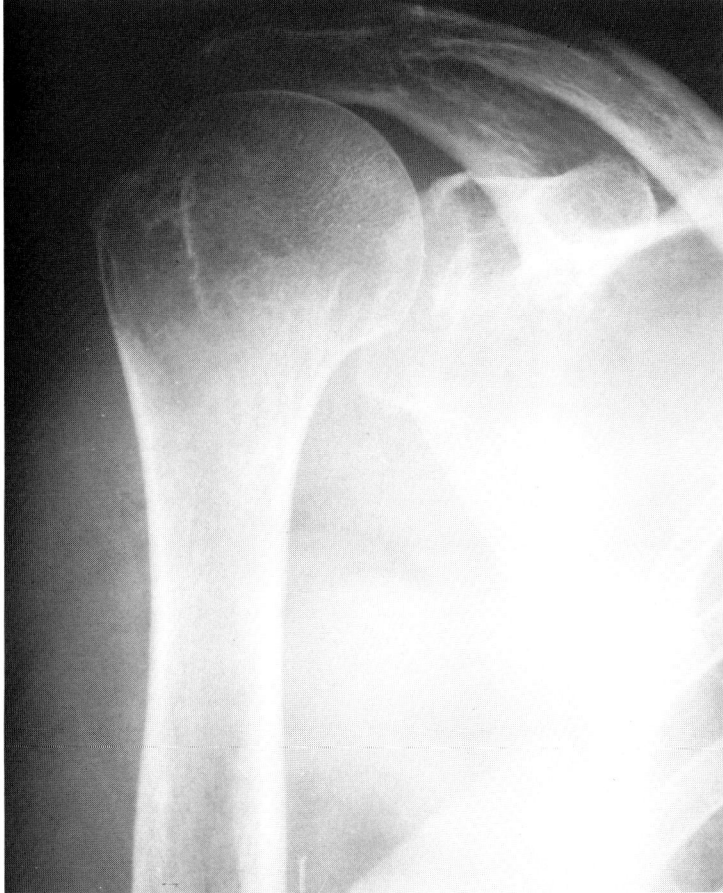

Figure 144

and rotation, both internal and external, is painful. You repeat the shoulder film (Fig. 144). Review his radiograph and suggest a further diagnostic procedure.

Sam's second radiograph shows slight superior migration of the humeral head in the glenoid fossa when compared with his first radiograph. A more extreme example is shown in Figure 145, in which the humeral head has impinged on the inferior aspect of the acromial process, producing a concave deformity. These changes are highly suggestive of a rotator cuff tear. The muscles may tear after acute trauma or chronic rotator cuff inflammation and strain or by destruction from some inflammatory arthritis, such as RA, in the shoulder. An arthrogram will reveal the tear. A normal arthrogram is shown in Figure 146. Note how the axillary pouch, the subcoracoid region and the sheath of the long head of the biceps are outlined by the injection of contrast medium into the shoulder joint. Compare this with Sam's arthrogram in Figure 147. Note in Figure 147 that contrast medium is present between the humeral head and the acromial process (arrows), with filling of the subacromial bursa, indicating a tear in the cuff with leakage of the contrast medium out of the confines of the normal shoulder capsule. It may be necessary to manipulate the joint to dem-

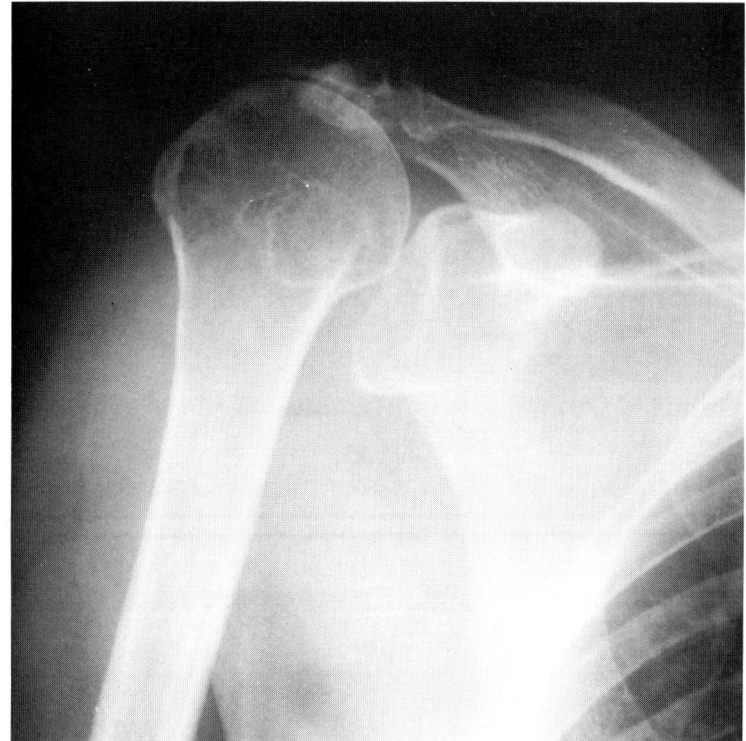

Figure 145

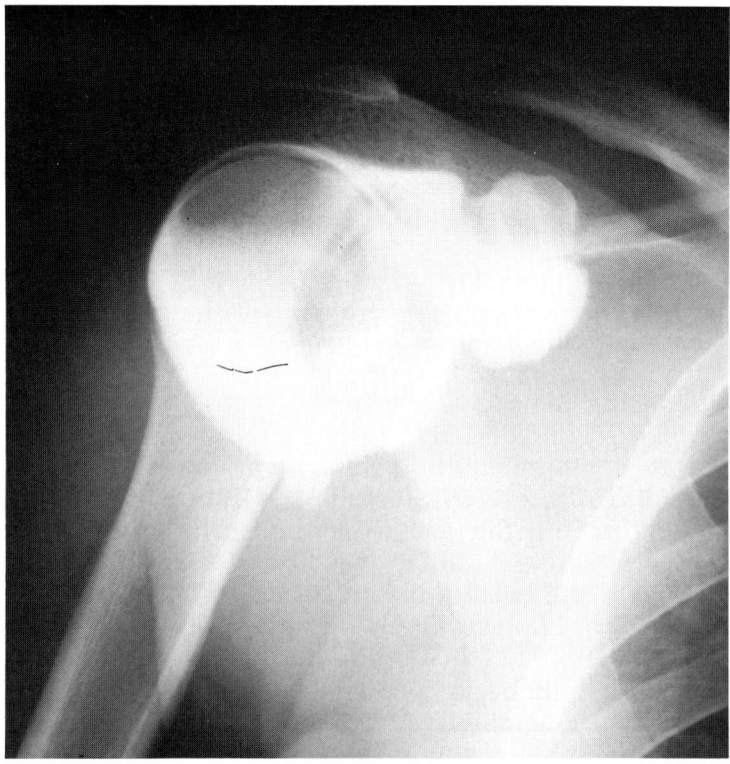

Figure 146

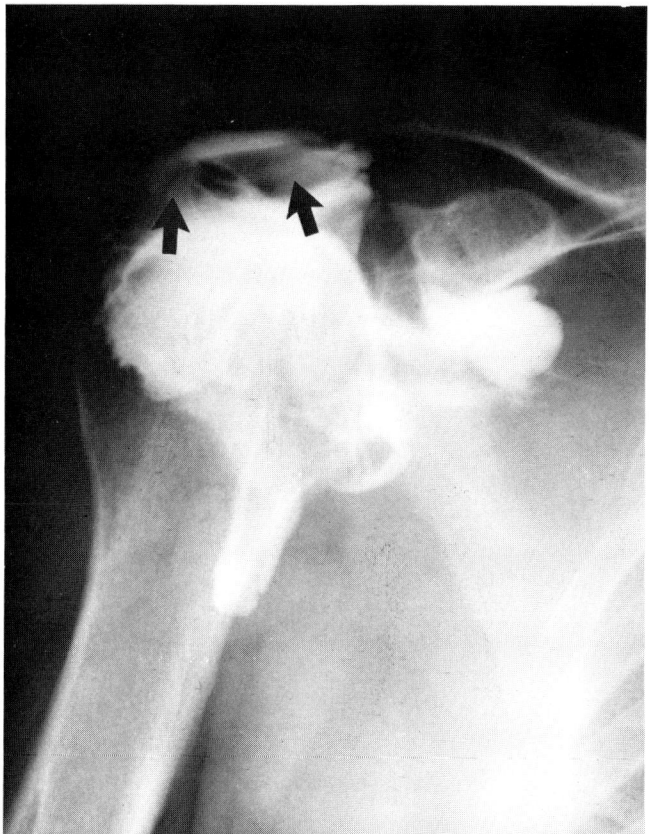

Figure 147

onstrate the leakage in some cases. Sam's torn rotator cuff was surgically repaired with good results.

Exercise 40

Robert was in a car accident 1 year ago. Since that time he has noted the gradual loss of motion in his right shoulder and pain on using it. His examination is identical to Sam's, except that his shoulder has limited range of motion and pain, both when he tries to move it and when you move it. The initial radiograph taken at the time of the accident was normal. Look at it now (Fig. 148) and suggest a further diagnostic procedure.

Robert's story sounds similar to Sam's of Figure 143. Robert's radiograph is still normal, but despite this an arthrogram was done to rule out a rotator cuff rupture. Robert's arthrogram (Fig. 149) reveals a small joint that leaks no contrast medium. In fact it will barely allow contrast medium to be ejected, taking only 8 ml instead of the normal 20 ml. Robert has an adhesive capsulitis, or frozen shoulder. Often seen after soft tissue trauma, in diabetic patients or idiopathically, the soft tissues of the shoulder capsule form scar tissue and contract, leaving a painful and immobile shoulder. Most seem to regain mobility with time, and range of motion exercises, physical modalities and local cortisone injections may hasten the recovery.

SECTION II—EXERCISES

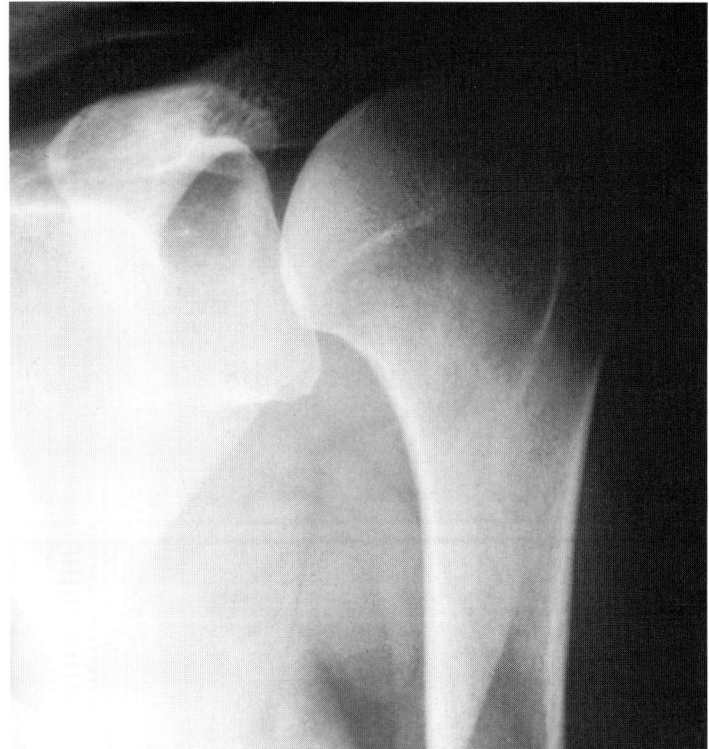

Figure 148

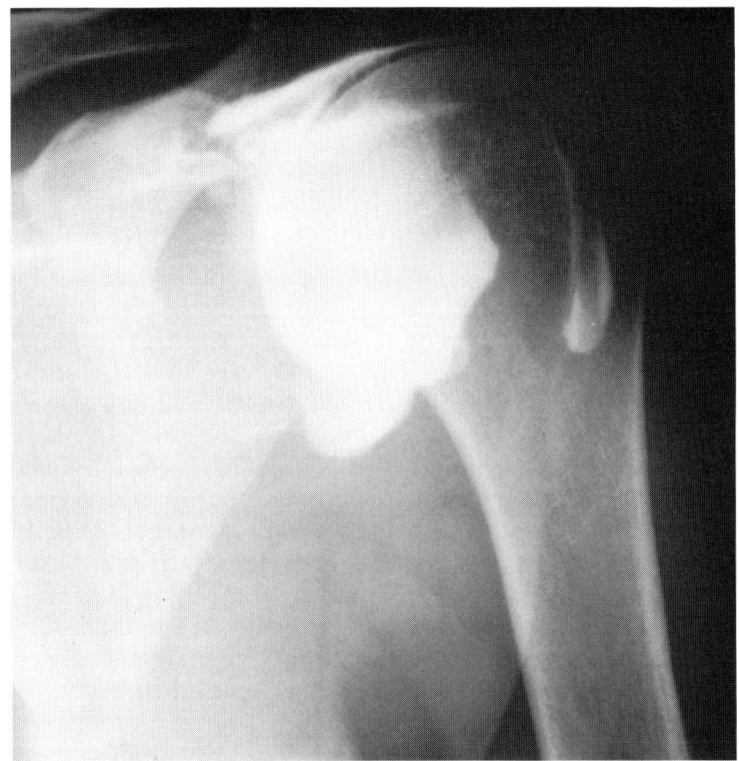

Figure 149

SECTION II—EXERCISES

Exercise 41

Henry is a tennis player. His favorite shot is an overhand slam. He injured his shoulder 2 years ago after such a shot, was told it was bursitis and responded to physical therapy and a cortisone injection. For the last 4 months he has noted persistent pain. On examination you are able to localize the area of tenderness to the acromioclavicular joint or biceps area. He has difficulty with abduction. His radiograph is shown here (Fig. 150). What do you think he injured before, what is hurting him now and what will you do about it?

Henry has narrowing and osteophyte formation in his acromioclavicular joint. There is no evidence of soft tissue calcification. He has degenerative arthritis of his acromioclavicular joint, which is the cause of his shoulder pain. The joint has a small meniscus in it that can be ruptured, leading later to degenerative changes. Henry's first episode of shoulder pain after a hard overhand smash was probably the tearing of the meniscus. His more chronic pain now is the result of the secondary degeneration. If nonspecific therapy does not help, a local injection of cortisone may be of benefit. If pain is persistent, resection of the clavicular end can be done.

Exercise 42

You are called on at a radiology conference to discuss the film shown in Figure 151. What do you say to the waiting group?

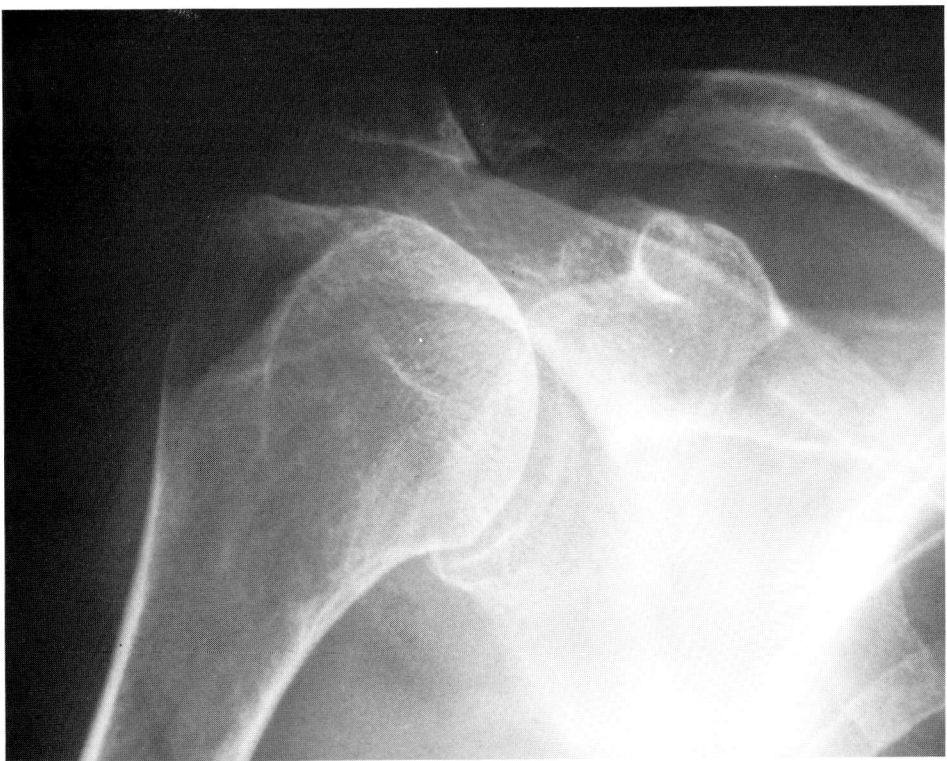

Figure 150

There is deformity and uniform narrowing of the glenohumeral joint without sclerosis or osteophytes. There is no collapse of the head of the humerus. There is no cartilage calcification (chondrocalcinosis). This suggests an inflammatory condition, in this case RA. Look also at the acromioclavicular joint, which demonstrates whittling without osteophytes. This is also typical of RA. If this is what you said, congratulations!

Spine

Exercise 43

Don, a gymnast, noted severe pain in his lower back radiating down the back of his right leg into his calf upon completion of his last triple back flip. Unable to straighten up, he hobbles into your office and you note a positive straight leg test result and absent Achilles tendon reflex on the right side. His spine radiograph is shown in Figure 152. Is this

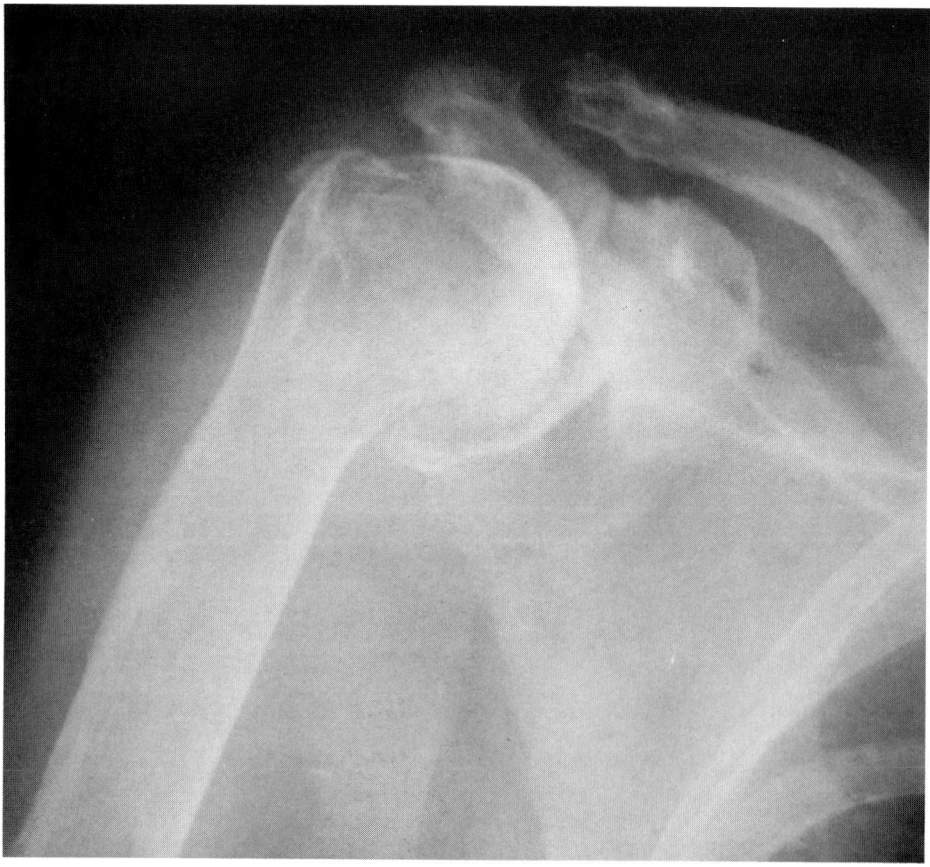

Figure 151

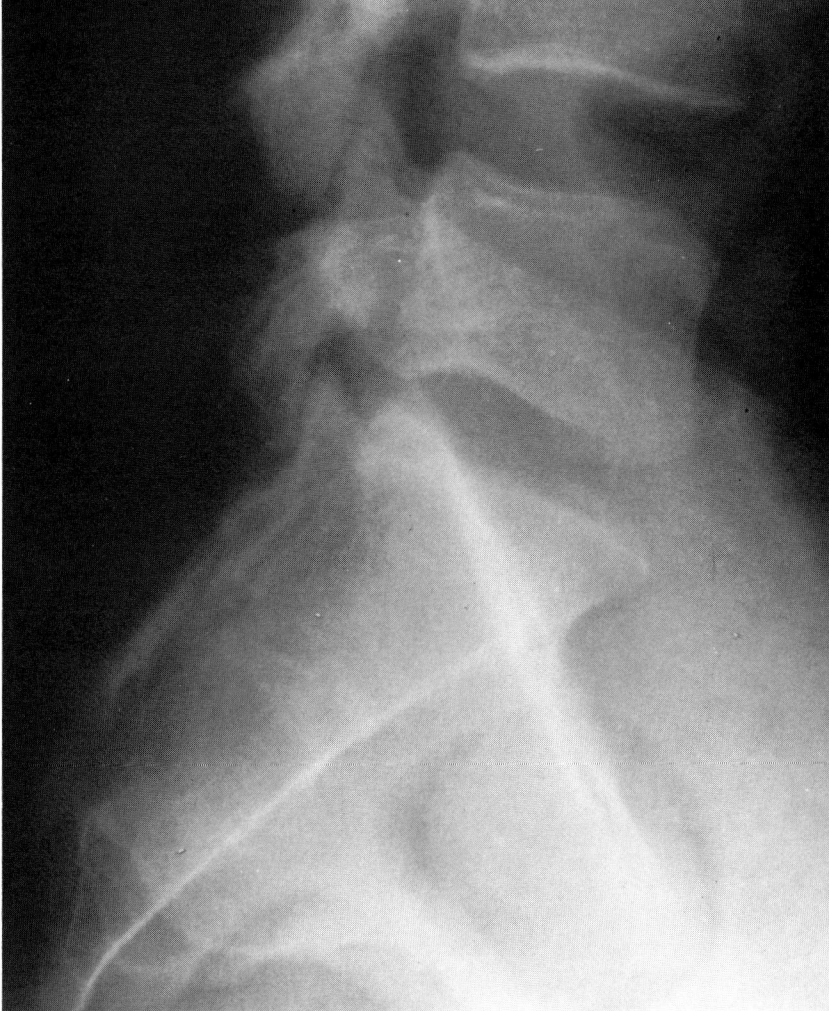

Figure 152

sufficient to confirm your clinical impression or do you require additional radiographic studies?

Don's spine radiograph is perfectly normal despite what sounds like a classic herniated disc. This is not unusual. If you expected to see disc space narrowing or osteophytes, you should remember that such changes represent chronic disc degeneration and not acute herniations. If you want to see Don's abnormal disc, you must image it in a different way. Figures 153 and 154 are CAT scans of the L4/L5 and L5/S1 disc spaces in this case. Note the herniated disc material filling the lateral foramina (arrow) in Figure 153 as compared with the normal space (arrow) in Figure 154. A myelogram, another way to image this, would likely have shown a filling defect in the nerve root sleeve in that area. An injection with chymopapain into the herniated disc completely relieved his symptoms.

144 SECTION II—EXERCISES

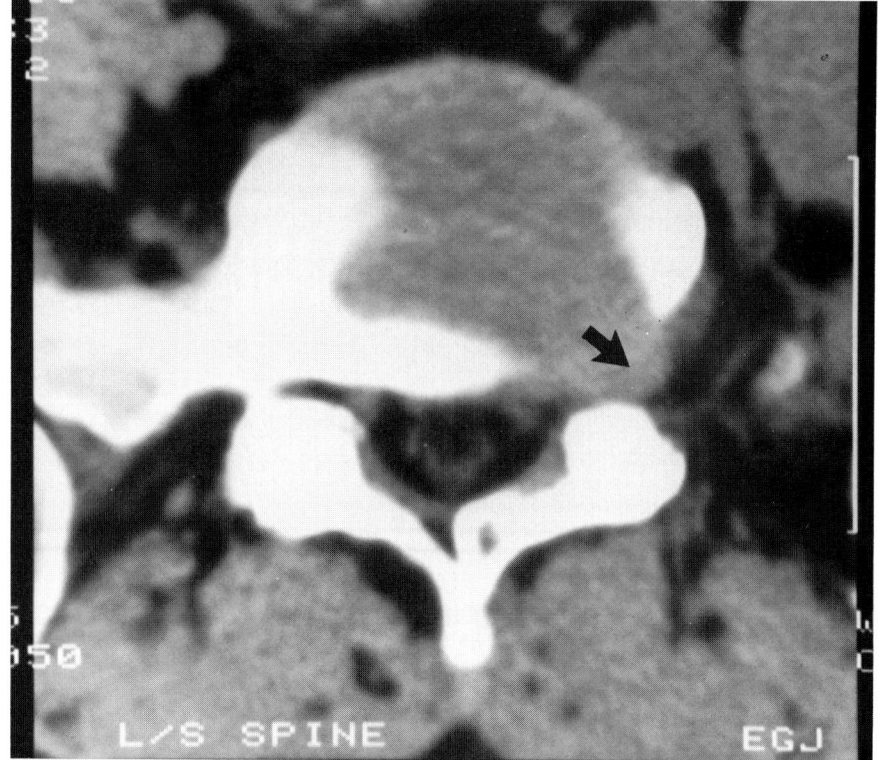

Figure 153

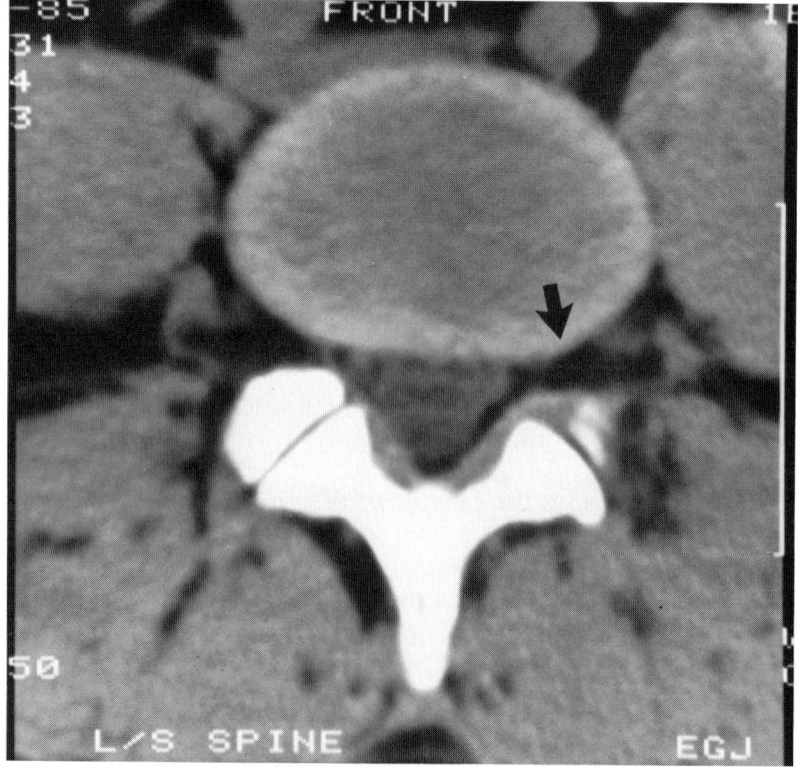

Figure 154

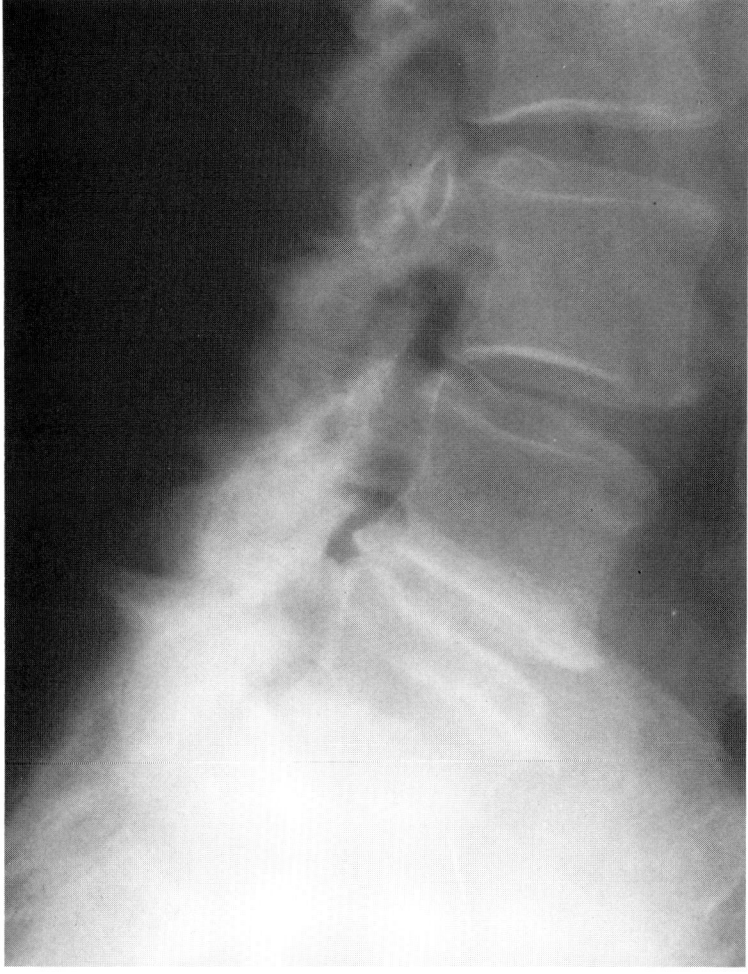

Figure 155

Exercise 44

Charles, 65 years old, has bilateral buttock and posterior thigh pain whenever he walks two blocks. In addition, the symptoms increase while going down stairs. Both pulses and reflexes in his lower extremities are normal, and the straight leg test results are negative. Look at his lateral spine radiograph (Fig. 155) and decide on your next diagnostic test.

Charles has a narrowed L4/L5 disc, with both anterior and posterior osteophytes present on his lateral spine films. His symptoms are those of spinal stenosis causing a neurogenic pseudoclaudication syndrome. The symptoms are due to encroachment of the lumbar spinal canal by some combination of herniated disc, osteophytes extending off the vertebral body or the apophyseal joints and hypertrophy of the ligamentum flavum. Spondylolisthesis, or slippage of one vertebra on another, may also narrow the canal, and may be seen in degenerative arthritis. Symptoms may mimic vascular claudication. Often, reflexes are normal

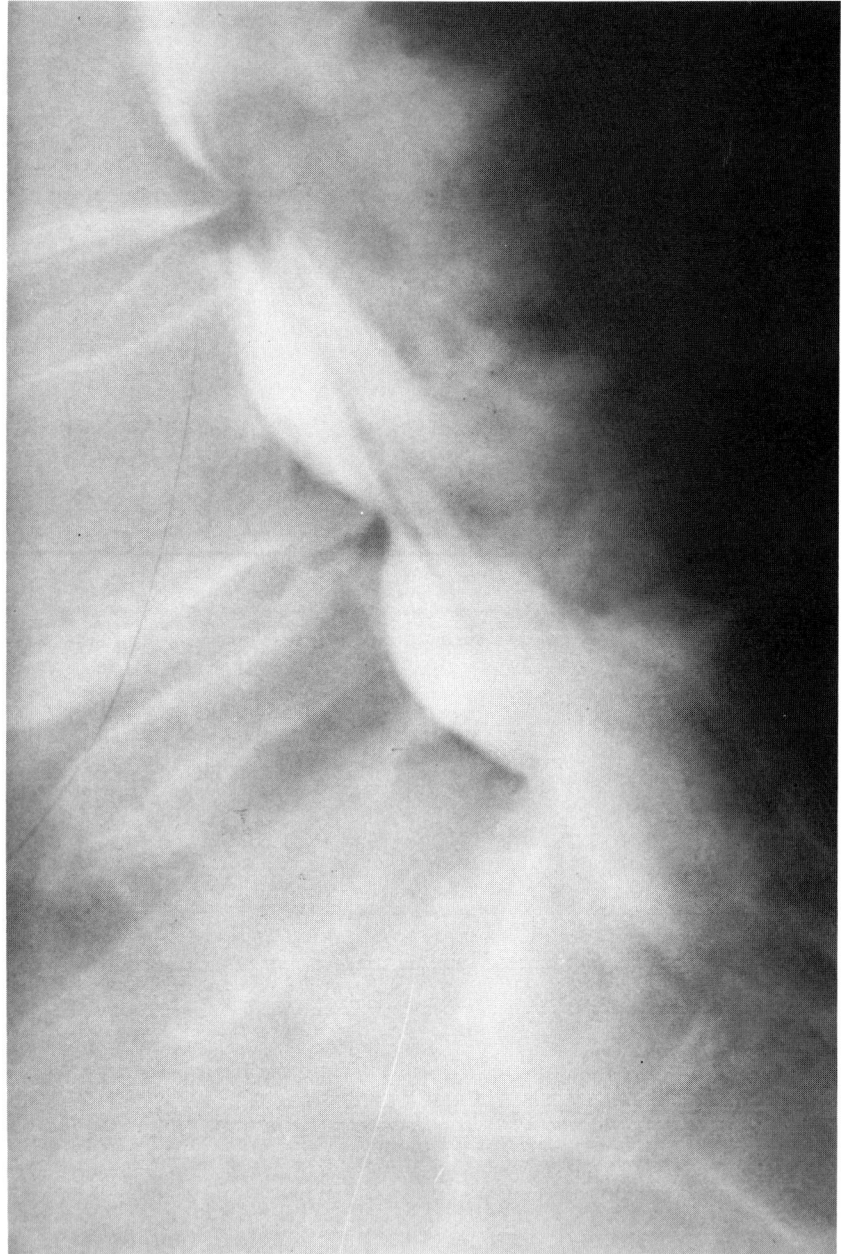

Figure 156

and straight leg testing results are negative. Look at his myelogram in Figure 156. It shows an incomplete block at the L4/L5 level, just around that posterior osteophyte. Surgery to decompress that area and remove the osteophyte gave him excellent relief.

Exercise 45

Jeremy, 73 years old, has noted stiffening of his lumbar and cervical spine over the last 4 years. The last time he had a chest radiograph, his doctor told him he had "severe arthritis of his spine." Look at his radiographs (Figs. 157 and 158) and decide the cause of his symptoms.

Jeremy has DISH syndrome or Forestier's disease, a hyperostosis of ligamentous attachments at the spine leading to flowing and bridging

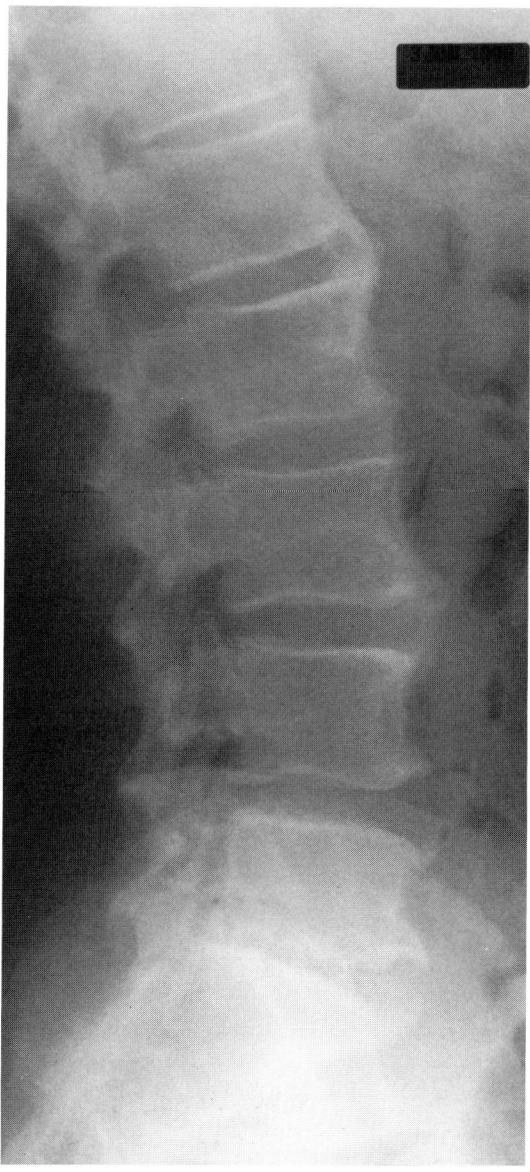

Figure 157

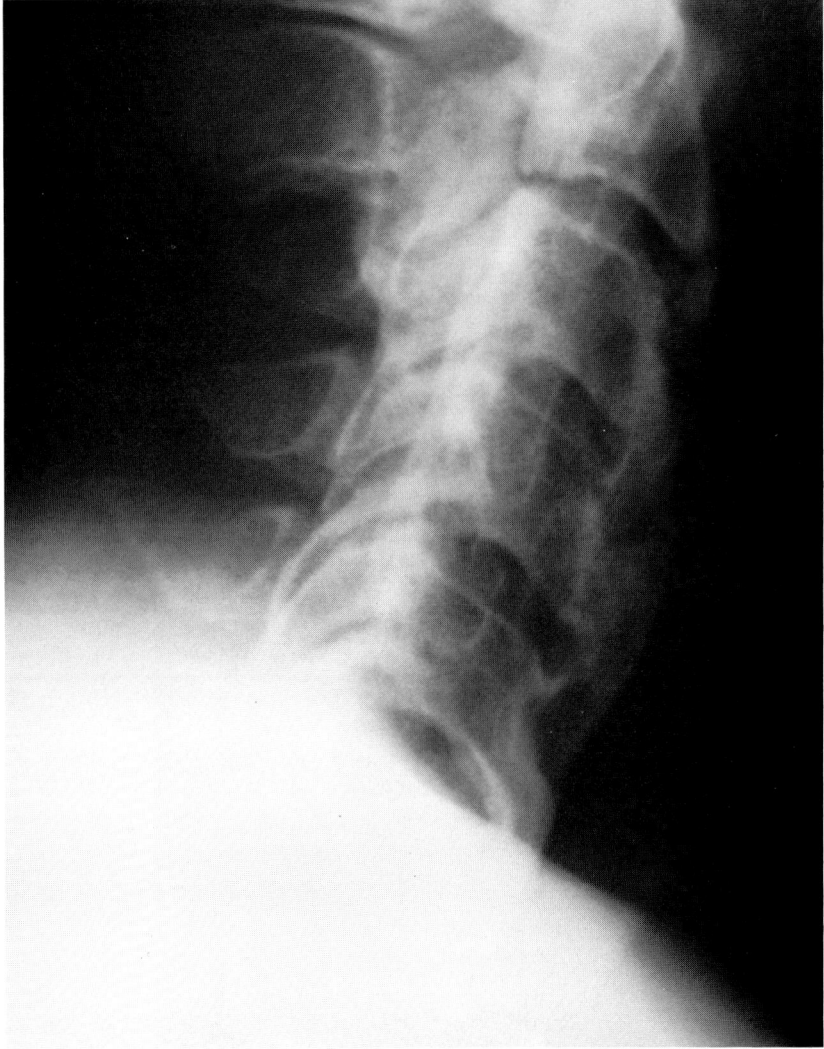

Figure 158

calcification across vertebral bodies. His radiographs demonstrate this extensive ossification involving the anterior spinal ligament and bridging multiple intervertebral disc spaces. Note also the sparing of the disc spaces and of the facet joints. The bridging ossification may superficially resemble the syndesmophytes of spondylitis, which are usually much thinner, do not arise from the body of the vertebra and are usually associated with squared vertebrae, abnormal facet joints and abnormal sacroiliac joints. They may also resemble the osteophytes of OA, but in general those of OA are more marginal and horizontal in nature and almost always associated with narrowed disc spaces. DISH syndrome is often asymptomatic except for some mild stiffness at the site of bridging of vertebral bodies. The ossification of DISH syndrome may also be seen at ligamentous attachments around the body, such as the Achilles tendon or pubic rami.

SECTION II—EXERCISES

Exercise 46

Tex, a 27 year old rodeo rider, has noted pain and stiffness in his low back over the last 4 years. Worse in the morning, he actually feels better while riding the bulls. He has taken several hard spills but as far as he knows has not broken anything. What do you think of the AP view of his lumbar spine (Fig. 159)?

Tex's pelvic radiograph demonstrates fusion of the sacroiliac joints. Tex has ankylosing spondylitis, which explains his morning stiffness and his improvement with use.

Exercise 47

Bob, a 24 year old heroin abuser, complains of lower back pain and right-sided buttock pain for 2 months. Look at his radiograph (Fig. 160) and decide what your next diagnostic move should be.

The radiograph reveals unilateral destruction of the right sacroiliac joint. The tomogram in Figure 161 shows this more clearly. The rapid destruction and the unilateral nature of the illness in the sacroiliac joint suggest an infection rather than an inflammatory spondylitis. An open biopsy specimen of his sacroiliac joint cultured a coagulase-positive *Staphylococcus*.

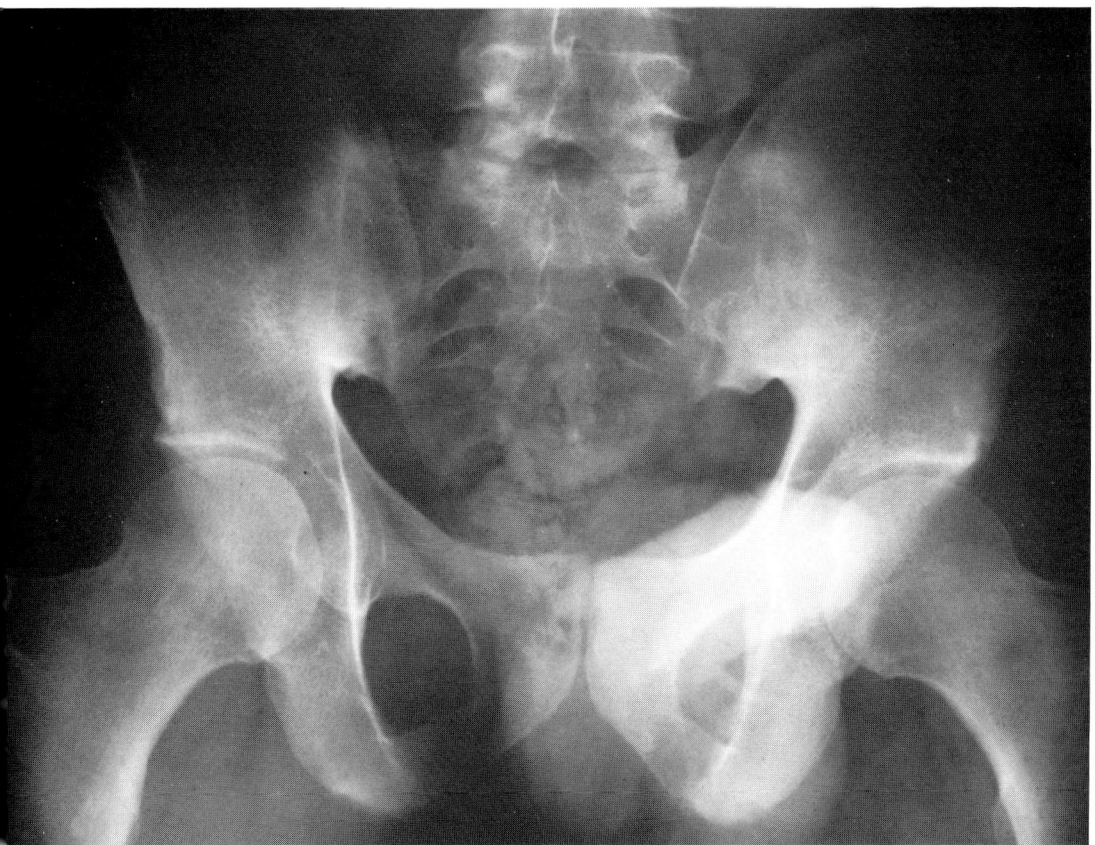

Figure 159

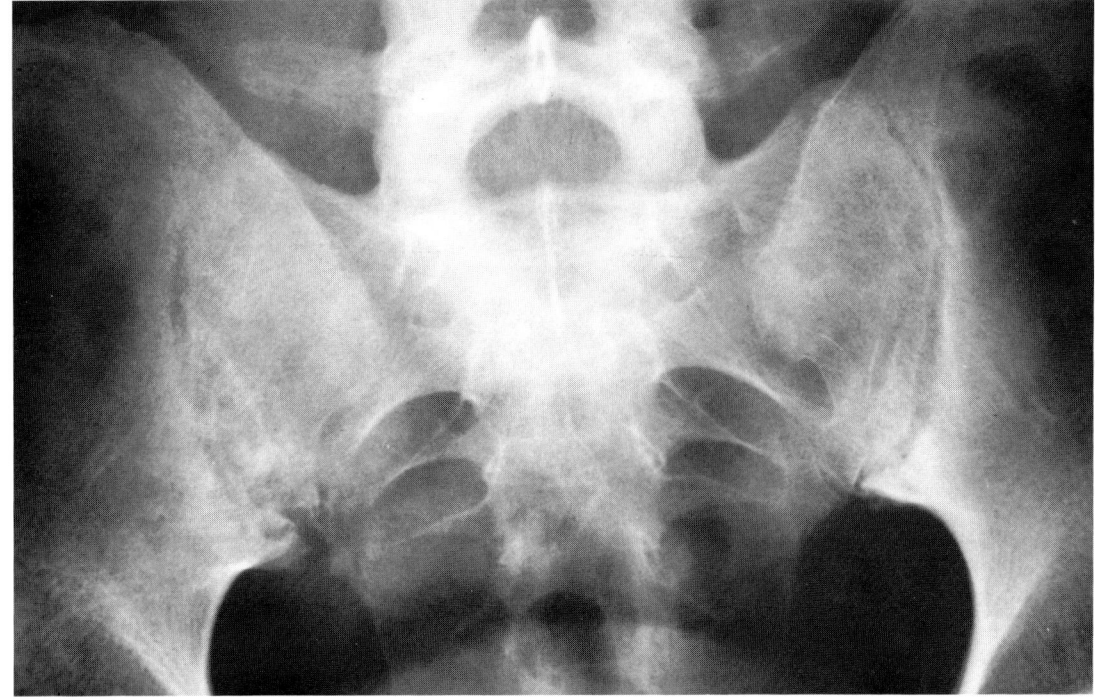

Figure 160

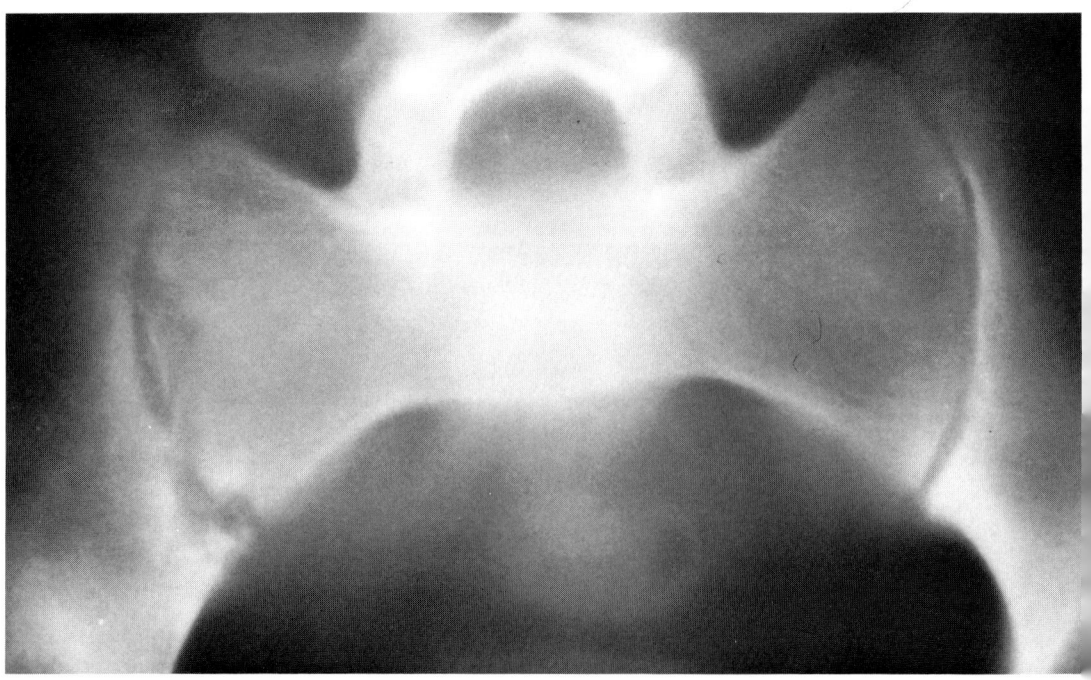

Figure 161

Exercise 48

Harvey, 44 years old, has had ankylosing spondylitis involving his lumbar, thoracic and cervical spine progressively for 20 years, and he has lost all motion except for slight movement in his cervical area. He has just slipped on the ice on the way to your office. When he gets there he relates to you that he now notes some increased motion in his thoracic spine that has not been present for years and is ecstatic at the news. You are not as thrilled and take a radiograph of his spine (Fig. 162). What do you find?

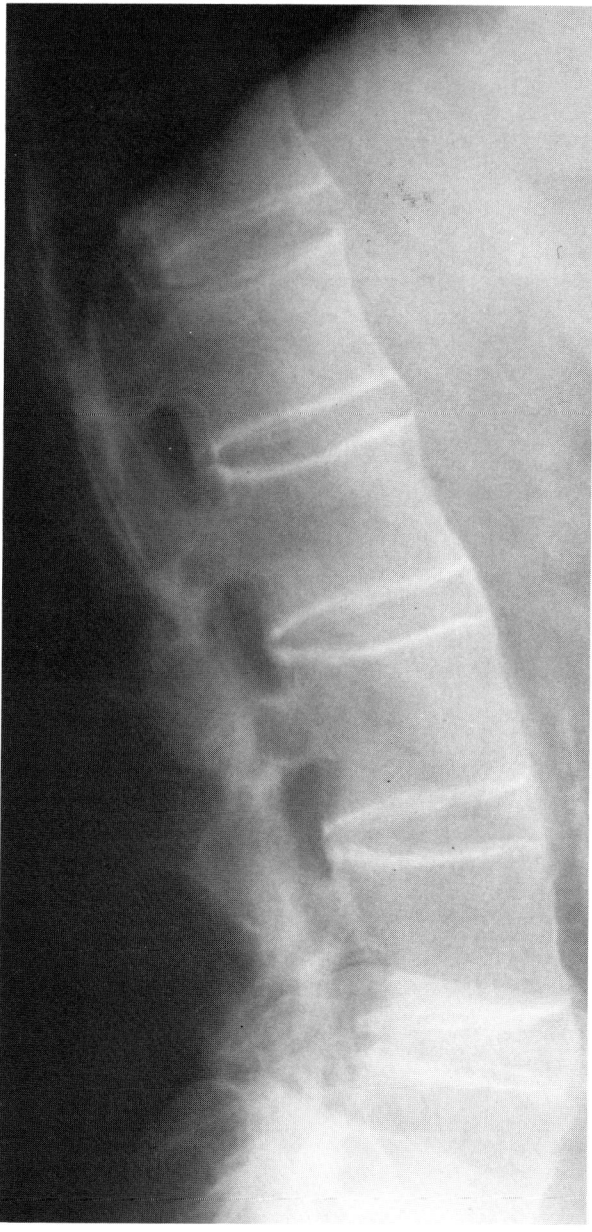

Figure 162

Harvey already has a "bamboo spine," or fusion of his entire spinal column by syndesmophytes. His radiograph shows an incomplete syndesmophyte across the T12/L1 interspace. Since he's had a complete fusion of his spine for years, this must represent a fracture. This would account for his increased motion, and is typical of the kind of reaction the weakened bone in ankylosing spondylitis has to minor trauma. Look at the tomogram in Figure 163, which shows the fracture more clearly. Since this is a transverse fracture through the whole spinal segment, his lower spinal cord is at risk for compressive injury. You immediately refer him to a neurosurgeon.

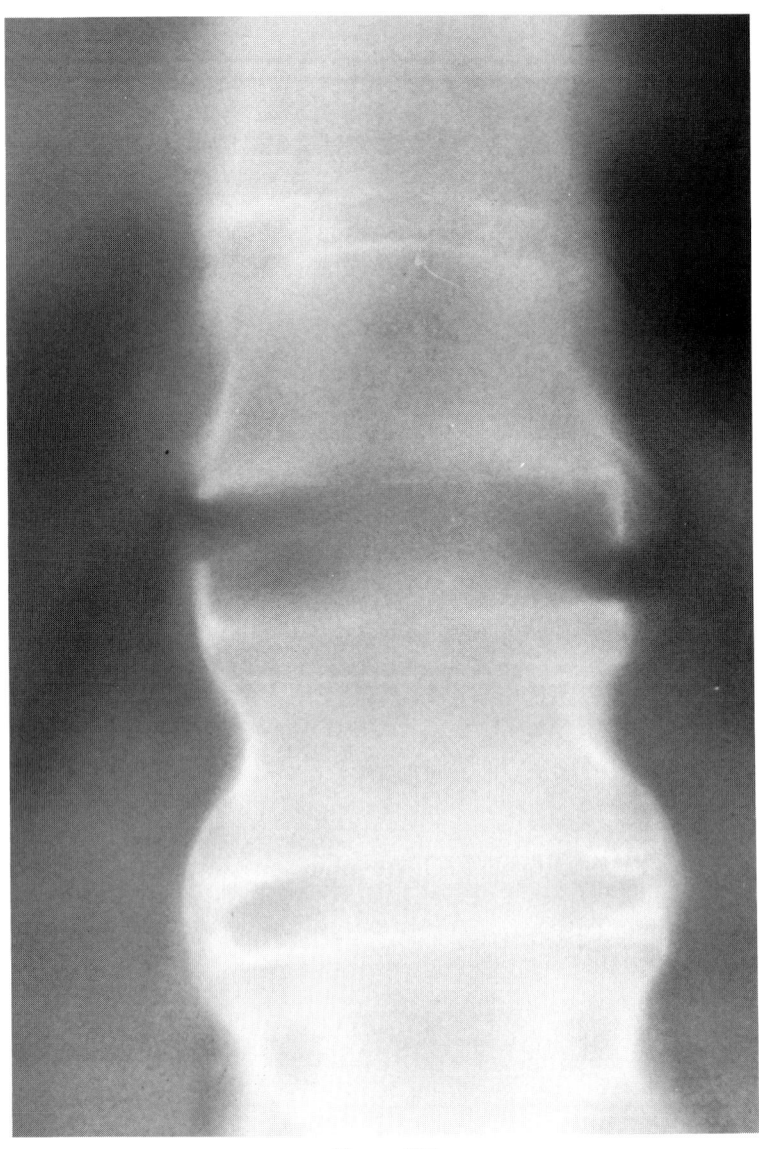

Figure 163

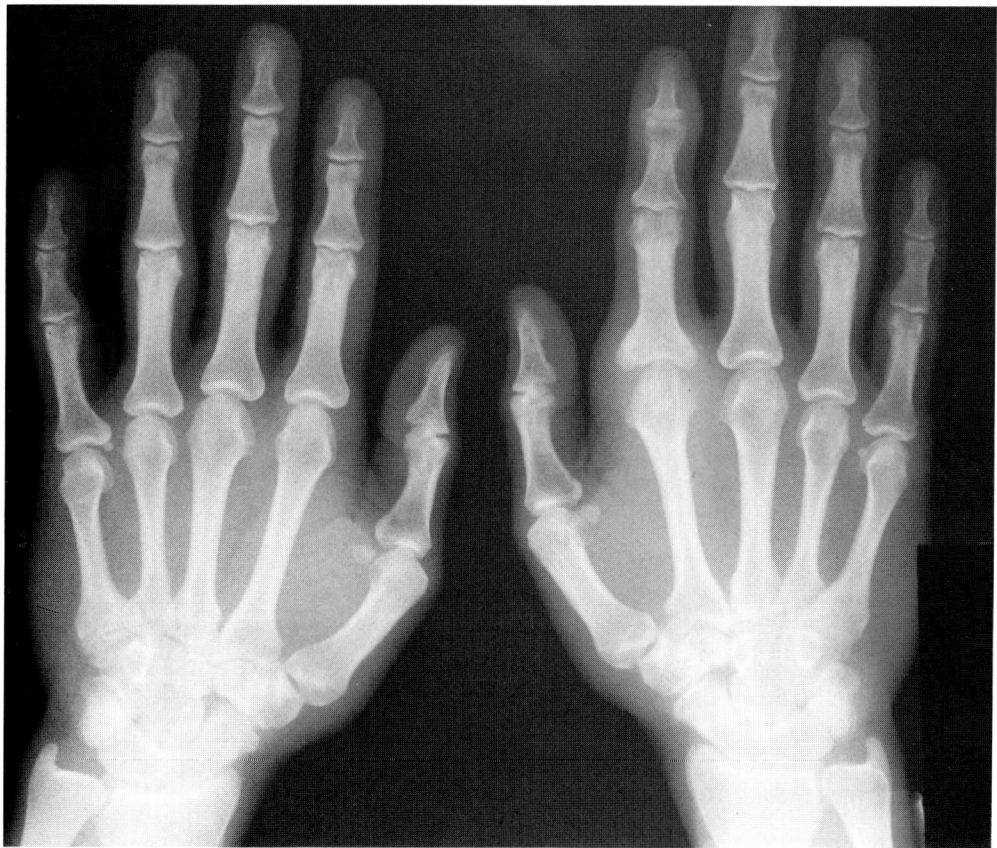

Figure 164

Exercise 49

Jed, 47 years old, has a 3 year history of pain and swelling in multiple PIP joints bilaterally. In addition, his whole right index finger is swollen up like a sausage. He complains of morning stiffness in his lower spine and has soreness when he steps on his big toe. His nails look ragged and irregular, and he has a rash. Does his hand radiograph (Fig. 164) tell you the kind of rash this is likely to be?

Jed's radiographs show changes consistent with an inflammatory arthritis. There is soft tissue swelling around all of the right PIP joints and around his second right MCP and DIP joints. There is a slight decrease in bone density in the right second digit; the rest of the hand is normal. Note the erosion around the second right MCP joint. Jed has psoriatic arthritis. The asymmetric arthritis coupled with the nail changes and rash are typical of this disease. Figures 165 and 166 show Jed's toe. Can you see why it hurts? The large erosion (arrow) in the first metatarsal head certainly explains his pain and is consistent with his disease elsewhere. Look at the radiographs of his pelvis and spine (Figs. 167 and 168); the right sacroiliac joint is abnormal, and a syndesmophyte is seen at T12 (arrow). Jed also has spondylitis associated with his psoriasis. It should be no surprise to learn that his HLA-B27 antigen test was positive.

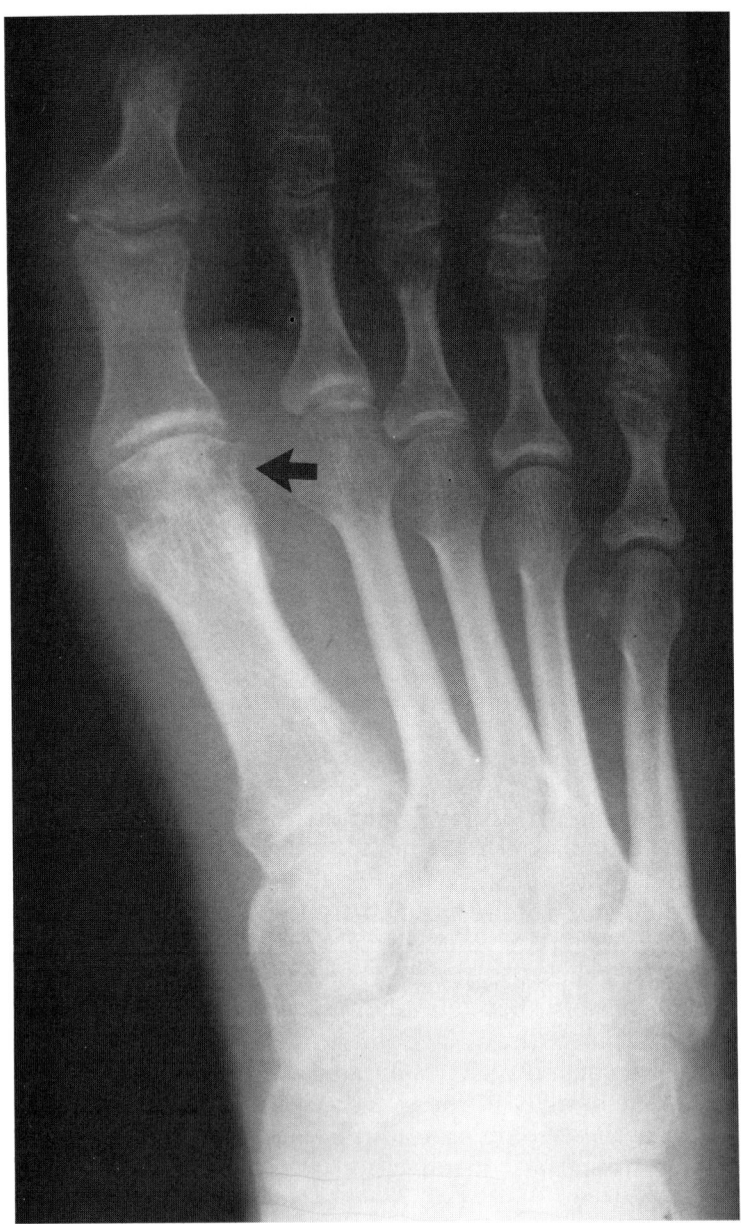

Figure 165

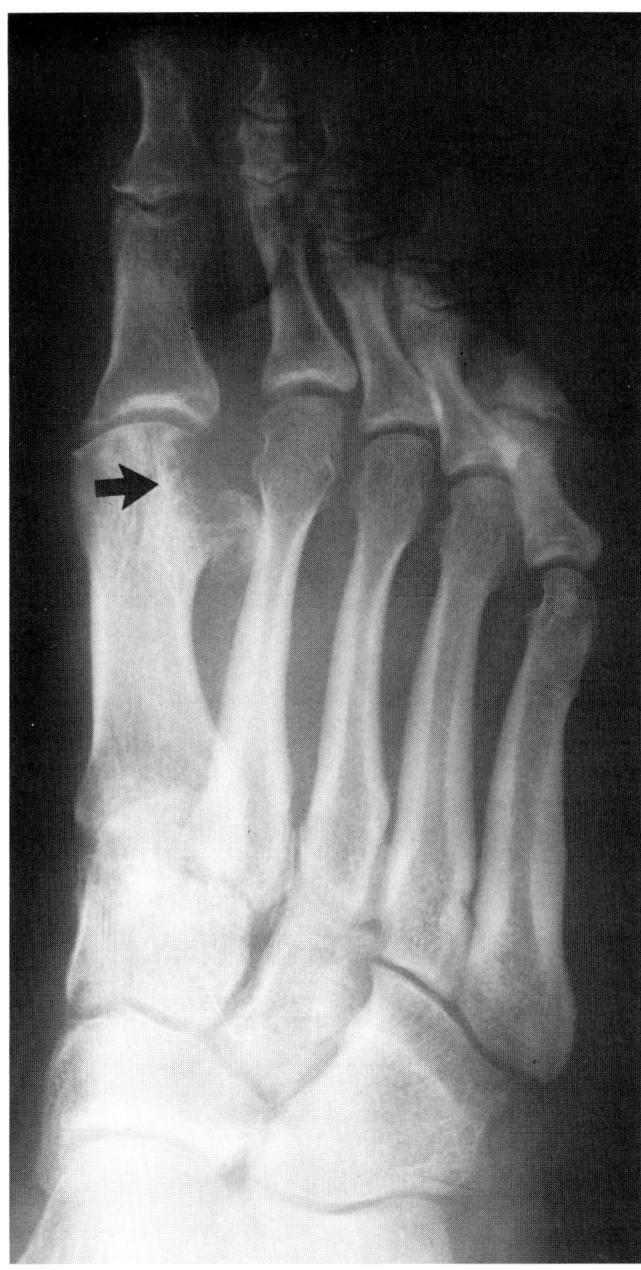

Figure 166

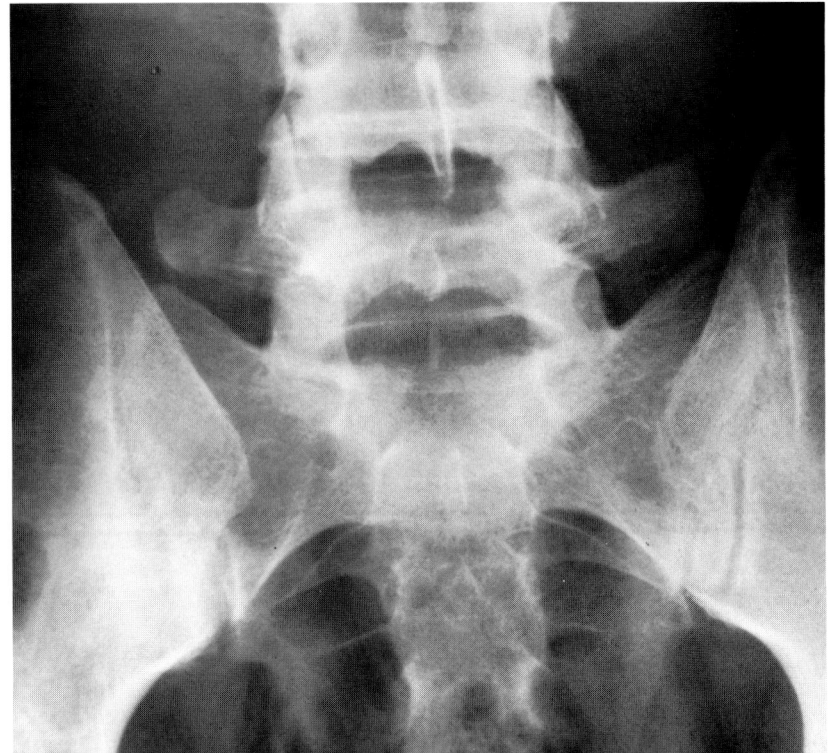

Figure 167

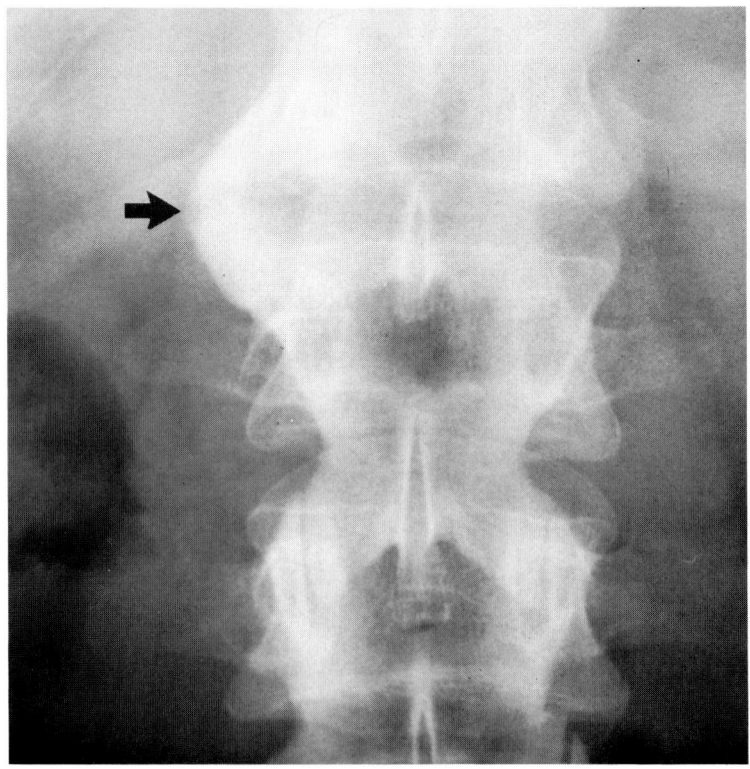

Figure 168

Exercise 50

Two months earlier, Melvin, 38 years old, underwent a routine appendectomy complicated by a urinary tract infection from catheter placement postoperatively. Since that time he has noted nonradicular lower back pain and a persistent low grade fever. One month ago his local physician took a radiograph (Fig. 169) but found little. You do a new one (Fig. 170) and compare them. What is your next diagnostic move?

Melvin's second radiograph reveals disc space narrowing and vertebral endplate osteoporosis and erosion consistent with a diagnosis of discitis. This is most likely a septic discitis, as no other illness will cause such a rapid destruction of the disc and vertebra. Biopsy of the disc cultured *Escherichia coli*, the same organism cultured from his urine during his previous hospitalization. The organism likely reached the spine via a paravertebral plexus of veins that drains from the pelvis along the spine to the base of the skull. This is a common pathway for pelvic disease to spread.

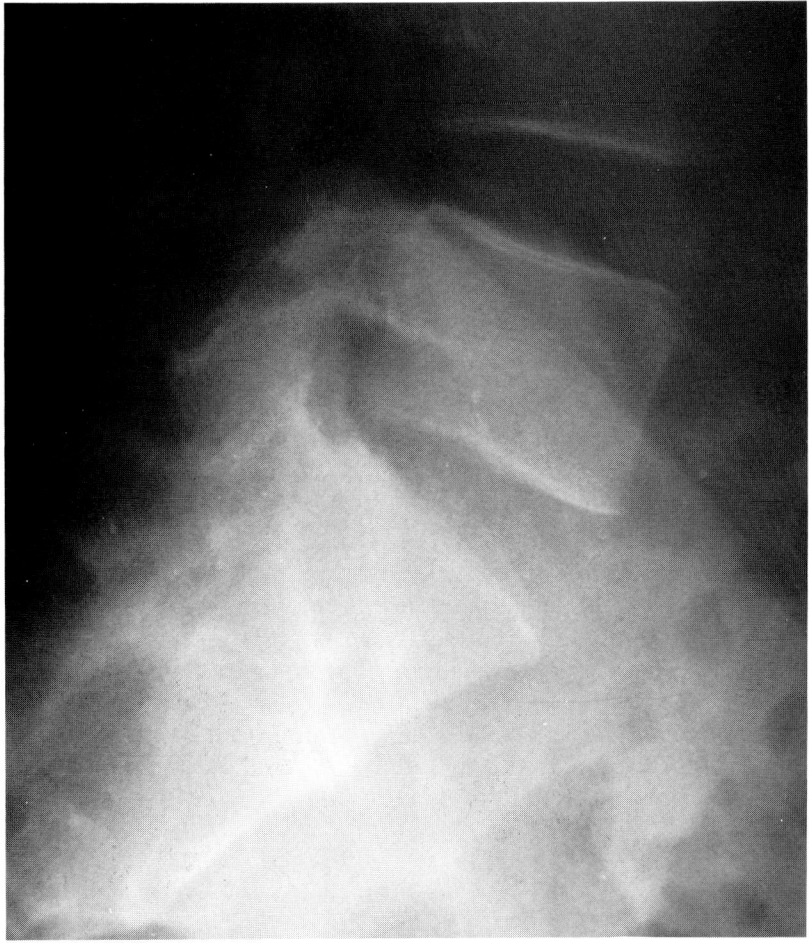

Figure 169

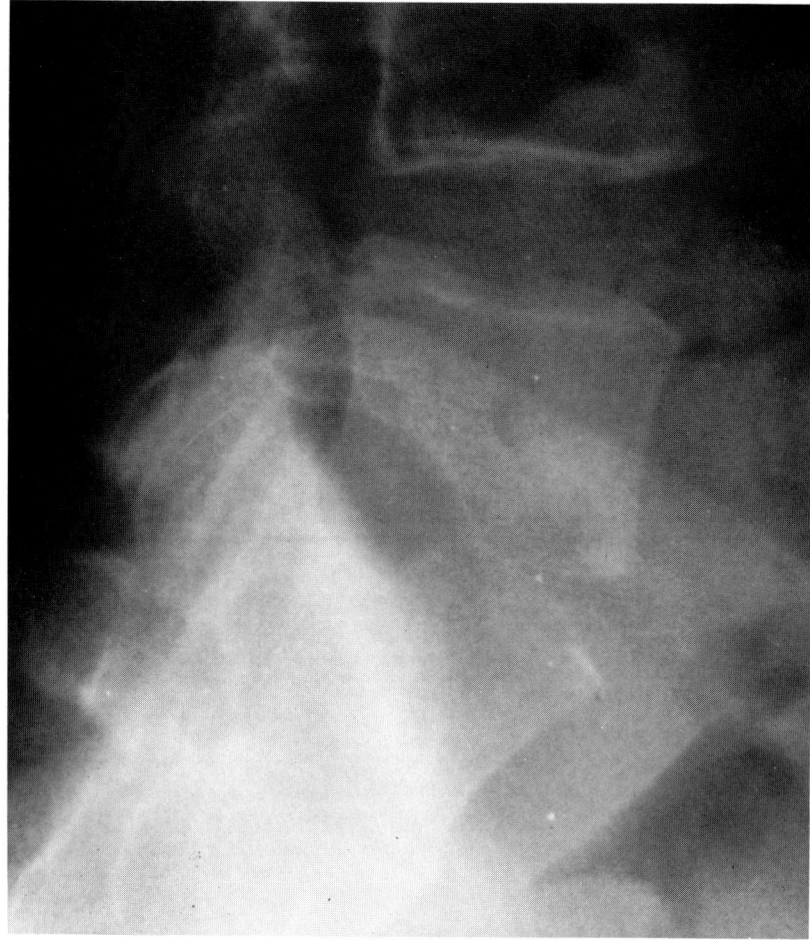

Figure 170

Exercise 51

Alice, 61 years old, has had nonradicular lower back pain for the last 3 years. Look at her spine radiographs (Figs. 171 and 172) and describe what you see.

You should notice that there is severe narrowing of multiple discs with vacuum signs at every level, indicating severe disc degeneration. However, the osteophytosis is minimal. Look at her knee film in Figure 173. Alice has chondrocalcinosis. There is calcification in the medial and lateral menisci. This represents CPPD deposition, which is likely to have become deposited in her disc spaces also, leading to the severe degeneration there. Careful evaluation revealed the CPPD deposition to be familial, being present in two siblings, and unassociated with an underlying defined metabolic process.

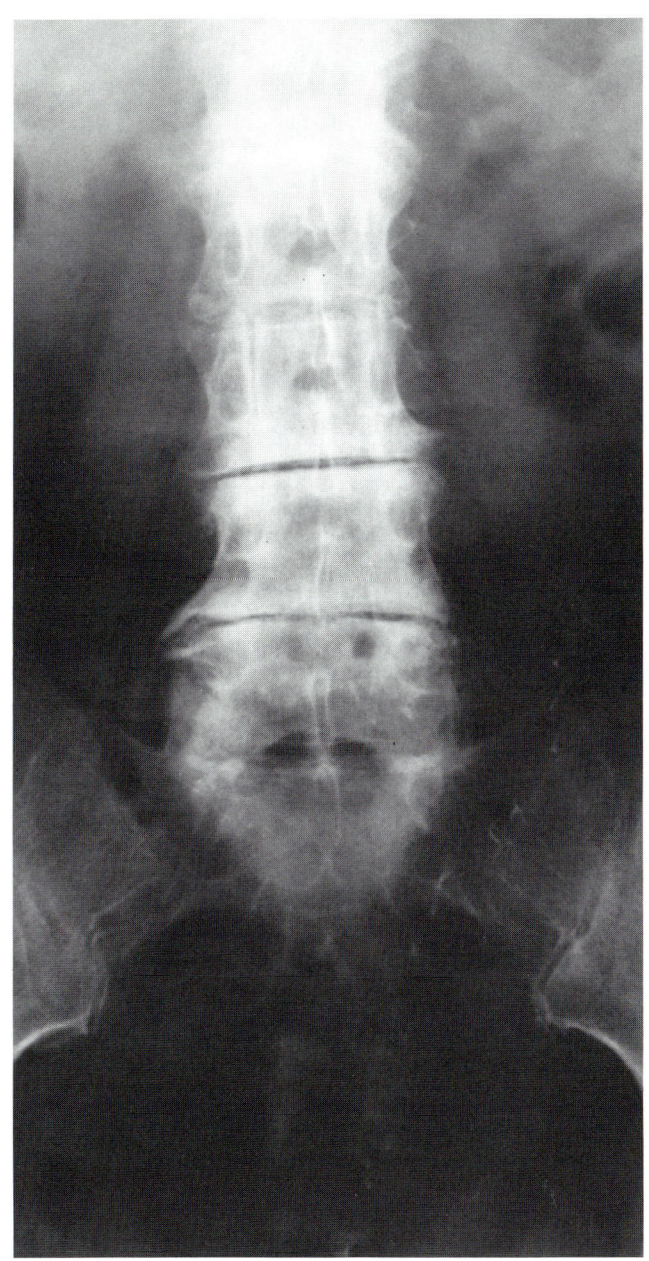

Figure 171

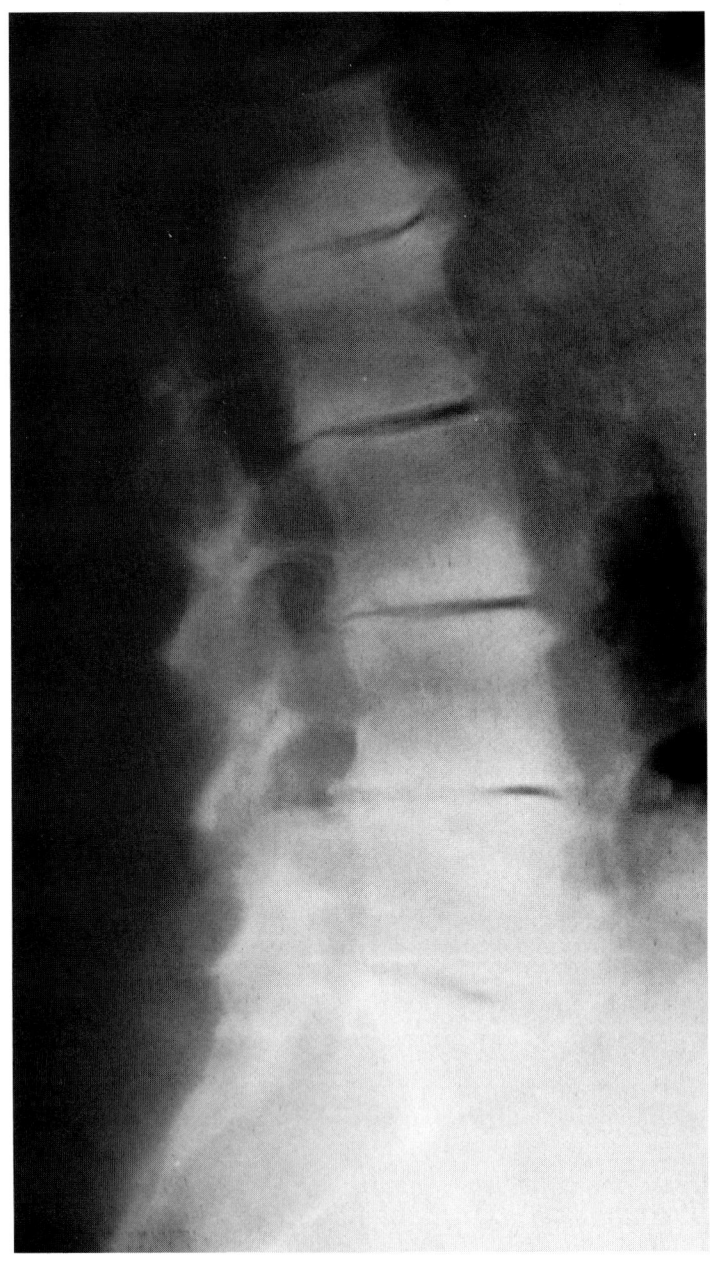

Figure 172

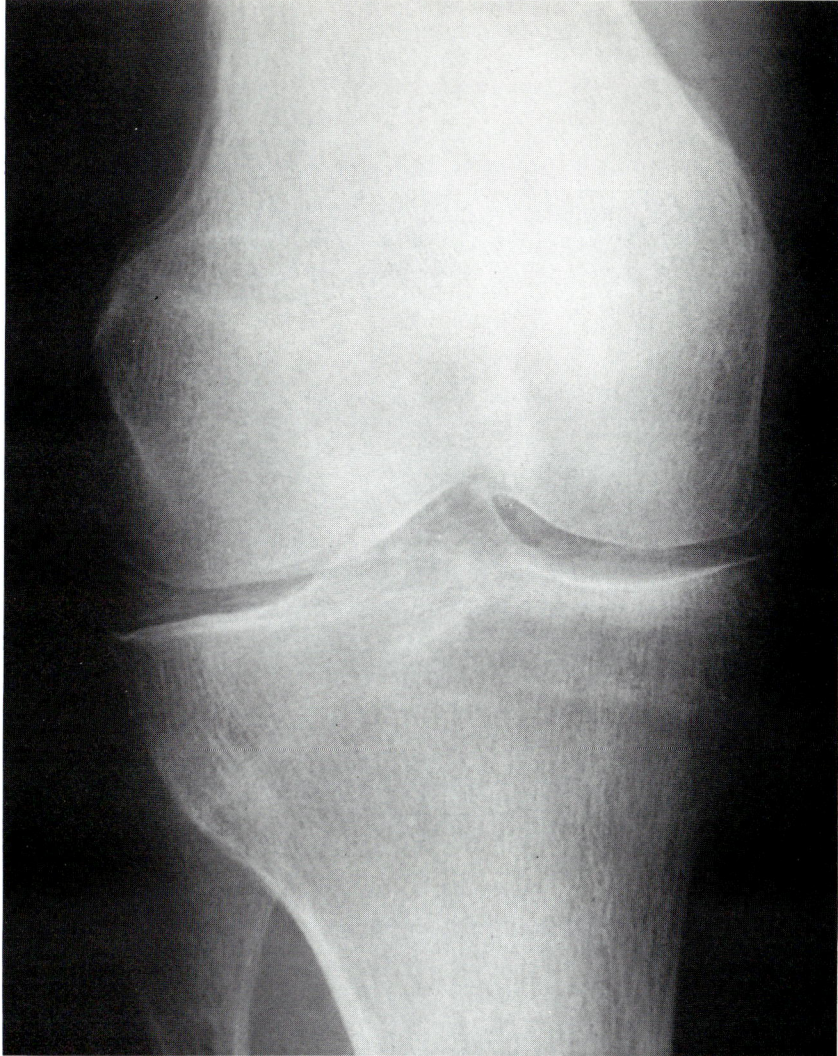

Figure 173

Exercise 52

Lisa, a college gymnast, has had complaints of lower back pain over the last few months. Look at her radiograph (Fig. 174) and decide what you think the cause of her pain is.

The lateral view of Lisa's lumbosacral spine shows slight displacement of L5 on S1 (spondylolisthesis) and a defect in the pars interarticularis (spondylolysis) as the cause of the displacement. Look at a closer view on the oblique film in Figure 175, in which the arrow highlights the defect at L5 and the arrowhead points to the normal pars interarticularis at L4. Compare this to Figure 25, in which the normal contour is outlined. Such injuries may be the result of stress fractures, and often occur in athletes. Lisa eventually needed a stabilization procedure to relieve her symptoms.

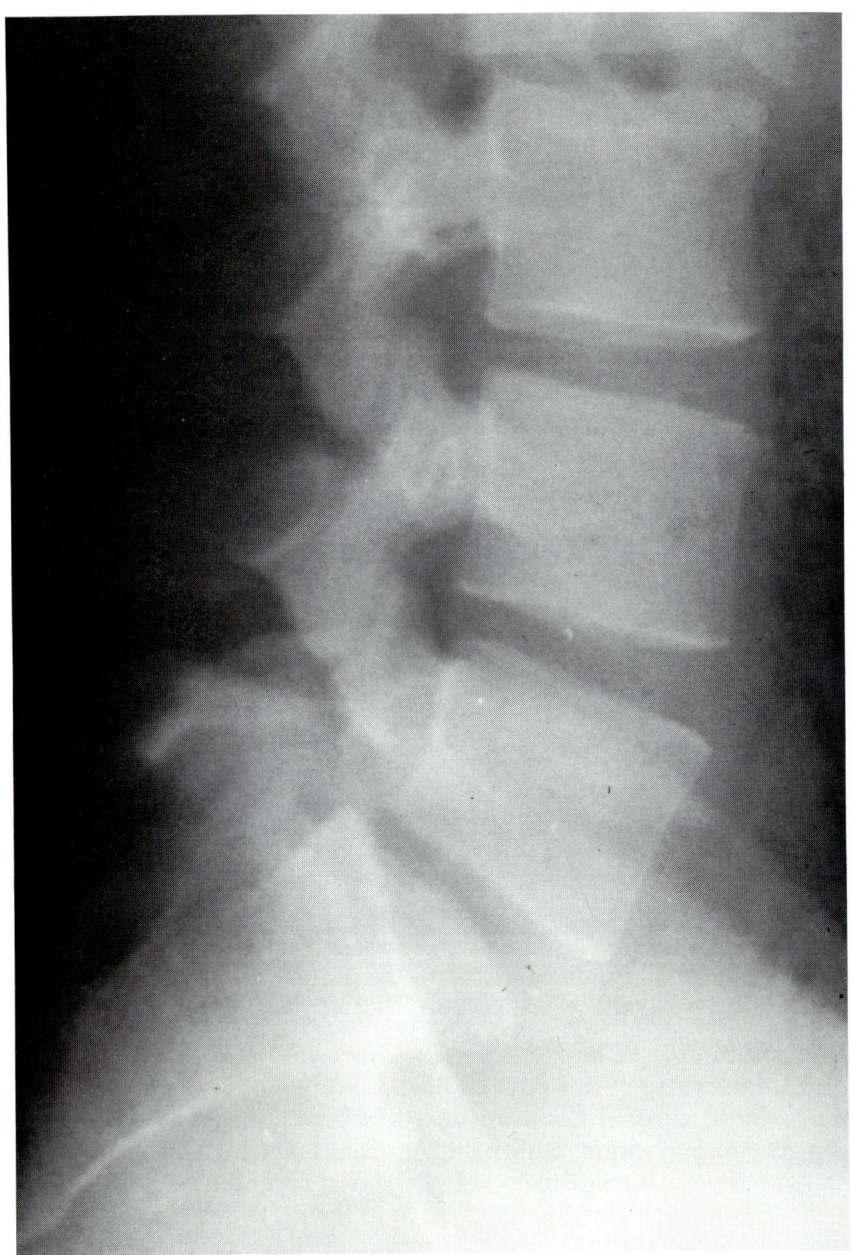

Figure 174

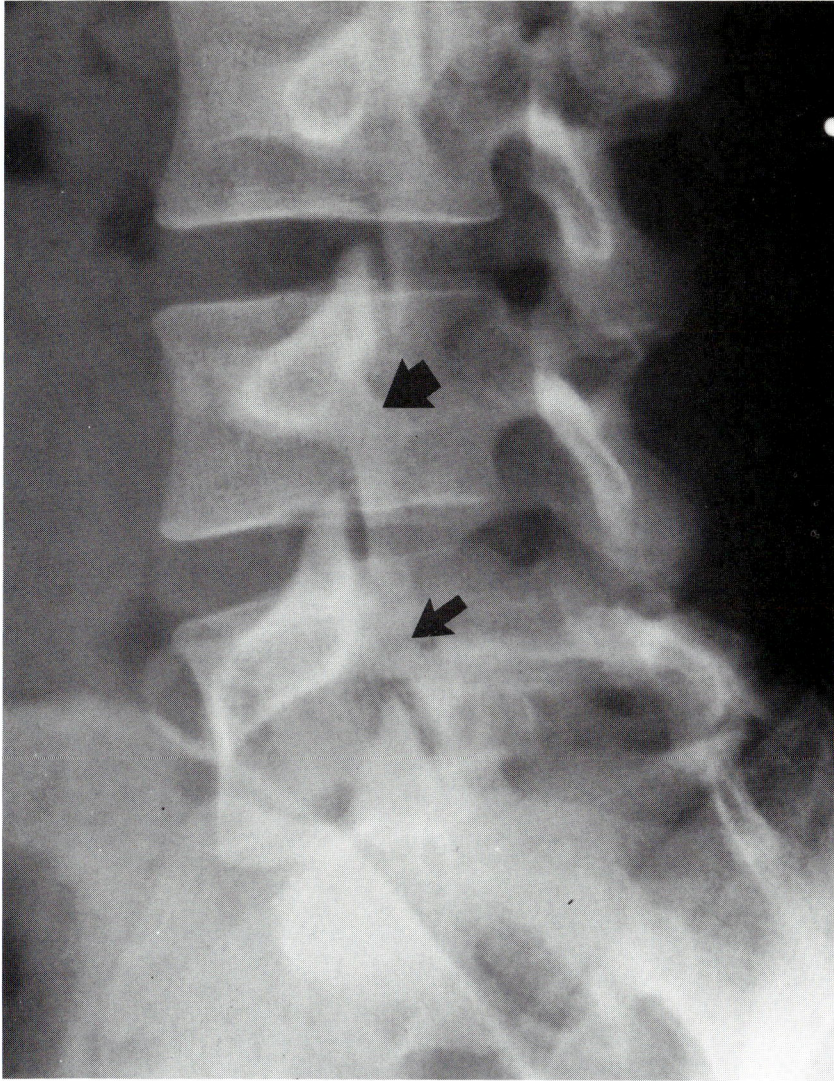

Figure 175

Exercise 53

Anne has had neck pain for years, and recently it has begun to radiate into her right trapezius muscle and down into her right arm. You note some weakness and reflex changes in her right biceps, and exacerbation of her symptoms occurs when she moves her cervical spine. Look at her radiographs and decide what she has.

The lateral view of the cervical spine (Fig. 176) demonstrates degenerative changes with narrowing of the C3/C4, C4/C5, and C5/C6 intervertebral disc spaces. Note the osteophytes at these levels. The oblique view (Fig. 177) further defines the illness by demonstrating encroachment of the neuroforamina by osteophytes arising from the joints of Lushka (arrow). Anne has a cervical radiculopathy resulting from root impingement caused by these changes, and she responded to therapy with traction and a cervical collar.

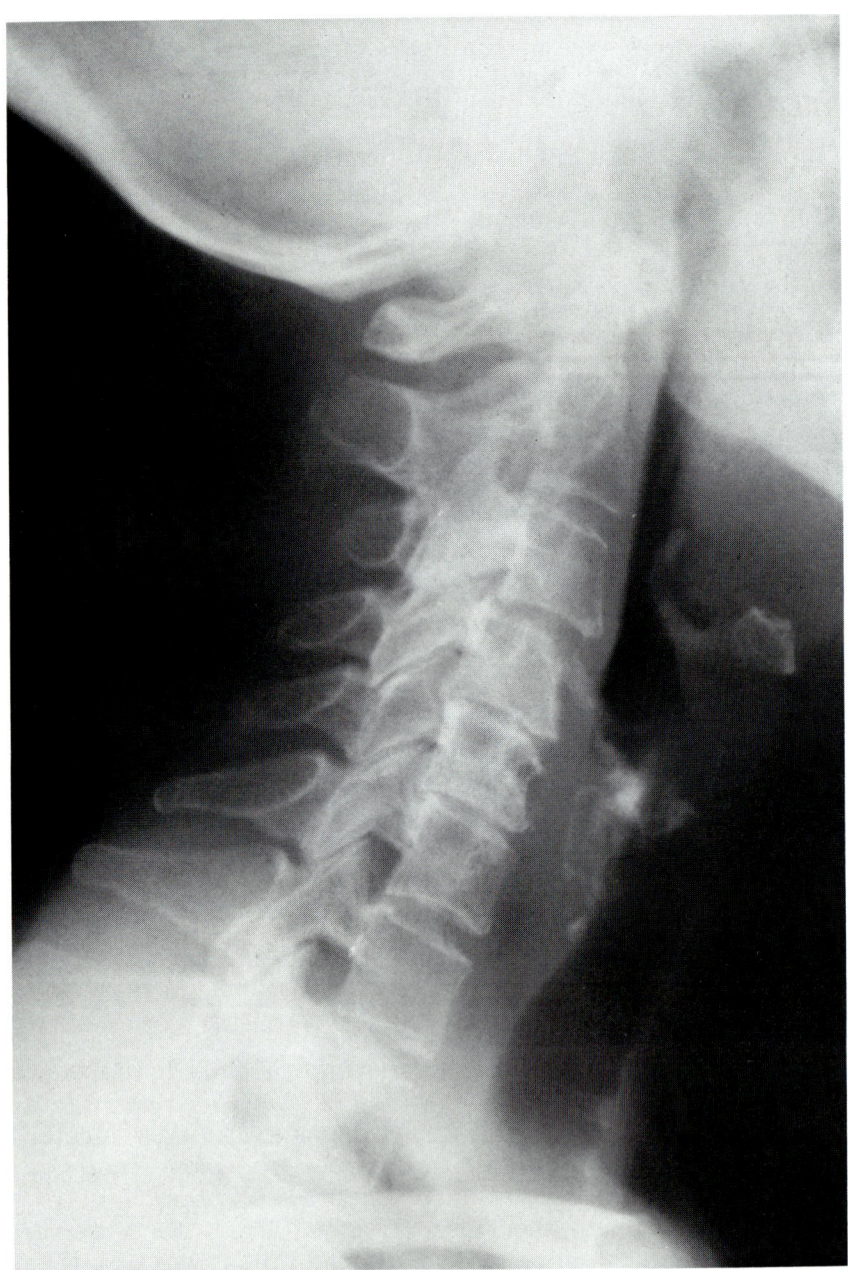
Figure 176

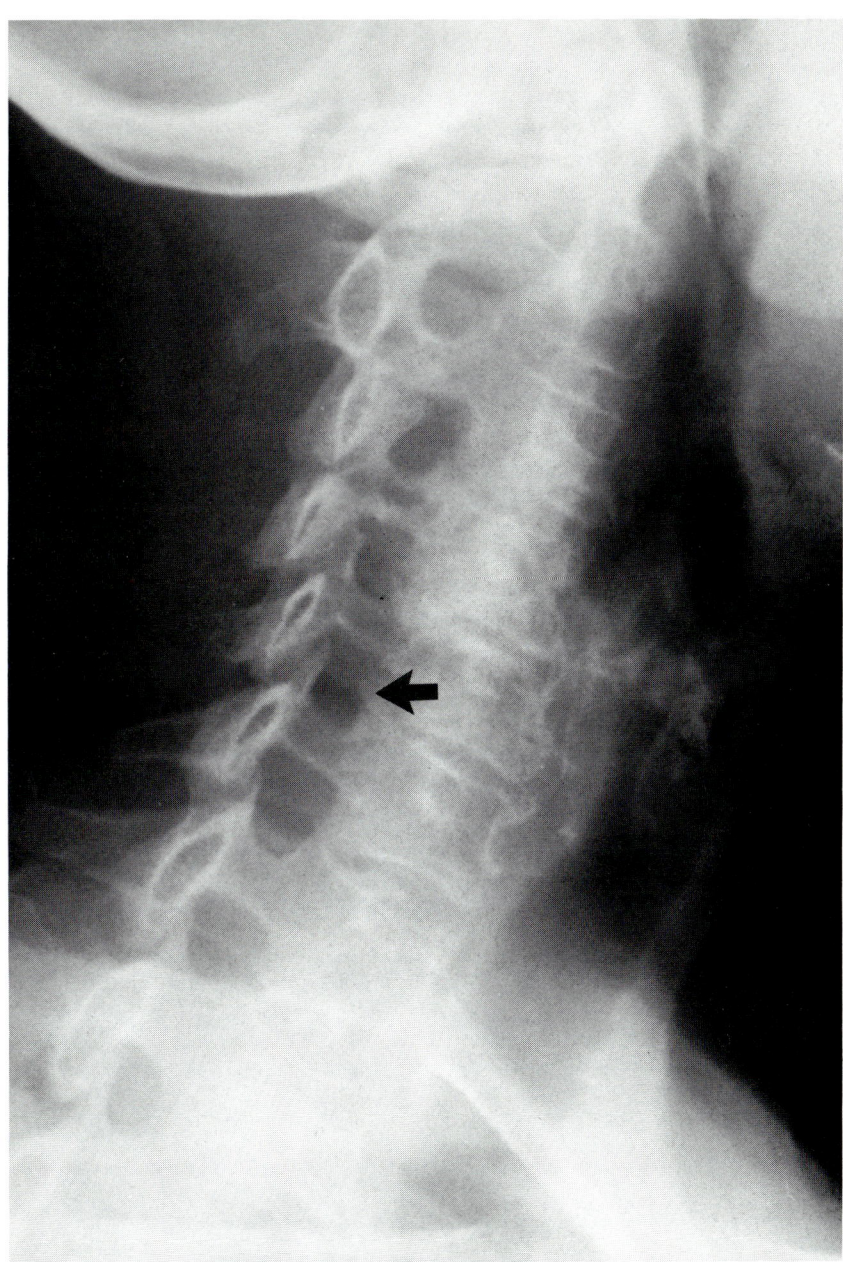

Figure 177

Exercise 54

This 40 year old man complains of neck pain in the morning and a decreasing ability to turn his head to the side while driving his car. Look at his radiograph (Fig. 178) and state your diagnosis.

There are thin syndesmophytes between C2/C3 and C3/C4 and an early one between C4/C5 with a small erosion anteriorly by C4, meaning

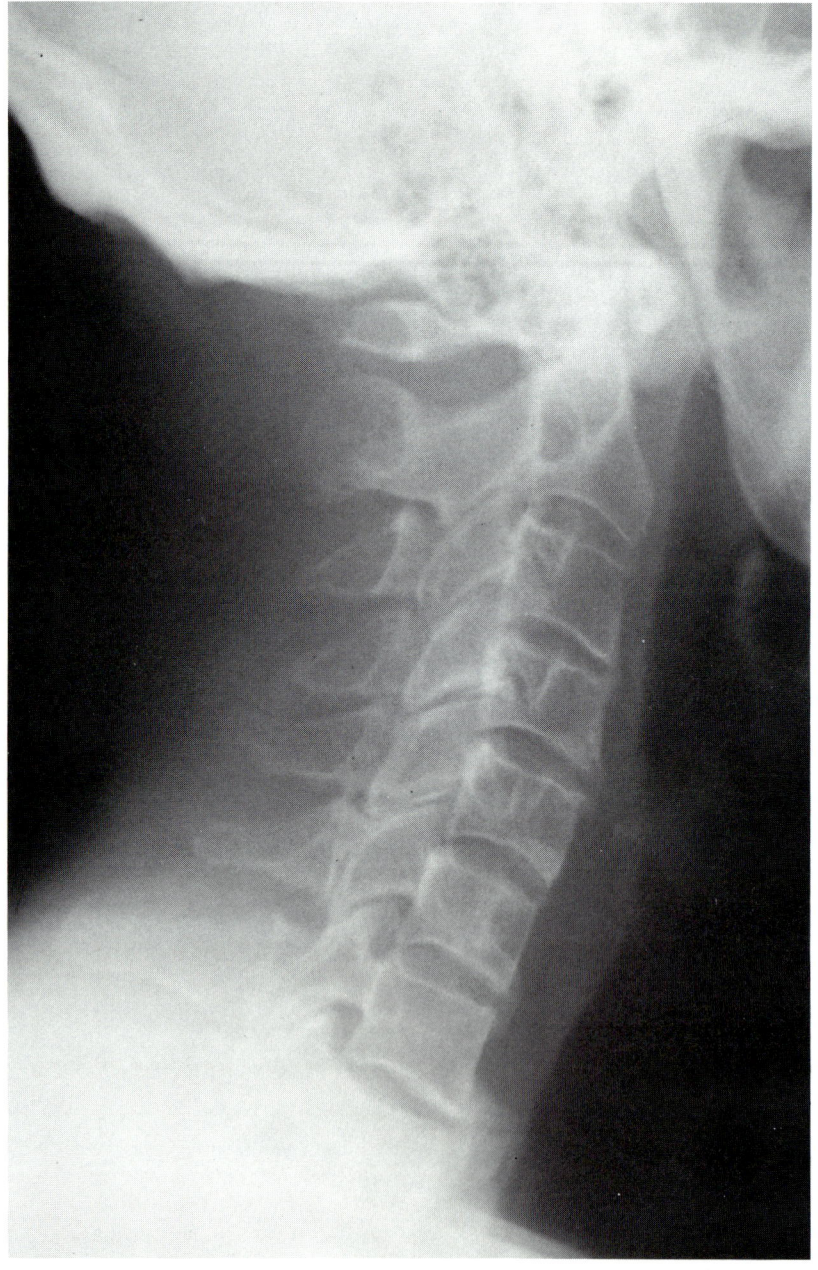

Figure 178

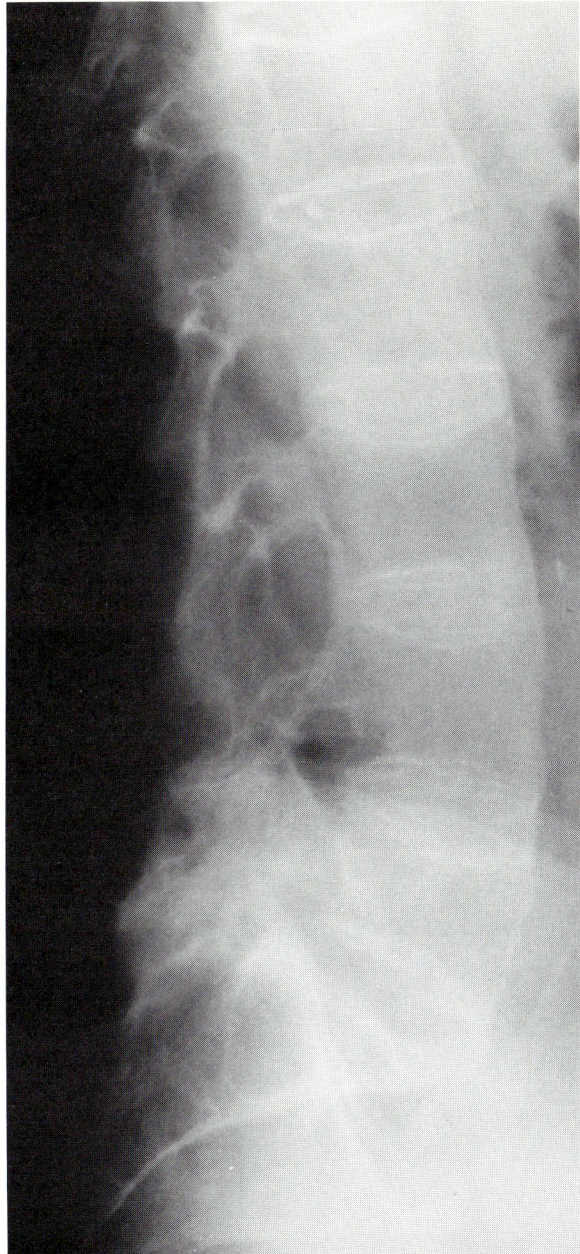

Figure 179

a spondylitis. Notice the loss of the normal concave form (squaring) of the C6 vertebral body. There is no disc space narrowing. This is early ankylosing spondylitis of the neck. A lateral view of the lumbar spine in this patient (Fig. 179) demonstrates squaring of the vertebral bodies, extensive syndesmophyte formation and fusion of the apophyseal joints characteristic of ankylosing spondylitis.

Exercise 55

Vince, 62 years old, has had RA for the past 16 years and despite therapy has developed multiple deformities of his peripheral joints. For the past 3 months, however, he has noted severe neck pain that radiates up his occiput, giving him headaches. On examination, you notice that his reflexes are hyperactive in his lower extremities and that clonus and a positive Babinski sign are present. Look at his neck films (Figs. 180 and 181) and explain these findings.

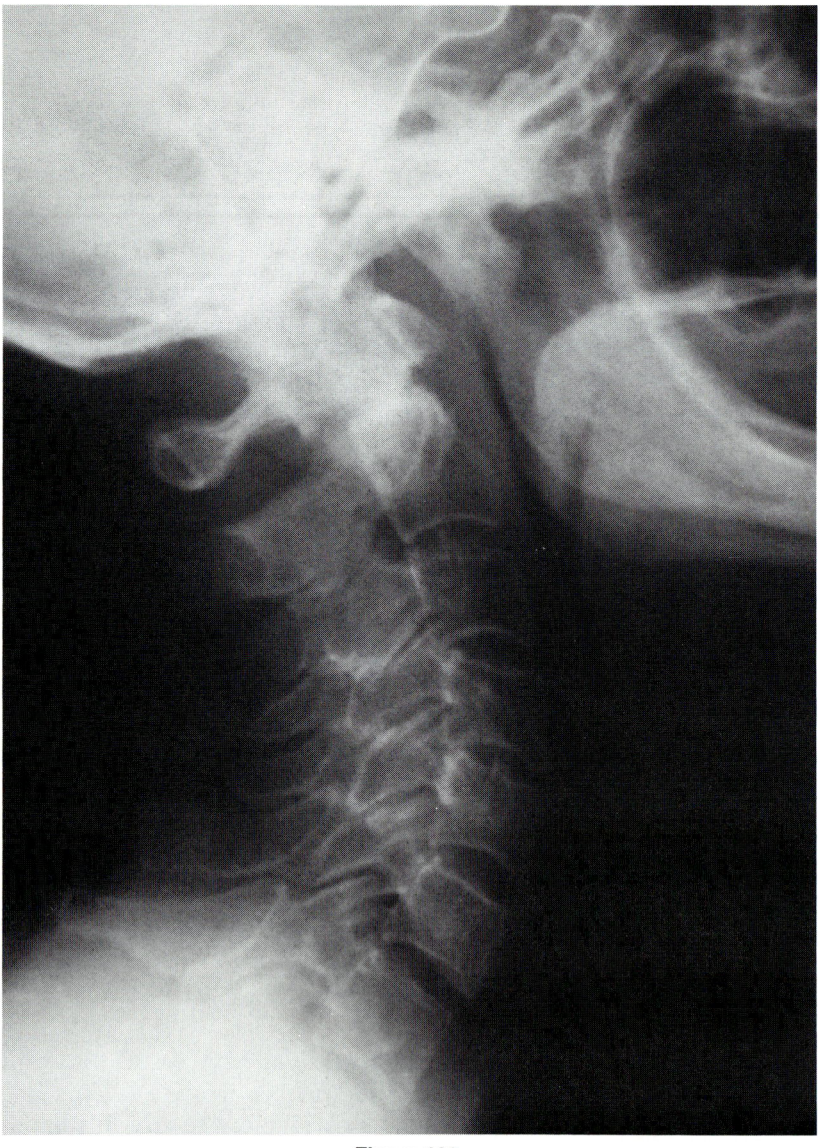

Figure 180

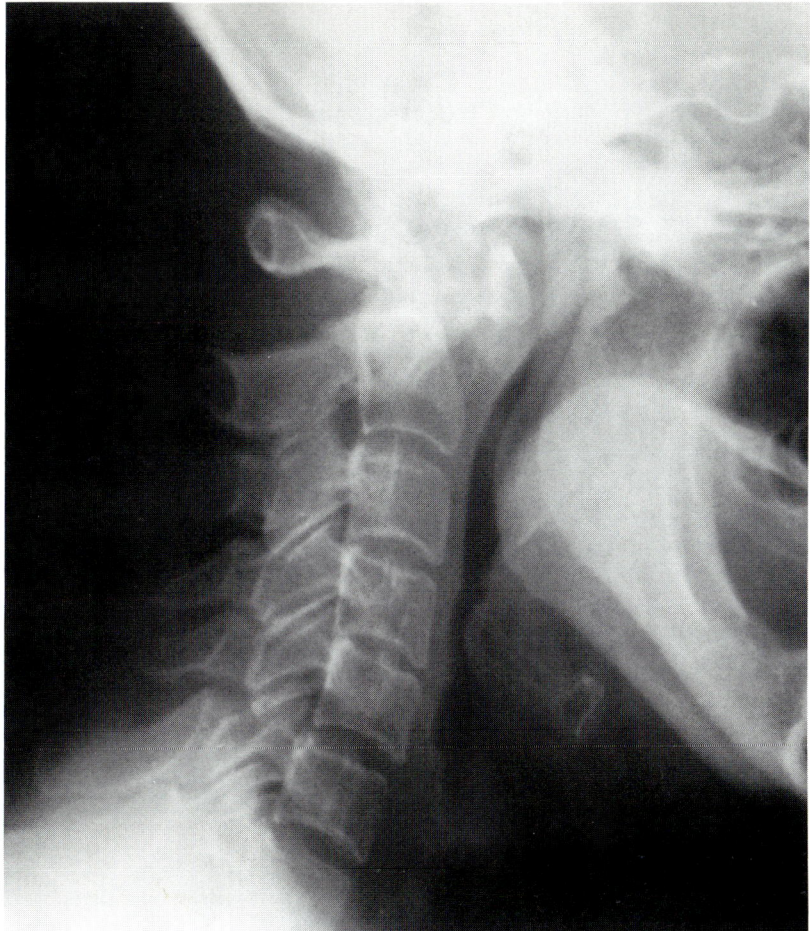

Figure 181

Notice the separation between the odontoid and the atlas (C2 and C1) on the flexion films of Figure 181, which are not present in Figure 180, when the patient is in extension. This is subluxation due to inflammation-induced ligamentous and joint destruction around the atlas and odontoid articulation, which is common in longstanding RA. Once free to migrate, the odontoid moves posteriorly into the anterior part of the spinal cord, giving long tract findings, as Vince demonstrates. Vince requires a fusion to protect his spinal cord from further slippage. Look at the films in Figures 182 and 183. This RA patient had symptoms similar to Vince, but his subluxation is in the lower cervical cord, leading to a "stepladder" deformity of one vertebra on another. It is especially important to know about such subluxations preoperatively so that special precautions can be taken to protect the neck during intubation.

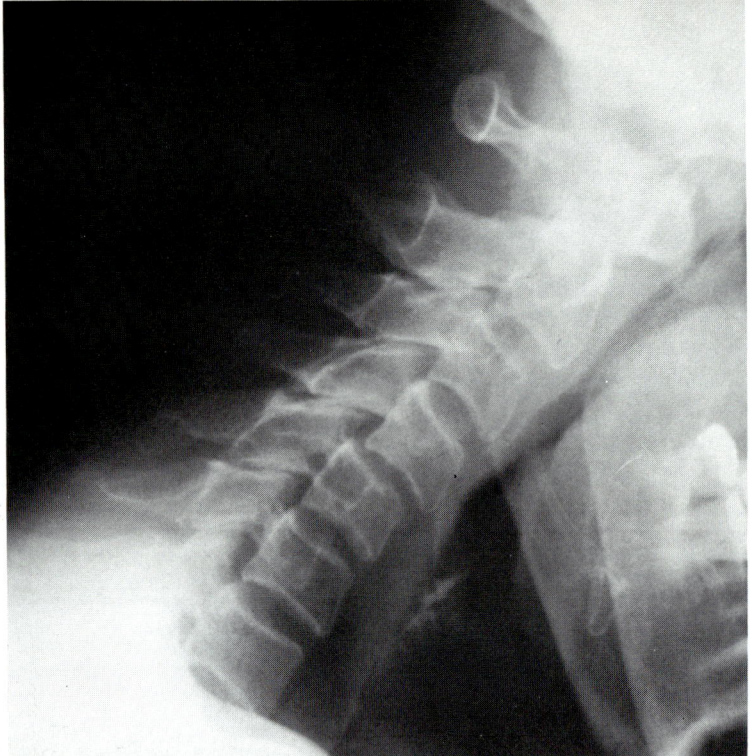

Figure 182

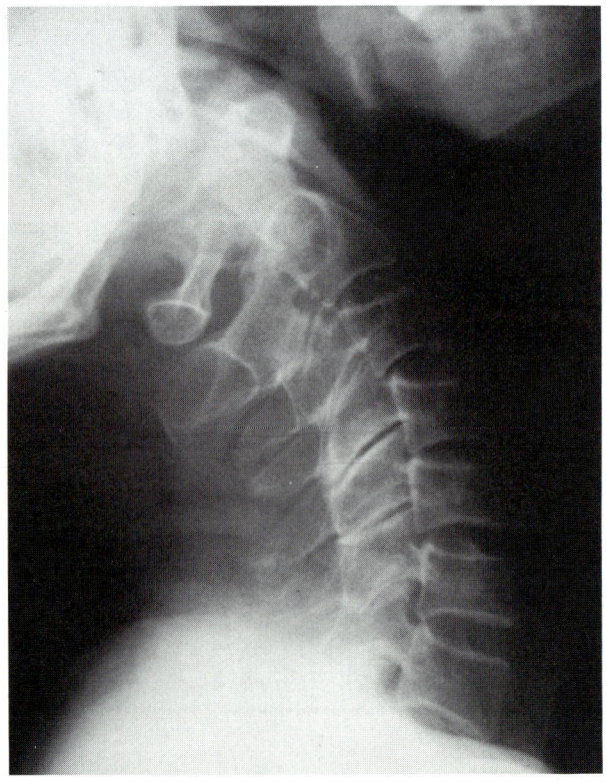

Figure 183

SECTION II—EXERCISES

Exercise 56

Look at Figures 184 to 187, all cervical spine radiographs, and decide what each reveals.

Figure 184 reveals syndesmophytes around all the cervical vertebrae and fused apophyseal joints, characteristic of ankylosing spondylitis. Compare this with Figure 185; note the apophyseal joint fusion around the C1/C2 area only, and no syndesmophytes are noted. This is typical of the changes seen in JCP. In addition, there is fusion of C1 to the occiput, also a common occurrence in JCP.

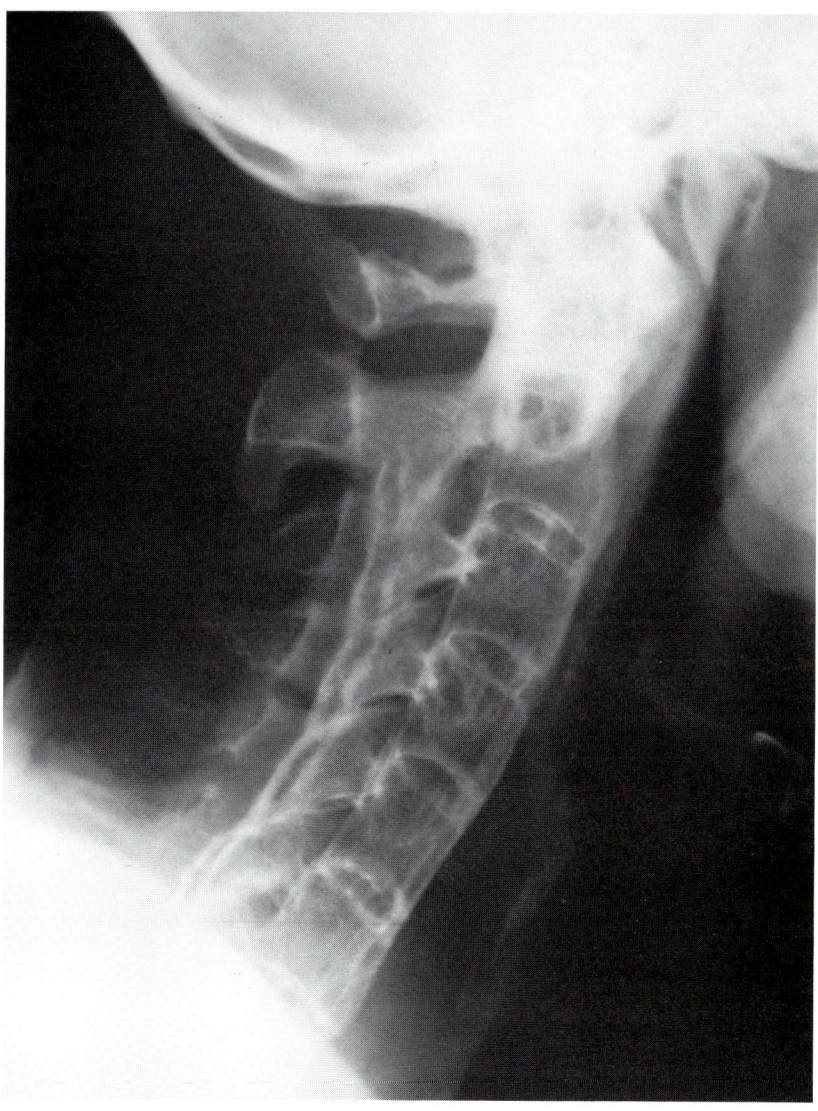

Figure 184

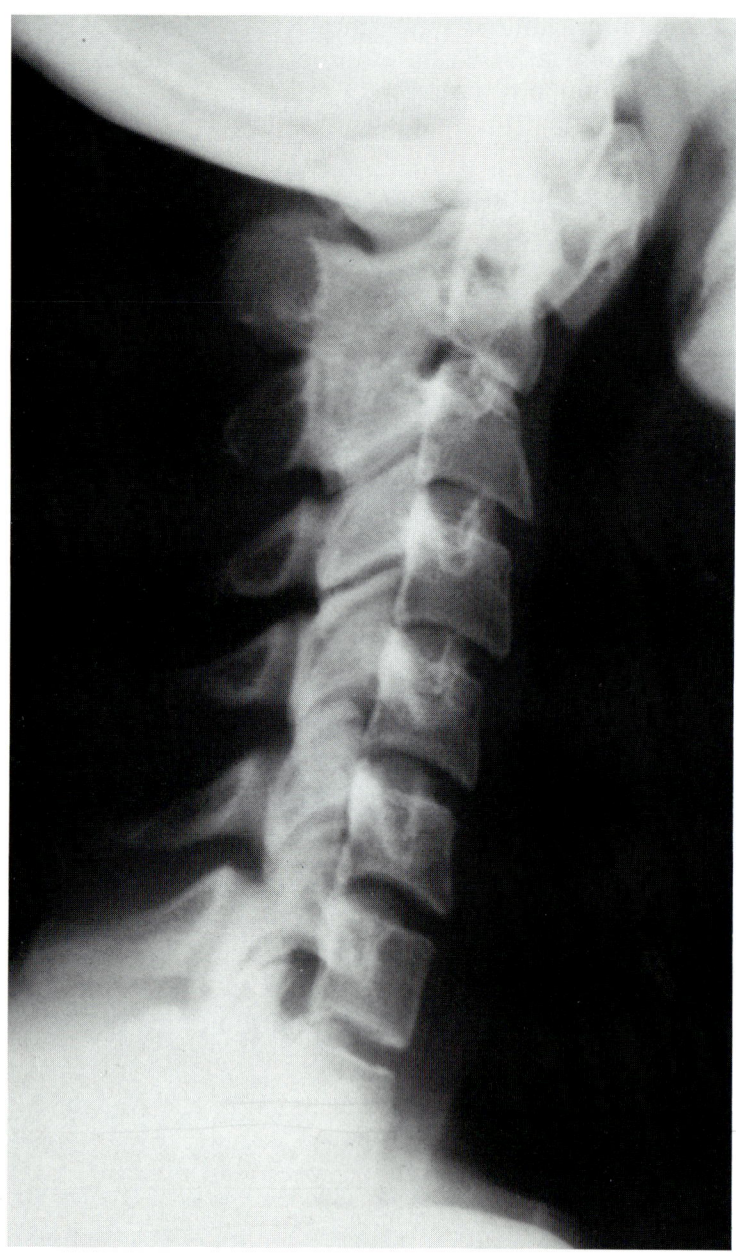

Figure 185

Figure 186 shows narrowed discs at several levels with osteophyte formation. This is OA, and in fact the patient had a cervical radiculopathy. Compare this with Figure 187; here the osteophytes are much larger, bridge the disc space and originate from the body of the vertebra. In addition, there is no disc space narrowing associated with these bony overgrowths. This is Forestier's disease, or DISH syndrome. This is the same patient as in Figure 157.

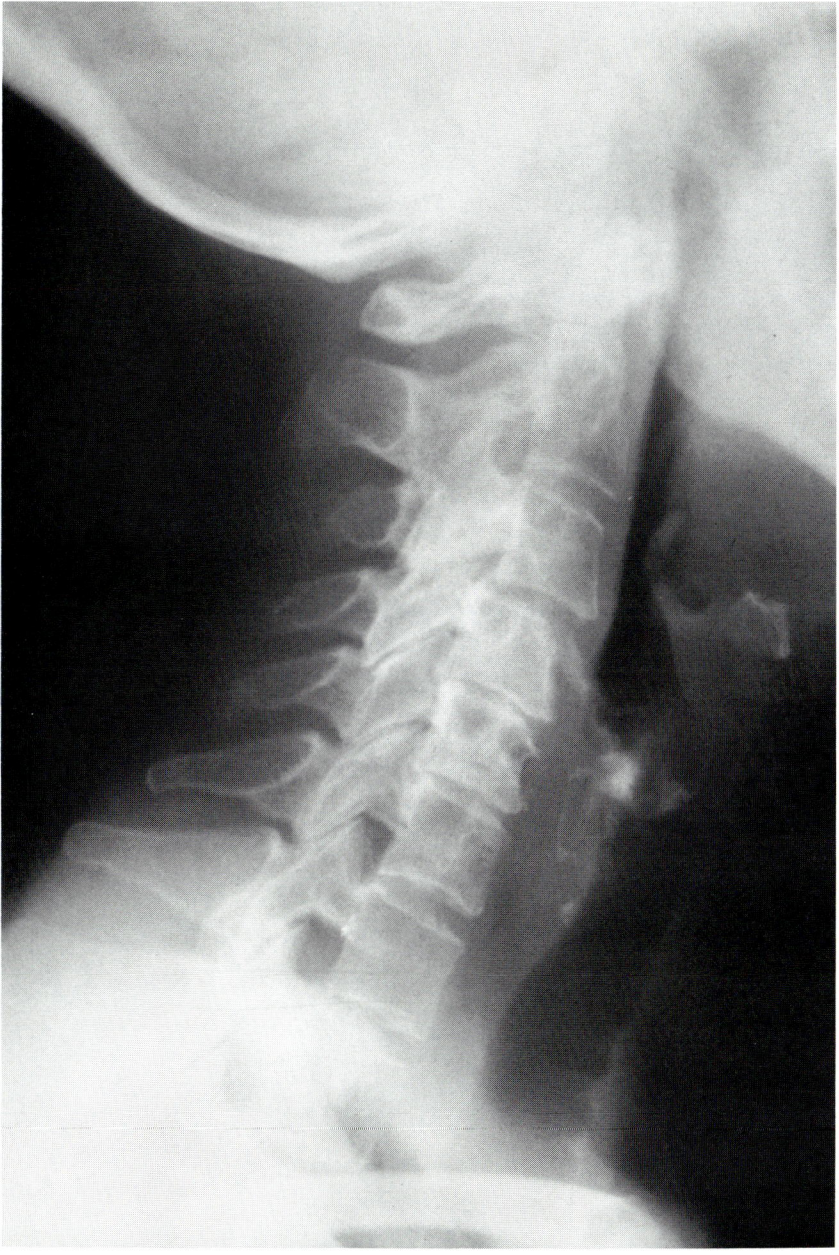

Figure 186

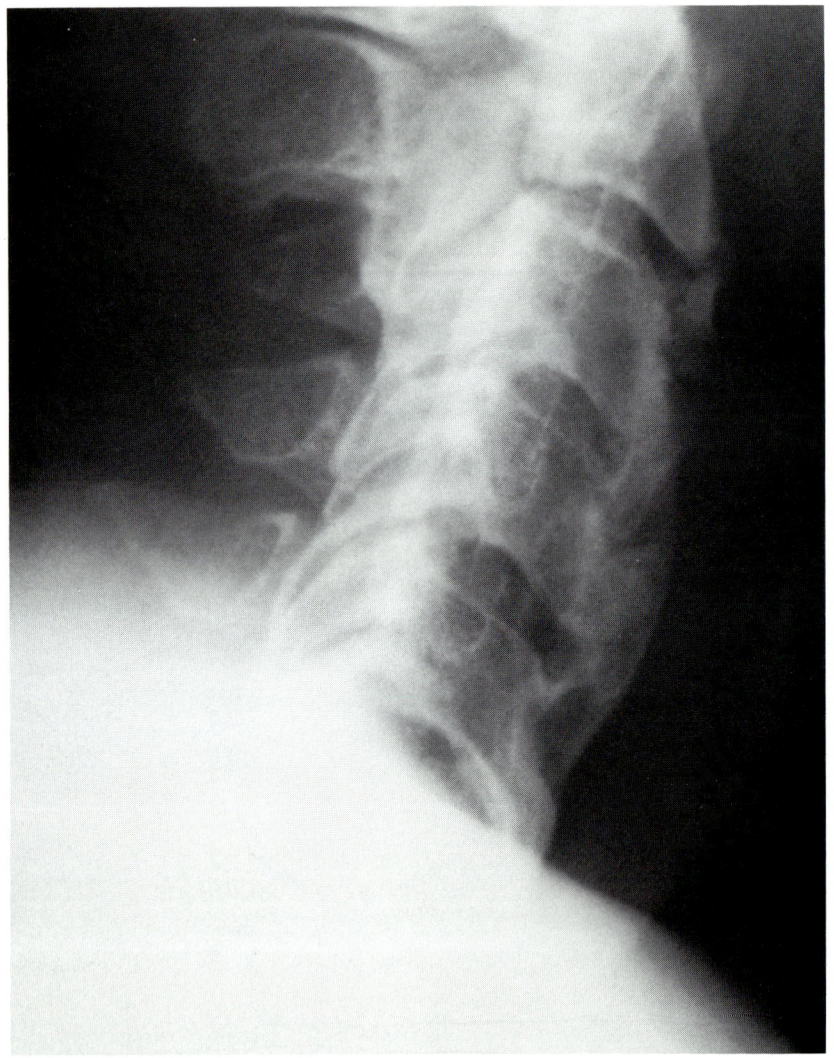
Figure 187

Exercise 57

Henry, 53 years old, complains of lumbar pain associated with night sweats. The pain radiates into his groin, and it is difficult for him to stand erect. A urinalysis reveals 15 red blood cells. You obtain an intravenous pyelogram (IVP) (Fig. 188). Look at the film and diagnose the cause of his problems.

The IVP reveals deviation of the right ureter and kidney medially with what seems to be a soft tissue mass overlying the psoas area. Did you notice, however, the destructive lesion in the inferior endplate of L1? Look at the tomogram in Figure 189, which more clearly demonstrates the narrowing of the L1/L2 disc space as well as destruction of the right side of the L1 vertebral body and irregularity of the inferior endplate of L1. This combination of findings is indicative of infection. The large associated psoas mass suggests this is more likely tuberculosis than a pyogenic infection. Open biopsy and drainage of the abscess revealed this to be true. Henry has Pott's disease, a psoas abscess from spread of a vertebral infection into the retroperitoneal area.

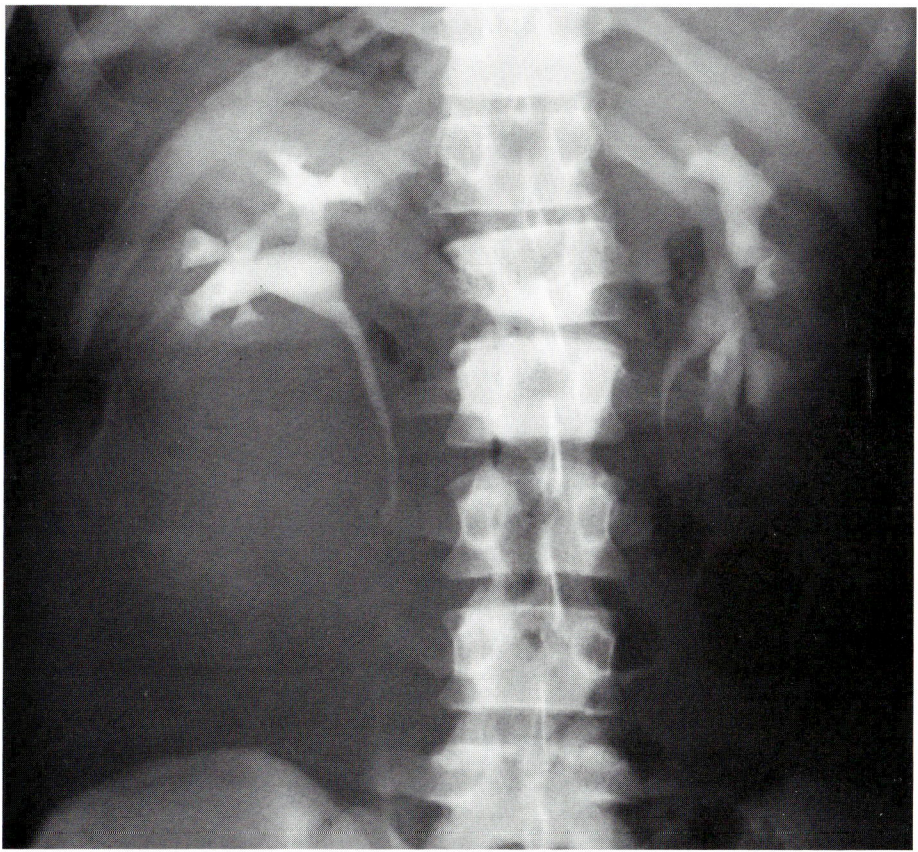

Figure 188

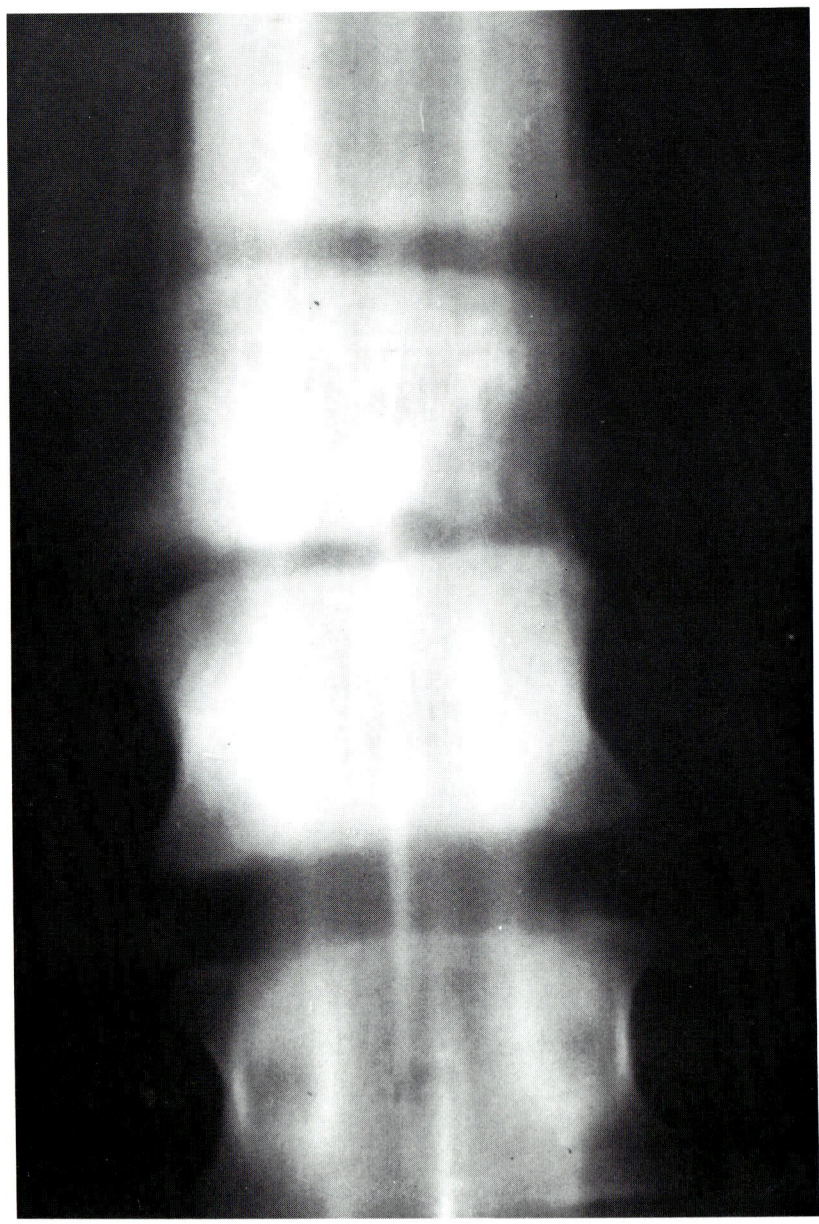

Figure 189

Exercise 58

Susan, 62 years old, has a history of polyarticular rheumatoid arthritis that has been treated with gold and prednisone for the last 5 years. While sitting down on a particularly low chair the other day she developed a sudden onset of intense lower back pain. Look at her radiograph (Fig. 190) and decide what you think has happened and why.

Susan has multiple compression fractures of the lumbar and thoracic spine. She has become osteoporotic from chronic steroid use, and her vertebrae have collapsed with only minimal trauma. It may be

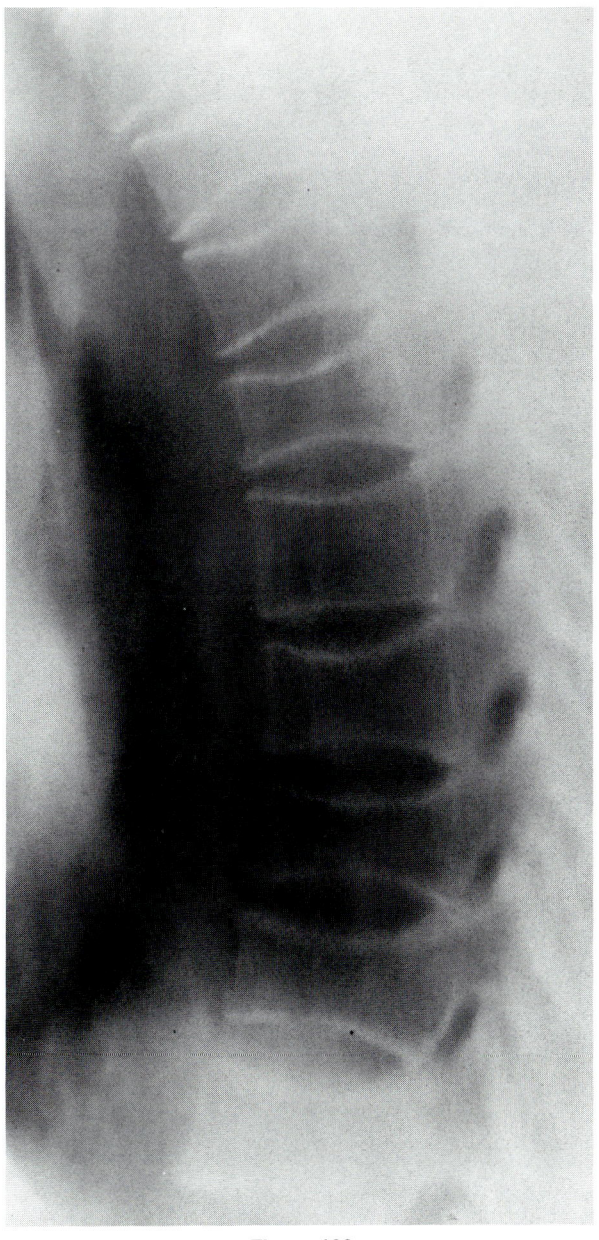

Figure 190

difficult to tell on such a radiograph what is an old or a new fracture. In this situation, a bone scan may be able to help; new fractures will show intense uptake, whereas old ones will be relatively less active. Other common places for osteoporotic fractures include the femoral neck and the distal radius.

Exercise 59

Look at this abdominal film (Fig. 191) and describe the likely cause of this man's diarrhea, weight loss and lower back pain.

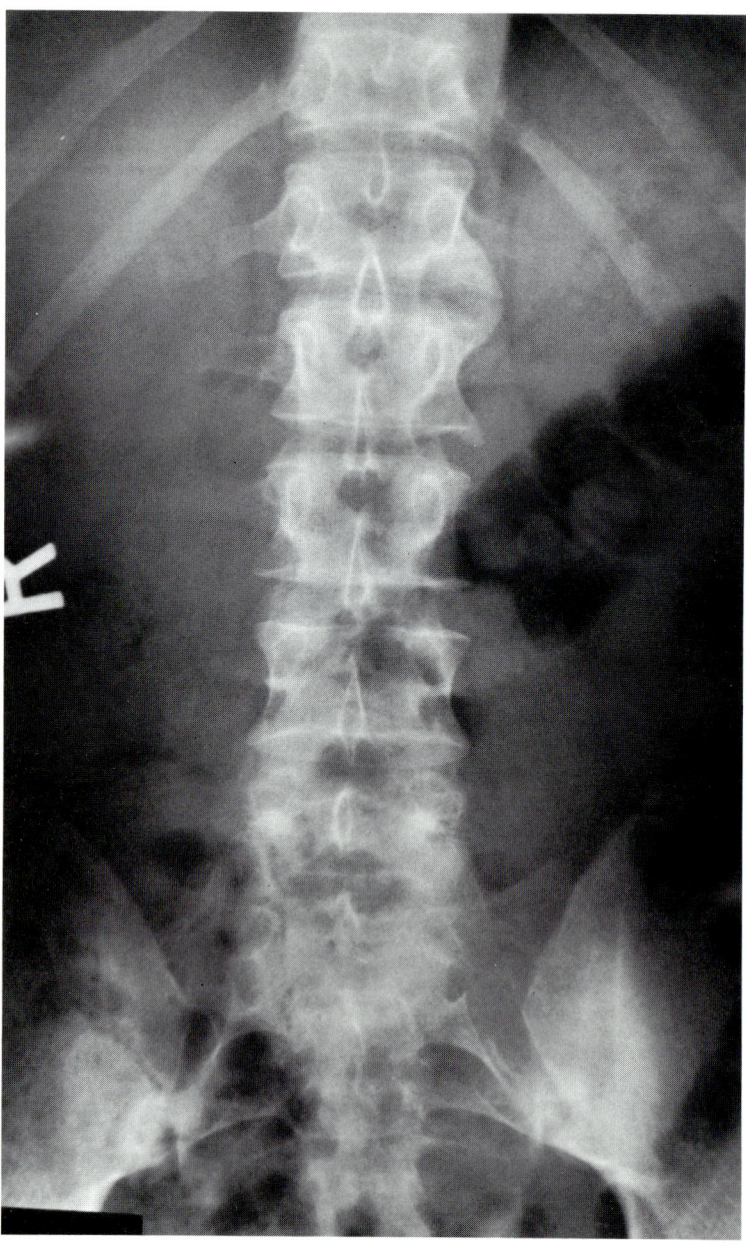

Figure 191

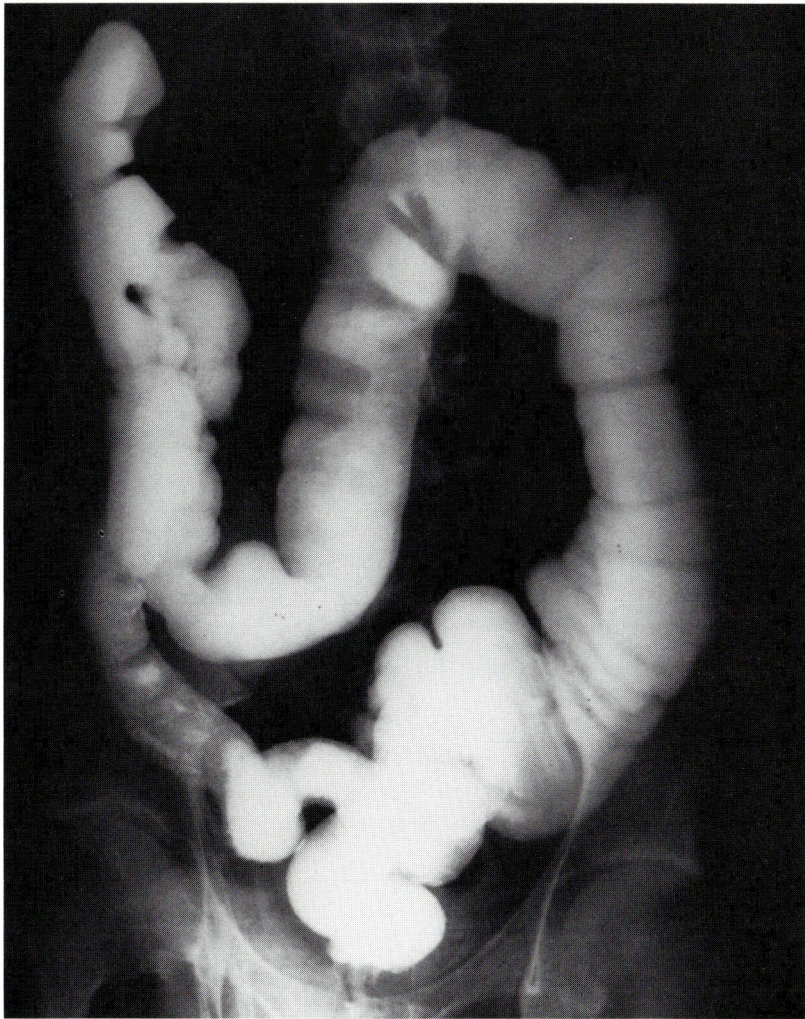

Figure 192

The abdominal radiograph reveals narrowing of the sacroiliac joints consistent with a spondylitis. Did you notice the thick syndesmophytes on the left at the L1/L2 level? This is further evidence of an inflammatory disease. It should not be confused with an osteophyte, which arises from the corner of the vertebral body and is oriented horizontally. This man has the spondylitis of Crohn's disease. Look at his barium enema study (Fig. 192), which demonstrates abnormality of the ascending colon. Similar osseous findings can be seen in ulcerative colitis.

INDEX

Note: Page numbers in *italics* refer to illustrations. Page numbers followed by t refer to tables.

Abscess, paraspinal, 39
   soft tissue, 38
Acetabulum, 78, *79, 80,* 80, *87,* 87, 91, *92,* 95, *96*
Acetylsalicylic acid, 131
Achilles tendon, 110, 121, 142, 148
Acromial process, 137, *138*
Acromioclavicular joint, 141, *142,* 142
Acro-osteolysis, 68, *69*
Adhesive capsulitis, 139
Aging, 9, 129, 131, 133
Alcohol abuse, 89
Ankle, 47, 101, 108, 125, 127, 131
   radiographs of, exercises in interpreting, 110–131
Ankylosing spondylitis, 31, *34,* 34, 35, *36,* 87, 87, *151,* 151, *152,* 152, *166, 167,* 167, *171,* 171
Antibiotic therapy, 95
Apophyseal joint, *31,* 31, *32,* 35, 36, 37, *38*
Appendectomy, 157
Arthritis, 121
   acute, 119, *120*
   degenerative. See *Degenerative arthritis.*
   erosive, 56, *58*
   infectious, 13, 20t, 27–48, 28t
   inflammatory, 9, 13, 14, 20t, 21t, 21–24, 27, 29, 52, *68,* 68, *83,* 84, 84, *85,* 85, *86,* 95, *96,* 97, *98,* 98, 110, *111, 112,* 119, *120, 133,* 133, 137, *138, 142,* 142, 153
   psoriatic, 21, *53,* 53–54, 56, *58,* 58, *66,* 66–67, *68,* 68, *70, 71,* 71, 98, *116,* 116, *118, 119,* 119, 153
   pyogenic, *28, 29, 30,* 29–30, 131
   reactive, 31
   rheumatoid. See *Rheumatoid arthritis.*
   septic, 131, *132*
   symmetric, 21
Arthrodesis, 110–113, *112*
Arthrogram, 137, 139
Arthropathy
   Charcot, *101,* 101
   crystal, 42
   hemophilia and, *85,* 85, *86*
   neuropathic, *101,* 101
   uric acid, 42, 44t

Articular surface changes, 3t, 4, 12–15
Aspirin, 82, 122, 123
Avascular necrosis, 87, *88,* 89, *90,* 91, 134, *135, 136*

Babinski sign, positive, 168
Baker's cyst, 102
"Bamboo spine," 34, 35, *36, 151, 152,* 152
Birefringent rhomboid-shaped crystals of CPPD, 80
Blocking agents, sympathetic, 124
Bone, changes in, 3t, 9–12
   contours of, changes in, 9
Bone alignment, 3t, 4, 16–20
Bone density, changes in, 3t, 3–4, 9–12, *10,* 52
   periarticular decrease in, 13–14, *13*
Bone growth, new, periosteal, 9, 11
Bone infarction, 9
Bone loss, periarticular, 9
Bone scan, 71, 72, 95, *96,* 178
Bouchard's nodes, 24
Boutonnière deformity, 16–18, *17, 19*
Bowlegged deformity, 77, *77*
Bunion, 114
Bursa, 47, 114
   subdeltoid, 133
Bursitis, 141
   acute, 9
   calcaneal, 129
   calcific, 133, *134*
   inflammatory, 47

Calcaneal bursitis, 129
Calcaneus, 121
Calcific bursitis, 133, *134*
Calcium deposits, 5, *8,* 8, 67, 133, *134*
Calcium hydroxyapatite (CHO) crystals, 42, 47–48, 133, *134*
Calcium pyrophosphate dihydrate (CPPD) disease, 42–47, 45t, 64, 80, 158, *161*
Capsular swelling, 5, *6*
Capsulitis, adhesive, 139

Carpal area, 9, *10*
Carpal bones, 102
Carpus, 97, *99*
CAT scan. See *Computed axial tomography scan.*
Cervical radiculopathy, 163, *173*, 173
Charcot arthropathy, *101*, 101
Charcot joint, 47, 126, *127*, 127, *128*
Chest, 73, 74
CHO crystals. See *Calcium hydroxyapatite crystals.*
Chondrocalcinosis, 45t, *45*, 45–46, 64, *65*, 80, *81*, 91, *93*, 142, 142, 158, *161*
Chondrocytes, 43–45
Chrondromatosis, synovial, 108
Chymopapain, 143
Clonus, 168
CMC joint, 52, *54*, 54
Colitis, ulcerative, 179
Computed axial tomography (CAT) scan, 37, 106, *107*, 143, *144*
Concave deformity, 137, *138*
Congenital hip disease, *80*, 80
Conjunctivitis, 121
Cortex, 9
Corticosteroid therapy, 9. See also *Steroid therapy.*
Cortisone, 47, 133, 139, 141
CPC joint, *56*, 56, *64*, 64, *65*
CPK. See *Creatine phosphokinase.*
CPPD disease. See *Calcium pyrophosphate dihydrate disease.*
Creatine phosphokinase (CPK), 106
"Crescent sign," 87, *88*, 89
Crohn's disease, *178*, *179*, 179
CRST syndrome, 8, 106
Crystal(s), birefringent rhomboid-shaped, of CPPD, 80
  calcium hydroxyapatite, 42, 47–48, 133, *134*
  calcium pyrophosphate dihydrate, 42–47, 45t, 64, 80, 158, *161*
  urate, 44t, 47, 68, 119
Crystal analysis of fluid, 68
Crystal arthropathies, 42
Crystal-induced arthritis, 20t
Crystal-induced synovitis, acute, 45
Cyst, Baker's, 102
  subchondral, 13, 14, *15*, 87, *87*, 97, *98*

Degenerative arthritis, 13, 20t, 24–27, 52, *113*, *114*, 114, 141, 145
  of CPPD, 46–47
  radiologic changes in, 24t
Degenerative destruction of joint space, 12
Degenerative disease with osteophyte formation, 42
Degenerative joint disease (DJD), 9, *51*, 51–52, *64*, 64, *65*
Dermatomyositis, 9, 106
Dermatopolymyositis, 48
Diabetes, 64, 101, 125, 127, 129, 139
Diarrhea, 95, 178
Diffuse idiopathic skeletal hypertrophy (DISH) syndrome, 34, 129, *147*, 147, *148*, 148, *173*, *174*
DIP joint. See *Interphalangeal joint, distal.*

Disc, herniated, *143*, 143, *144*, 145
Disc space infection, 39
Discitis, *157*, 157, *158*
  inflammatory, 38–39
  noninfectious traumatic, 38–39
  septic, 39, *40*, 157, *158*
DISH syndrome. See *Diffuse idiopathic skeletal hypertrophy syndrome.*
DJD. See *Degeneative joint disease.*
Dystrophy, reflex sympathetic, 124

Elbow, 60, *61*, *62*, 119, *120*, 127
  replacement of, 60, *63*
Erosion of joint, 13, *53*, 53, 54, 58, *59*, *68*, 68, *70*, *71*, 71, 78, *78*, 91, *93*, 95, *96*, 97, *98*, 98, *99*, 102, 110, *111*, *112*, *115*, 115, *116*, 116, *117*, *118*, *119*, 119, *123*, 123, 129, *130*, *131*, 131, *132*, *133*, 133, 153, 157, *158*, *166*, 166
Erosive arthritis, 56, *58*
Erosive osteoarthritis, 14, *15*
Escherichia coli, 157
Extensor tendon synovitis, 6

Facet joint, 31, *33*, 36
Factor VIII replacement, 85
Femoral condyles, 78, *78*
Femoral head, *80*, 80, 87, *88*, 89, 91, *92*, *93*, 95, *96*, 97, *98*
  collapsed, 89
Femoral neck, 178
  fracture of, 89
Femur, 78, *79*, 87, *87*
Fever, rheumatic, 82, 84
Finger, index, *66*, 66, 67, *70*, 70, *71*, 153
Finger tuft, 8, 8, 68, *69*
Foot, 47, 97, 98, *99*, 101, 115, *116*, 116, *118*, *119*, *123*, 123, *124*, 124, *125*, 125, *126*, 127
  radiographs of, exercises in interpreting, 110–131
Foreign bodies, 5
Forestier's disease, *147*, 147, *148*, *173*, *174*
Fracture, 9
  femoral neck, 89
  spinal, *151*, *152*, 152, *153*, 153, *154*, *155*, *156*
  spondylolysis and, 31
Fracture healing, 9
"Frog leg view," 87, *88*
Frozen shoulder, 139
Fungal infections, 27, 38
Fusiform swelling, 5, 5, 6

Glenohumeral joint, *133*, 133, 142
Glenoid fossa, *133*, 133, *137*, 137
Gold therapy, 123
Gout, 6, 7
  acute, 42, 44t, 47
  tophaceous, 43, *44*, 67, *67*, *68*, 68, 119, *120*

Hammer toes, *116*, 116
Hand, 8, *8*, *66*, 66, *67*, *68*, *69*, *70*, 70, *71*, 97, *99*, 115, 116, *117*, *122*, 122, 131, *153*, 153
 normal, *3*, 3, *4*
 radiographs of, exercises in interpreting, 51–76
Headaches, 168
Heart, 64
Heart failure, 73, 74
Heberden's nodes, 24, 53
Heel, 121, 129, *130*, *131*
 "lover's," 129
Hemarthrosis, 85
Hemochromatosis, *64*, 64, 65
Hemophilia arthropathy, *85*, 86, *86*
Hepatitis, chronic active, 134
Herniated disc, *143*, 143, *144*, 145
Hips, 23, 58, *60*, 60, *80*, 80, *87*, 87, *88*, *89*, 91, *92*, *93*, *95*, 95, *96*, *97*, 97, *98*, 98, *99*, *100*, 100, *101*, 101, *106*, 106, *107*, *108*, 108, *109*, *110*, 127
 congenital disease of, *80*, 80
 intracapsular infection of, 89
 prosthetic, *94*, 94
 radiographs of, exercises in interpreting, 77–109
 replacement of, 60, 78, 89, 100, 101
HLA-B27 antigen test, 153
HLA-B27–related illnesses, 129
Honeycombing, 73, 74
Humerus, capitellum of, 89
 head of, *133*, 133, *137*, 137, *138*
Hypercalcemia of renal failure, 106
Hyperparathyroidism, 9
Hypertrophic disease, *39*, 39
Hypertrophic osteoarthropathy, 9

Index finger, *66*, 66, *67*, *70*, 70, *71*, 153
Indomethacin, 121
Infarction, bone, 9
Infection, 9, 21, 39, 175
 disc space, 39
 fungal, 27, 38
 nonpyogenic, 27, 38, 132
 peripheral joint, 38
 pyogenic, 175
 septic disc, 38
 tuberculous, 38
Infectious arthritis, 13, 20t, 27–48, 28t
Infiltrative marrow diseases, 9
Inflammation, 9
Inflammatory arthritis, 9, 13, 14, 20t, 21t, 21–24, 27, 29, 52, *68*, 68, *83*, *84*, 84, *85*, 85, *86*, 95, *96*, 97, *98*, 98, 110, *111*, *112*, 119, *120*, *133*, 133, 137, *138*, *142*, 142, 153
Inflammatory bowel disease, 31
Inflammatory bursitis, 47
Inflammatory destruction of joint space, 12
Inflammatory discitis, 38–39
Inflammatory noninfectious arthritis, 27
Inflammatory spinal arthritides, 31
Inflammatory spondylitis, 149, *150*
Inflammatory spondyloarthropathy, 34
Inflammatory synovitis, chronic, 85

Intercarpal joint, 97, *99*
Interphalangeal joint, distal, *6*, 6, 14, *15*, *18*, 18, *19*, 21, 24, *51*, 51, 52, *53*, 53–54, *55*, 56, *58*, *64*, 64, *65*, *66*, 66, *67*, 67, *68*, 68, *70*, *71*, 71, *115*, 115, *116*, 116, *117*, *118*, *119*, 123, *123*, 153
 proximal, *5*, 6, 5–6, 9, *10*, 14, *15*, *18*, 18, *19*, 21, 24, *51*, 51, 52, *52*, 54, *55*, *64*, 64, *65*, *66*, 66, *67*, 67, *68*, 68, *70*, 70, *71*, 73, *73*, 102, *115*, 115, 116, *117*, *122*, 122–123, 153
Interstitial infiltrate of lungs, diffuse, 73, 74
Intertarsal joint, 110, 113
Intervertebral disc, 46
Intracapsular hip infection, 89
Intracondylar notch, *78*, 78
Intravenous pyelogram, *175*, 175

Joint(s), *3*, 3, 64. See also individual joints.
Joint disease, degenerative, 9, *51*, 51–52, *64*, 64, 65
Joint erosion, 13, *53*, 53, 54, 58, *59*, *68*, 68, *70*, *71*, 71, *78*, 78, 91, *93*, *95*, *96*, *97*, *98*, 98, *99*, 102, 110, *111*, *112*, *115*, 115, *116*, 116, *117*, *118*, *119*, 119, *123*, 123, 129, 130, 131, *131*, *132*, *133*, 133, 153, 157, *158*, *166*, 166
Joint infection, peripheral, 38
"Joint mice," 89
Joint pain, polyarticular, 9
Joint space, narrowing of, 12, 18, *20*, *68*, 68, *78*, 78, *80*, 80, *83*, *84*, 84, *85*, 85, *86*, *87*, 87, 91, *92*, *95*, *97*, 97, *98*, *100*, 100, 102, 110, *111*, *112*, *113*, *114*, 114, *115*, 115, *116*, 116, *122*, *123*, 129, *131*, *133*, 133, *143*, 143, 157, *158*, 158, *159*, *160*, 163, *165*, *166*, 167, *173*, 173, *174*, 175, *176*, *178*, 179
Juvenile rheumatoid arthritis (JRA), *83*, *84*, 84, 85, 123, 171, *172*

Knee, 18, *20*, 23–24, *26*, *27*, *28*, 28, *29*, 29, *30*, *64*, 64, 65, 77, *78*, 78, 80, *81*, *82*, 82, *83*, *84*, 84, *85*, 85, *86*, 89, *90*, *91*, 101, *102*, 102, *104*, 108, 121, *127*, 127, 128, 131
 radiographs of, exercises in interpreting, 77–109
 replacement of, *84*, 84, 85, 87

Lesion, lytic, from tumors, 9
Lips, overhanging, 43, 67, 119, *120*
Liver, 64
"Lover's heel," 129
Lumbar radiculopathy, 37
Lumbosacral spine, 127
Lung, diffuse interstitial infiltrate in, 73, 74
 rheumatoid, 73, 74
 tumor of, 9
Luschka, joints of, 163, *165*
Lytic lesions from tumors, 9

Magnetic resonance imaging, 37
Menisci, 80, *81*, 141
Metastases, 9
Metacarpal bones, 9, *11*
Metacarpophalangeal (MCP) joint, 5, 6, 9, 10, *14*, 14, *16*, 16, 21, 24, 47, *51*, 51, 52, 54, *55*, 56, *58*, 58, *59*, 64, 64, *65*, *66*, 66, *68*, 68, *70*, 70, *71*, 71, 102, *115*, 115, 116, *117*, *122*, 122, 153
Metatarsal heads, 98, *99*
Metatarsal joint, 113
Milwaukee shoulder, 48
MIP joint, 43, *44*, 98, *99*, *113*, *114*, 114, *116*, 116
MTP joint, 114, 116, *118*, *119*, 119, *120*, *123*, 123
Myelogram, 37, 143, *146*
Myeloma, multiple, 9
Myelopathy, 36
Myositis ossificans, 48, 106

Nails, *70*, *71*, 71
  pitting of, 58
  ragged, 52, 53, 153
Neck, 163, *164*, *165*, *166*, 166, *167*, 167, *168*, 168, *169*, 169, *170*
Necrosis, avascular, 87, *88*, 89, *90*, *91*, 134, *135*, *136*
Neural foramina, 37, 42
Neurogenic pseudoclaudication syndrome, 145
Neuropathic arthropathy, *101*, 101
Neuropathic joint, 47, 126, 127
Nitrogen toxicity, 89
Nodes
  Bouchard's, 24
  Heberden's, 24, 53
Nodular swelling, 5, 6
Nodule, 119, *120*
  rheumatoid, 6, *52*, 52
  soft tissue, 6
Noninfectious traumatic discitis, 38–39
Nonpyogenic infections, 27, 38, 132
Nonrheumatoid inflammatory illnesses, 12
Norgaard view, 54, *55*

Os calcis, 110, 121
Osteoarthritis, 14, *15*, 34, 36, 45, 53, *54*, 54, *55*, *56*, 56, 77, *77*, 78, 79, 91, *93*, 148, *173*, 173
  erosive, 14, *15*
  peripheral joint, 35
  primary, 24, 46, 47
  secondary, 24
  spinal, 35–36, *37*, 37
Osteoarthropathy, hypertrophic, 9
Osteochondritis dessicans, 89, *90*, *91*
Osteomalacia, 9
Osteomyelitis, 9, 127
  contiguous vertebral, 38
  periarticular, 27
Osteopenia, *83*, *84*, 84, *85*, 85, *86*, 95, *96*, 97, *98*, *122*, 122
  diffuse, 73, *73*
  periarticular, *53*, 53, *54*, *55*, 58, *59*, *60*, 64, *68*, 68, *70*, 70, 71, 102, *133*, 133

Osteophyte, 5, 13, 14, *15*, 35, 36, *37*, 37, 42, 43, 51, *53*, 53, *54*, 58, *64*, 64, *65*, 67, 77, *77*, 78, *78*, 79, *83*, *84*, 84, 87, 87, 91, *93*, 97, *98*, *100*, 100, 102, *113*, *114*, 114, *116*, 116, 119, *120*, *133*, 133, 142, 142, *143*, 143, 145, *146*, 146, 148, 163, *165*, *173*, 173, *174*, 179
Osteophytosis, 158, *159*, 160
Osteoporosis, 9, *124*, 124, 126, 157, *177*, 177, 178
Overhanging lips, 43, 67, 119, *120*

Paget's disease, 9
Pain, polyarticular, 9
Pancreas, 64
Paraspinal abscess, 39
Pars articularis, 31, 33
Pelvis, *60*, 60, *80*, 80, 129, *131*, 153, *156*
"Pencil and cup" configuration, *66*, 66, 98, *99*
Penicillamine, 177
Penicillin, 131
Phalanges, 6, 7, 9, *11*
PIP joint. See *Interphalangeal joint, proximal.*
Plantar fascia, 121, 129
Pneumococcal pneumonia, 131
Pneumonia, pneumococcal, 131
  staphylococcal, 131
Polyarthritis, *80*, 80, 102, *103*
Polyvinyl chloride, exposure to, 68, *69*
Prednisone, 134, 177
Proprioception, loss of, 101, 127
Prosthesis, 56, 57
  hip, *94*, 94
  wrist, 73, *75*, *76*
Protrusio acetabuli, *60*, 60, *80*, 80
Pseudofracture line, 87, *88*, 134, *135*, *136*
Pseudogout, 45, 80, *81*, 94
  acute, 47, 64
Psoas mass, *175*, 175
Psoas muscle, 38
Psoriasis, *58*, 58
Psoriatic arthritis, 21, *53*, 53–54, 56, *58*, 58, *66*, 66–67, *68*, 68, *70*, *71*, 71, 98, *116*, 116, *118*, *119*, 119, 153
Psoriatic spondylitis, 31
Psoriatic spondyloarthropathy, *35*, 35
Pubic rami, 148
Pubic symphysis, *60*, 60
Pyelogram, intravenous, *175*, 175
Pyogenic arthritis, 28, *29*, *30*, 29–30, 131
Pyogenic infection, 175

Radiculopathy, 36
  cervical, 163, *173*, 173
  lumbar, 37
Radiocarpal joint, 51, *52*, 97, *99*, *122*, 123
Radiologic examination, approach to, 3–20
Radioulnar joint, 97, *99*
Radius, distal, 97, *99*
Rales, 73, 74
Rash, 52, 56–58, 106, 153
Reactive arthritis, 31
Reflex sympathetic dystrophy, 124
Reiter's syndrome, 31, 121, 129, *131*

Renal dialysis, 48
Renal failure, hypercalcemia of, 106
Rheumatic fever, 82, 84
Rheumatoid arthritis, 6, 14, *16*, 16, 18, 21,
  23, *23–24*, 52, 54, 56, 58, *59*, *60*, *61*,
  62, *63*, 64, *65*, *68*, 68, 73, *73*, *78*,
  78, *80*, 80, 91, *92*, 97, *98*, 98, *99*, 102,
  110, *111*, *112*, *133*, 133, 137, *138*, *142*,
  142, *168*, 168, *169*
  nodules and, *52*, 52
  polyarticular, 177
Rheumatoid disease, early, 9
Rheumatoid factor, 133
Rheumatoid lung, 73, *74*
Rheumatoid nodules, 6
Rheumatology, diagnostic radiology and,
  1–48
  exercises in, 49–179
Rotator cuff tear, 47, *48*, 137, *138*, 139
Rott's disease, 175

Sacroiliac joint, *34*, 34, 35, *36*, *87*, 87,
  121, 149, *150*, 153, *156*
Sacroiliitis, 34
Salmonella, 95
"Sausage" digit, *66*, 67
Sclerodactyly, 68, *69*
Scleroderma, 8, *8*, 48, 68, *69*, 106
Sclerosis, 36, 38, 68, *69*, 77, *77*, 78, *79*,
  91, *93*, *100*, 100, *113*, *114*, 114, *116*,
  116, 134, *135*, *136*, *142*, 142
  subchondral, 9, *56*, 56, *64*, 64, *65*, *78*,
  78, *83*, *84*, 84, *87*, 87, 97, *98*, 102,
  119, *120*, *133*, 133
Septic arthritis, 131, *132*
Septic disc infections, 38
Septic discitis, 39, *40*, 157, *158*
Serum uric acid, 119
Shoulder, 23, 48, 121, 127, 131, *133*, 133,
  134, 134, *135*, *136*, *137*, 137, *138*, *139*,
  139, *140*, *141*, 141
  frozen, 139
  Milwaukee, 48
  radiographs of, exercises in interpreting,
  131–142
  replacement, 134, *136*
Skin, 64, 70, *71*, 71
SLE. See *Systemic lupus erythematosus*.
Soft tissue abscess, 38
Soft tissue changes, 3t, 3, 4, 4–9, 5
Soft tissue nodules, 6
Soft tissue swelling, 4–5, *5*, 6, 14, *51*, 51,
  52, 52, *53*, 53, 58, *59*, *66*, 66, 97, *99*,
  115, 115, *122*, 122, *153*, 153
Spinal osteoarthritis, 35–36, *37*, 37
Spinal stenosis, 37, *38*, 145
Spine, 30, 31, *31–33*, *35*, 35, 39, *39–43*,
  121, 142, 143, *143–148*, 145–149,
  150–179, 151–153, 157, 158, 161, 163,
  166–169, 171, 173, 175, 177–179
  bamboo, 34, 35, *36*, *151*, *152*, 152
  fracture of, *151*, *152*, 152, *153*, 153, *154*,
  155, *156*
  lumbosacral, 127
  radiographs of, exercises in interpreting,
  142–179

Spondylitis, 121, 148, 153, *166*, 167, *178*,
  179
  ankylosing, 31, 34, 34, 35, *36*, *87*, 87,
  151, 151, *152*, 152, *166*, *167*, 167, *171*,
  171
  Crohn's disease and, *178*, *179*, 179
  inflammatory, 149, *150*
  inflammatory bowel disease and, 31
  psoriatic, 31
Spondylitis deformans, *37*, 37
Spondyloarthropathy, 31, 39
  inflammatory, 34
  psoriatic, 35
Spondylolisthesis, 36, 145, 161, *162*
Spondylolysis, 161, *162*
  and fractures, 31
Squared vertebrae, 34
Staphylococcal pneumonia, 131
Staphylococcus, 149
Staphylococcus aureus, 29, 149
Stenosis, spinal, 37, *38*, 145
"Stepladder" deformity, 169
Steroid therapy, 9, 89, 124, 134, 177
Straight leg test, 142, 145, 146
Subchondral cyst, 13, 14, *15*, *87*, 87, 97,
  98
Subchondral sclerosis, 9, *56*, 56, *64*, 64,
  65, *78*, 78, *83*, *84*, 84, *87*, 87, 97, *98*,
  102, 119, *120*, *133*, 133
Subdeltoid bursa, 133
Subtalar joint, 110–113, *112*
Suprapatellar pouch, 46
Swan-neck deformity, *18*, 18, *19*
Swelling, asymmetric, 5, 6
  capsular, 5, 6
  fusiform, 5, *5*, 6
  nodular, 5, 6
  periarticular, 5
  soft tissue, 4–5, *5*, 6, 14, *51*, 51, *52*, 52,
  53, 53, 58, *59*, *66*, 66, 97, *99*, *115*,
  115, *122*, 122, *153*, 153
  synovial, 5
Symmetric arthritis, 21
Symphysis pubis, 46
Syndesmophytes, 34, *35*, 35, *36*, 148, 152,
  153, *156*, *166*, 166, *167*, 167, *171*, 171,
  178, 179
Synovectomy, 108
Synovial chondromatosis, 108
Synovial joint, 31–34
Synovial swelling, 5
Synovitis, chronic inflammatory, 85
  extensor tendon, 6
Synovium, 64, 108
Syringomyelia, 127
Systemic illnesses, 9
Systemic lupus erythematosus, 21, 54, *55*,
  89
Systemic tumor, 9

Tabes, *127*, 127, *128*
Tabes dorsalis, 101
Talus, 89
Tan, 64
Tarsal-metatarsal joint, *125*, *126*, 126
Tendon, Achilles, 110, 121, 142, 148
Tendonitis, 9

Thumbs, 18, *19*, *56*, 56, *57*, *68*, 68, *69*, *115*, 115
Tibial plateaus, *78*, 78
Tibiotalar joint, 110
Toe, 47, *113*, 113, *114*, 119, *120*, *123*, 123, 153
  hammer, *116*, 116
Tomogram, *152*, 175, *176*
Tophaceous deposits, chronic, 42, 43, *44*, 44t
Tophaceous gout, 43, *44*, *67*, 67, *68*, 68, 119, *120*
Tophi, 6, 43, 67
Trabeculae, 9
Tuberculosis, 27, 175
Tuberculous infections, 38
Tumor, 9

Ulcerative colitis, 179
Ulna, 9, *11*, 67, 67, *68*, 68

Ulnar styloid, *6*, 6, 97, *99*, 102
Urate crystals, 44t, 47, 68, 119
Urethritis, 121
Uric acid, serum, 119
Uric acid arthropathy, 42, 44t
Urinary tract infection, 157

"Vacuum disc" phenomenon, 36
Valgus deformity, 18, *20*, 114
Varus deformity, 18, *20*, 77, *77*
Vertebrae, squared, 34
Vertebral osteomyelitis, contiguous, 38

Wrist, 24, *46*, 46, 47, *47*, 51, 52, 54, *55*, 56, 58, *59*, 64, *64*, *65*, *66*, 66, *68*, 68, *70*, *71*, 71, 73, *73*, *82*, 82, *83*, 84, *84*, *122*, 122, 131
  prosthesis, 73, *75*, *76*